# Study Guide for Medical-Surgical Nursing
## Concepts for Clinical Judgment and Collaborative Care

### Eleventh Edition

**Donna D. Ignatavicius,**
**MS, RN, CNE, CNEcl, ANEF, FAADN**
Speaker and Nursing Education
    Consultant;
Founder, Boot Camp for Nurse Educators®;
President, DI Associates, Inc.
Littleton, Colorado

**Nicole M. Heimgartner,**
**DNP, RN, CNE, CNEcl, COI, FAADN**
Subject Matter Expert and Nursing
    Education Consultant;
Associate Professor of Nursing,
    Galen College of Nursing
Louisville, Kentucky

**Cherie R. Rebar,**
**PhD, MBA, RN, CNE, CNEcl, COI,**
    **FAADN**
Subject Matter Expert and Nursing
    Education Consultant
Beavercreek, Ohio;
Professor of Nursing, Galen College
    of Nursing
Louisville, Kentucky

T0195100

## Study Guide prepared by

**Donna D. Ignatavicius,**
**MS, RN, CNE, CNEcl, ANEF, FAADN**

**Cherie R. Rebar,**
**PhD, MBA, RN, CNE, CNEcl, COI,**
    **FAADN**

Elsevier
3251 Riverport Lane
St. Louis, Missouri 63043

---

**Notice**

Practitioners and researchers must always rely on their own experience and knowledge in evaluating and using any information, methods, compounds, or experiments described herein. Because of rapid advances in the medical sciences, in particular, independent verification of diagnoses and drug dosages should be made. To the fullest extent of the law, no responsibility is assumed by Elsevier, authors, editors, or contributors for any injury and/or damage to persons or property as a matter of products liability, negligence or otherwise, or from any use or operation of any methods, products, instructions, or ideas contained in the material herein.

---

**Previous editions copyrighted 2021, 2018, 2016, 2013, 2010, 2006, 1999, 1995, and 1991.**

*Executive Content Strategist:* Lee Henderson
*Senior Content Development Specialist:* Rebecca Leenhouts
*Publishing Services Manager:* Deepthi Unni
*Project Manager:* Sheik Mohideen K
*Design Direction:* Gopalakrishnan Venkatraman

Printed in Canada

Last digit is the print number: 9 8 7 6 5 4 3 2 1

Working together
to grow libraries in
developing countries

www.elsevier.com • www.bookaid.org

# Preface

The *Study Guide for Medical-Surgical Nursing: Concepts for Clinical Judgment and Collaborative Care,* eleventh edition, is a companion publication for Ignatavicius, Rebar, and Heimgartner's *Medical-Surgical Nursing: Concepts for Clinical Judgment and Collaborative Care,* eleventh edition. This Study Guide, written by Donna Ignatavicius and Cherie Rebar, will help to ensure mastery of the textbook material and help you learn about collaborative practice in the care of the adult medical-surgical patient.

The eleventh edition has been carefully revised and updated for an increased emphasis on utilization of clinical judgment skills.

The overall organization of the *Study Guide for Medical-Surgical Nursing: Concepts for Clinical Judgment and Collaborative Care* directly corresponds to the unit/chapter name and number in the textbook so that you or your instructor can readily select the corresponding learning exercises in the Study Guide. Chapters contain:

- **Learning Outcomes** that mirror those in the textbook
- **Preliminary Reading** to help you focus on knowledge needed to complete the activities in the *Study Guide*
- **Chapter Review** activities geared to provide review of key information in the textbook; examples of activities included are matching terms, fill-in-the-blank phrases, "hot spot" identification on pictures, true and false, and short answer (and others!).
- **Learning Assessment** NCLEX-RN®–style questions that are designed to encourage prioritizing, use of clinical judgment, participation in interprofessional collaboration, and application of the steps of the nursing process. Questions have been created to emphasize the NCLEX-RN® priorities of safety, patient-centered care, and evidence-based practice.

Answers and rationales to the Study/Review Questions are provided for each chapter.

The *Study Guide for Medical-Surgical Nursing: Concepts for Clinical Judgment and Collaborative Care* is a practical tool to help you prepare for classroom examinations and standardized tests as well serve as a review for clinical practice. This improved format will help you review and apply medical-surgical content and help you prepare for the Next-Generation NCLEX® Examination.

# Contents

# 1 CHAPTER

# *Overview of Professional Nursing Concepts for Medical-Surgical Nursing*

## LEARNING OUTCOMES

1. Differentiate the six core Quality and Safety Education for Nurses (QSEN) competencies that professional nurses need to provide safe, coordinated patient-centered care.
2. Describe two examples of how nurses can promote effective teamwork and interprofessional collaboration.
3. Explain the relationship between evidence-based practice and clinical judgment.
4. Identify the nurse's role in systems thinking and the quality improvement process to ensure patient safety.

5. State three ways that informatics and technology are used in health care.
6. Explain why selected populations are at risk for health equity issues, including social determinants of health.
7. Identify the major ethics principles that help guide professional nursing practice.
8. Describe how to promote well-being to prevent moral distress in professional nursing practice.

## Preliminary Reading

Read and review Chapter 1, pp. 1–20.

## Chapter Review

### Activity #1

Medical-surgical nurses practice in four "spheres" of health care delivery. Match each sphere in Column A with a health care setting in Column B where medical-surgical nurses may practice.

**Sphere of Care (A)**

___1. Disease prevention/promotion of health
___2. Chronic disease care
___3. Regenerative or restorative care
___4. Hospice/palliative/supportive care

**Example of Health Care Setting (B)**

A. Tertiary care center
B. Long-term care facility
C. Ambulatory care clinic
D. Rehabilitation facility

### Activity #2

List three examples of common errors nurses make that can jeopardize patient safety.

1. _____

2. _____

3. _____

**Activity #3**

Match each professional nursing concept with its description/definition.

<u>Professional Nursing Concept</u>

____1.  Patient-Centered Care

____2.  Safety

____3.  Teamwork and Collaboration

____4.  Evidence-Based Practice

____5.  Informatics

____6.  Quality Improvement

____7.  Clinical Judgment

____8.  Health Equity

____9.  Systems Thinking

___10.  Ethics

<u>Definition of Concept</u>

A.  The observed outcome of critical thinking and decision making

B.  A theoretical and reflective domain of human knowledge that addresses issues and questions about morality in human choices, actions, character, and ends

C.  The integration of the best current evidence and practices to make decisions about patient care

D.  The ability to recognize differences in the resources and/or knowledge needed for individuals to fully participate in health care and achieve optimal outcomes

E.  The process of accessing and using information and electronic technology to communicate, manage knowledge, prevent error, and support decision making

F.  The ability to recognize the patient or designee as the source of control and full partner in providing compassionate and coordinated care based on respect for the patient's preferences, values, and needs

G.  The process in which indicators (data) are used to monitor care outcomes and develop solutions to change and improve care

H.  The ability to recognize, understand, and synthesize the interactions and interdependencies in a set of components designed for a specific purpose

I.  The ability to keep the patient and staff free from harm and minimize errors in care

J.  The ability to function effectively within nursing and interprofessional teams, fostering open communication, mutual respect, and shared decision making to achieve quality patient care

**Activity #4**

List at least three issues that affect the health of veterans.

1. _____

2. _____

3. _____

## Activity #5
Fill in the blank with one of the appropriate ethical principles that nurses use as a guide for nursing practice.

1. Patient _____ is also referred to as self-determination.

2. _____ emphasizes the importance of preventing harm and ensuring the patient's well-being.

3. _____ refers to the agreement that nurses will keep their obligations or promises to patients to follow through with care.

4. _____ is a principle in which the nurse is obligated to tell the truth to the best of his or her knowledge.

## Activity #6
List at least four social determinants of health that can negatively impact health equity.

1. _____

2. _____

3. _____

4. _____

## Learning Assessment

### NCLEX Examination Challenge #1
The nurse requests analgesia from the primary health care provider for an alert and oriented client experiencing breakthrough cancer pain. Which ethical principle does this nursing action represent?
A. Veracity
B. Fidelity
C. Autonomy
D. Beneficence

### NCLEX Examination Challenge #2
The nurse is working with a team to review the evidence about best practices to reduce falls among older clients in a long-term care facility. What is the best source of evidence to include in this review?
A. Facility policies and procedures
B. Research studies
C. Consultant's expert opinion
D. Facility data on the incidence of falls

### NCLEX Examination Challenge #3
The nurse checks on an immobile client to determine if the client was turned by the assistive personnel to relieve sacral pressure. Which right of delegation is the nurse demonstrating?
A. Right communication
B. Right circumstance
C. Right supervision
D. Right task

# 2
CHAPTER

# *Clinical Judgment and Systems Thinking*

## LEARNING OUTCOMES

1. Discuss elements of critical thinking, clinical reasoning, and clinical judgment.
2. Identify cognitive skills within the National Council of State Boards of Nursing Clinical Judgment Measurement Model.
3. Differentiate environments of care and roles of health care providers within the health care system.
4. Describe the process of incorporating nursing knowledge into systems thinking.
5. Connect the importance of applying appropriate clinical judgment to systems thinking.

## Preliminary Reading

Read and review Chapter 2, pp. 21–34.

## Chapter Review

### Activity #1

Fill in the blank from the Key Term bank below. Not all Key Terms will be used.

> **clinical judgment**
> **clinical reasoning**
> **critical thinking**
> **Evidence-Based Practice**
> **Informatics**
> **Patient-Centered Care**
> **Quality and Safety Education for Nurses (QSEN)**
> **Quality Improvement (QI)**
> **Safety**
> **systems thinking**
> **Teamwork and Collaboration**

1. The use of _____ and _____ leads to _____, which is the observed outcome of these two underlying mental processes.
2. Which term refers the use of best evidence, the nurse's clinical expertise, and patient preferences? _____
3. The key way in which the interprofessional team functions is defined by the QSEN competency of _____.

4. Use of data, information, and technology to develop solutions to improve care based on data is reflected in the QSEN competencies of _____ and _____.

5. The nurse has undergone training at national nursing conference regarding interventions that prevent transmission of COVID-19. After the conference, the nurse returns to the hospital environment. When entering a patient's room, the nurse uses these interventions to prevent transmission of infection to a specific patient. This is an example of _____.

## Activity #2
Match the Key Term with its components.

1. Clinical judgment
2. Critical thinking
3. Informatics
4. Quality Improvement
5. Systems thinking
6. Patient-Centered Care

A. Use of logic and reasoning applied to clinical practice
B. Observed outcome of critical thinking and decision making
C. Understanding that the patient is in control of their care
D. Synthesis of patterns, interactions, and interdependencies
E. Use of technology and information in planning care
F. Use of indictors to monitor outcomes and improve care

## Activity #3
Match the factors that influence health equity and patient outcomes with their description.

| Factors That Influence Health Equity/ Patient Outcomes | Description |
|---|---|
| Behavioral and social determinants of health | A. Use of new technologies to assess health risks and implement treatment plans based on personal factors |
| Evolving approaches to population health management | B. Involvement, coordination, and respect of all members of the health care team to provide competent, precise, and personalized care |
| Policy and health care reform | C. Evidence-based methods to reduce health inequities and improve health using methods of data collection and analysis |
| Available and emerging technologies | D. Recognition that health care maintenance, activities, and interventions do not occur in isolation and that a systems approach to prevention and care is more likely to have positive health outcomes than actions taken by a single provider |
| Interprofessional practice with an emphasis on patient-centered care | E. Viewpoint that health care is a right rather than a privilege and that individuals should be active participants in their own health choices and actions |
| Shift toward systems thinking | F. What "health" means to each person within the context of their culture and what actions they are willing or able to take to achieve or maintain it |

## Activity #4
Fill in the blank from the Nurse's documentation below to complete each sentence.

1. When documenting components of **Recognize Cues,** the nurse's documentation will say _____.

2. When documenting components of **Analyze Cues,** the nurse's documentation will say _____.

3. When documenting components of **Take Action,** the nurse's documentation will say _____.

4. When documenting components of **Evaluate Outcomes,** the nurse's documentation will say _____.

| | **Nurse's Documentation** |
|---|---|
| A. | "Fever decreased from 103.4°F to 101.2°F (39.6°C to 38.4°C) in 2 hours post administration of acetaminophen." |
| B. | "Reports history of hypertension and type 2 diabetes in addition to today's symptoms of sore throat, fever of 103.4°F (39.6°C), and cough. Lung sounds with crackles bilaterally." |
| C. | "Was exposed to several people at a concert last week that now have tested positive for influenza B." |
| D. | "Placed in droplet isolation, administered acetaminophen as ordered. Diet order placed." |

## Learning Assessment

**NCLEX Examination Challenge #1**

Which barriers to successful implementation of community health care exist? **Select all that apply.**

A. Shortages in the workforce
B. Discrimination against people
C. Insurance coverage maximizes benefits
D. Insufficient personal finances for health care
E. Lack of understanding of social determinants of health

**NCLEX Examination Challenge #2**

Which individual is recognized as an advanced practice nurse (APRN)?

A. Registered nurse
B. Clinical nurse educator
C. Licensed practical nurse
D. Certified nurse practitioner

# 3

CHAPTER

# Overview of Health Concepts for Medical-Surgical Nursing

## LEARNING OUTCOMES

1. Plan collaborative interventions with the interprofessional team to help patients meet basic nutrition, elimination, and tissue integrity needs.
2. Plan nursing interventions to manage pain and promote comfort.
3. Assess risk factors that may result in altered sexuality.
4. Plan nursing interventions to promote cognition, mobility, and sensory perception and to maintain safety.
5. Differentiate the concepts of inflammation, immunity, and infection.
6. Describe common physiologic consequences when a patient has impaired acid-base balance and/or impaired fluid and electrolyte balance.
7. Describe how to determine a patient's perfusion, gas exchange, and clotting status.
8. Plan patient-centered nursing interventions to help patients meet selected physiologic health needs related to cellular regulation and glucose regulation.

Read and review Chapter 3, pp. 35–57.

## Chapter Review

### Activity #1

The scope of the concept of cognition can be viewed as a continuum with adequate cognition on one end and severe cognitive impairment on the other as shown in the figure below:

**Continuum of the Concept of Cognitive**

<————————————————————————————————————————————>

**Adequate Cognition**                                                                 **Severe Impaired Cognition**

For each of these patients below, indicate their cognitive status on the continuum using the number of the patient scenario. Use your personal device to look up any information you don't know.
1.   Older adult who has moderate-stage Alzheimer's disease and lives in an assisted living facility
2.   Four-week-old full-term healthy newborn baby living at home with parents
3.   Adolescent who was recently diagnosed with depression and anxiety and lives with grandparents
4.   Middle-aged adult who had a severe hemorrhagic stroke and is unable to communicate
5.   Young adult who experienced a severe traumatic brain injury from a motorcycle crash

## Activity #2

List at least five complications (physiologic consequences) of impaired mobility or immobility.

1. _____

2. _____

3. _____

4. _____

5. _____

## Activity #3

For inflammation in an extremity, best practice interventions include the use of **R-I-C-E**. Fill in the blank with what each of these interventions are.

R = _____
I = _____
C = _____
E = _____

## Activity #4

List at least three factors that place individuals at risk for decreased immunity.

1. _____

2. _____

3. _____

## Activity #5

Nurses assess and care for patients who have impaired gas exchange. State at least three physical assessment techniques that help to identify a patient's gas exchange status.

1. _____

2. _____

3. _____

## Activity #6

Match the risk factor in Column A with the concept for which the risk factor is most associated in Column B.

| Column A | Column B |
|---|---|
| ___1.   Immune compromise | A.   Pain |
| ___2.   Food insecurity | B.   Tissue integrity |
| ___3.   Osteoarthritis | C.   Infection |
| ___4.   Diabetes mellitus | D.   Nutrition |
| ___5.   Urinary incontinence | E.   Perfusion |

## Learning Assessment

### NCLEX Examination Challenge #1

1. The nurse is assessing a client for the risk for increased clotting. Which assessment findings may place the client at risk for this health problem? **Select all that apply.**
   A. Smoking
   B. Diabetes mellitus
   C. Immobility
   D. Advanced age
   E. Pressure injury

### NCLEX Examination Challenge #2

The nurse is caring for a postoperative client recently diagnosed with impaired cognition. The client was alert and oriented before surgery. What condition would the nurse suspect as the cause of the client's impaired cognition?
A. Depression
B. Delirium
C. Dementia
D. Delusion

### NCLEX Examination Challenge #3

The nurse assesses an older adult's sensory perception status. What normal physiologic change of aging would the nurse expect is related to sensory perception?
A. Presbycusis
B. Increased sense of smell
C. Numbness in feet
D. Minimal sense of taste

# 4 CHAPTER

# *Concepts of Care for Older Adults*

## LEARNING OUTCOMES

1. Describe evidence-based fall risk and prevention interventions for older adults that promote safety and maintain mobility.
2. Plan health teaching about lifestyle practices to promote health in older adults.
3. Discuss how to conduct a medication assessment for all older adults to ensure safety and quality care.
4. Identify social determinants of health that impact health equity within the older-adult population.
5. Differentiate the 3Ds of impaired cognition commonly associated with older adults.
6. Explain factors that contribute to decreased nutrition and elimination changes among older adults in the community and inpatient facilities.
7. Summarize the core elements of the 4Ms of an Age-Friendly Health System that help ensure patient-centered care for older adults in any setting.

## Preliminary Reading

Read and review Chapter 4, pp. 58–74.

## Chapter Review

### Activity #1

During the COVID-19 pandemic, older adults, especially those residing in care facilities, experienced more hospitalizations and deaths than any other group. Within this population, older adults of color were affected more often than Whites because of many contributing factors, particularly social determinants of health (SDOH). List at least four SDOH experienced by older adults of color that help to explain these clinical outcomes when compared with other groups.

1. _____

2. _____

3. _____

4. _____

## Activity #2
For each statement below, specify if the statement is **true (T)** or **false (F)**.

_____1.  One of the benefits of maintaining physical activity for older adults is to improve their well-being and self-esteem.

_____2.  Swimming is an appropriate exercise for older adults to help prevent osteoporosis (bone loss).

_____3.  Medicare B pays for inpatient hospital ___ and skilled care for a limited time for qualifying older adults.

_____4.  Older adults usually have more difficulty adapting to major changes when compared with younger and middle-aged adults.

_____5.  The Beers criteria help determine the appropriateness of specific medications for older adults.

_____6.  Family caregivers are the most frequent abusers of older adults because they feel burdened by the care they need to provide.

_____7.  If a court determines that an older adult is not legally competent, a guardian is typically appointed to make health care decisions.

_____8.  Depression is one of the most common mental health disorders experienced by older adults.

_____9.  Older adults need to keep up to date with their immunizations, including a Tdap every 10 years.

_____10.  Older adults need to increase their intake of fiber-containing foods and grain products.

_____11.  The Timed Up and Go (TUG) test for older adults should take less than 18 seconds.

_____12.  If a home care nurse suspects elder abuse or neglect, Adult Protective Services should be contacted.

## Activity #3
Nurses need to assess the medication profile for older adults for whom they provide care. List at least three recommended interview questions related to the medication assessment.

1.  _____

2.  _____

3.  _____

## Activity #4
Match the glossary term below with its definition/description.

### Glossary Term
___1.  Dementia
___2.  Neglect
___3.  Delirium
___4.  Geriatric syndrome
___5.  Presbyopia
___6.  Depression

### Definition/Description of Glossary Terms
A.  Farsightedness that worsens with aging
B.  Failure of a caregiver to provide for a person's needs
C.  Chronic, progressive, and global impairment of intellectual function
D.  Major health issue associated with late adulthood
E.  Mood disorder that has cognitive, affective, and physical manifestations
F.  Acute, fluctuating cognitive disorder that can be hypo- or hyperalert

**Activity #5**
List the patient-centered elements of the 4Ms of an Age-Friendly Health System used in inpatient health care settings today.

1. _____

2. _____

3. _____

4. _____

**Activity #6**
List at least five of the eight evidence-based risk factors identified as essential to predicting falls.

1. _____

2. _____

3. _____

4. _____

5. _____

## Learning Assessment

**NCLEX Examination Challenge #1**
The nurse is planning care for a hospitalized older adult who has a history of falls at home. Which nursing action is **most** important to help reduce falls for this client?
A. Inform the family that they need to take turns staying with the client.
B. Place the client in a reclining chair close to the nurses' station.
C. Identify current factors that increase the client's risk for falls.
D. Reorient the client each time when entering the client's room.

**NCLEX Examination Challenge #2**
The nurse is assessing medications being taken by an older adult who lives in the community. For which medication would the nurse contact the client's primary health care provider?
A. Lorazepam
B. Amlodipine
C. Simvastatin
D. Famotidine

**NCLEX Examination Challenge #3**
The nurse is assessing an older adult using the Confusion Assessment Method (CAM) and finds that the client meets the required criteria. Which condition would the client **most likely** have?
A. Depression
B. Dementia
C. Anxiety
D. Delirium

# 5 CHAPTER

# *Concepts of Care for Transgender and Nonbinary Patients*

## LEARNING OUTCOMES

1. Plan collaborative care with the interprofessional team to provide evidence-based care to transgender and nonbinary patients.
2. Explain the role of the nurse in providing high-quality care and improving health equity for transgender and nonbinary patients.
3. Discuss appropriate use of culturally sensitive terminology when providing care for transgender and nonbinary patients.
4. Identify major sources of stress that contribute to health issues experienced by transgender and nonbinary patients.
5. Prioritize evidence-based care for transgender and nonbinary patients who are taking hormone therapy and/or are having gender-affirming surgery.
6. Identify appropriate health care resources for transgender and nonbinary patients.

## Preliminary Reading

Read and review Chapter 5, pp. 75–92.

## Chapter Review

### Terminology Review

#1.   Match the Key Term in Column A with its definition in Column B.

| Column A | Column B |
|---|---|
| ____1.   Cisgender | A.   Distress caused by an incongruence between someone's sex assigned at birth and gender identity |
| ____2.   Gender dysphoria | |
| ____3.   Gender identity | B.   Adjective used to describe persons who self-identify as the opposite gender or another gender |
| ____4.   Genderfluid | |
| ____5.   Intersex | C.   Adjective used to describe people who have a chromosomal pattern, reproductive system, or sexual anatomy that does not fit the sex assigned at birth binary |
| ____6.   MtF | |
| ____7.   Nonbinary | D.   Steps a person takes to bring congruence in their gender |
| ____8.   Sex | E.   Adjective used to describe people whose gender identity is in alignment with their sex assigned at birth |
| ____9.   Sexual orientation | |
| ___10.   Transgender | F.   Physical, emotional, romantic, or sexual attraction to another person |
| ___11.   Transition | G.   Adjective describing people whose gender changes dynamically rather than remaining static |
| | H.   Person's genital anatomy present at birth |
| | I.   A synonym for transwomen |
| | J.   Umbrella term for gender identities that are not male or female, that are between or beyond genders, or that are agender |
| | K.   Person's inner sense of being male, female, neither, or an alternative gender |

**Review of Nursing Care for Transgender and Nonbinary Patients**

#2. For each statement below, specify if the statement is **true (T)** or **false (F).**

_____1. Nonbinary people have gender identities that are not exclusively male or female or that are between and beyond genders or they are without a gender.

_____2. Gender identity is always related to reproductive anatomy.

_____3. Transition is a process that must include surgical alteration of the patient's genitalia.

_____4. The population of people who are transgender is extremely diverse.

_____5. Gender is a social construct that helps people to explain the world around them.

_____6. It is appropriate to ask patients which pronouns they use.

_____7. Vaginoplasties are uncomplicated surgical procedures with few adverse effects.

_____8. The patient using transdermal estrogen should remove one patch before applying another.

_____9. Allow patients to identify the people who they consider to be part of their family.

____10. Monitor the patient taking spironolactone carefully for signs of hypertension.

## Activities

### Activity #1

List three ways that the nurse can provide a safe environment of care for a patient who is transgender or nonbinary.

1. _____

2. _____

3. _____

### Activity #2

A MtF patient has just been prescribed the drugs listed. After the nurse has completed teaching, the client is asked to restate the purpose of these drugs. Which client statements indicate an understanding of these drugs?

1. Estrogen _____

_____

2. Spironolactone _____

_____

3. Cyproterone acetate _____

_____

4. Finasteride _____

_____

## Activity #3

Match the surgical terminology in Column A with the procedure description in Column B.

| Column A | | Column B | |
|---|---|---|---|
| ____1. | Labiaplasty | A. | Creation of a small penis |
| ____2. | Penectomy | B. | Removal of the penis |
| ____3. | Vaginoplasty | C. | Fatty tissue removal |
| ____4. | Scrotectomy | D. | Creation of a small scrotum |
| ____5. | Mammoplasty | E. | Urethra creation |
| ____6. | Liposuction | F. | Vocal feminizing surgery |
| ____7. | Reduction thyroid chondroplasty | G. | Creation of a vagina and surrounding parts |
| ____8. | Scrotoplasty | H. | Removal of the testes |
| ____9. | Ureteroplasty | I. | Removal of the vagina |
| ___10. | Metoidioplasty | J. | Genital area contouring |
| ___11. | Vaginectomy | K. | Creation of labia minora |
| ___12. | Monsplasty | L. | Removal of scrotal tissue |
| ___13. | Orchiectomy | M. | Changing appearance of breast tissue |

## Activity #4: Fill in the blank from the choices below to complete the sentence. Not all choices will be used.

Review the nurse's documentation below and assign a number to each phrase.

1. A client tells the nurse, "I recently transitioned from male to female."
   o The nurse will document this information by recording, "client states they are _____, having recently transitioned from male to female."

2. The nurse has assessed a client who says, "I don't have a gender."
   o When documenting the client's gender identity, the nurse will use the term _____.

3. The nurse is caring for a client who says, "Some days I feel very masculine and other days I feel more feminine."
   o When documenting the client's gender identity, the nurse will use the word _____.

4. A client tells the nurse, "I was born with reproductive anatomy that has characteristics that are both male and female."
   o The nurse will use the term _____ to document this information.

5. When taking a sexual history, a client reports having intercourse with people assigned male at birth and people assigned female at birth.
   o The nurse will use the term _____ to document this information.

| Word Bank | |
|---|---|
| A. | Agender |
| B. | Androgynous |
| C. | Asexual |
| D. | Bisexual |
| E. | Cisgender |
| F. | Genderfluid |
| G. | Genderqueer |
| H. | Intersex |
| I. | Nonbinary |
| J. | Transgender |

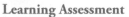 

## Learning Assessment

### NCLEX Examination Challenge #1

A client who is being seen at the primary health care provider's office tells the nurse, "My name is Shawn." When the client's health record shows "Mary" as the first name, which nursing response is appropriate?

A. "Hello, Shawn, it is nice to see you today."
B. "Mary, we need to bring your name up to date."
C. "I'm confused because your health record says your name is Mary."
D. "Why did you change your name from Mary to Shawn?"

### NCLEX Examination Challenge #2

Which health teaching will the nurse include when caring for a FtM client who has had no surgical intervention? **Select all that apply.**

A. Schedule a prostate examination.
B. Routine Pap examinations are recommended.
C. Use condoms when having sexual intercourse.
D. Talk with your provider about having mammograms.
E. Oocyte freezing is available if you are interested in this option.

### NCLEX Examination Challenge #3

The nurse is caring for a MtF client who has just had a vaginoplasty. Which action will the nurse take when the client returns to the floor from the postanesthesia care unit (PACU)? **Select all that apply.**

A. Begin daily dilation regimen.
B. Remove the urinary catheter.
C. Check capillary refill in extremities.
D. Monitor for the return of movement in the legs.
E. Assess the surgical dressing for bright red blood.

### NCLEX Examination Challenge #4

When a client who is nonbinary asks if surgical procedures are available, which response will the nurse provide? **Select all that apply.**

A. "Why do you want to have surgery?"
B. "Nullifying surgery can be done to flatten the chest."
C. "There are no procedures available for nonbinary clients."
D. "Have you considered asking your provider about a phalloplasty?"
E. "Modified genital surgery is something you may wish to consider."

# 6 CHAPTER

# Assessment and Concepts of Care for Patients with Pain

## LEARNING OUTCOMES

1. Identify the role of the nurse as an advocate for patients with acute pain or persistent (chronic) pain.
2. Plan collaborative care with the interprofessional team to promote comfort in patients with pain.
3. Teach the patient and caregiver(s) about drug therapy and complementary and integrative therapies for pain management.
4. Plan patient- and family-centered nursing interventions to decrease the psychosocial impact caused by pain.
5. Use knowledge of anatomy and physiology to perform an evidence-based assessment for a patient with pain.
6. Organize care coordination and transition management for patients with pain.
7. Use clinical judgment to plan evidence-based nursing care to promote comfort and prevent complications in patients with pain.
8. Incorporate factors that affect health equity into the plan of care for patients with pain.

## Preliminary Reading

Read and review Chapter 6, pp. 93–119.

## Chapter Review

### Activity #1
Define each type of pain.

1. Acute pain _____

   _____

2. Breakthrough pain _____

   _____

3. Nociceptive pain _____

   _____

4. Persistent pain _____

   _____

## Activity #2

For each scenario, specify if the patient most likely has:

A. Acute pain
B. Breakthrough pain
C. Persistent pain

_____1. Patient with joint pain for 7 years related to rheumatoid arthritis
_____2. Patient who just fell in a ski accident and has a broken ankle
_____3. Patient with a new onset of severe back pain who has been taking oxycodone for chronic back pain
_____4. Patient who experienced a second-degree burn earlier this evening while cooking
_____5. Patient with ongoing pain for the past 6 months due to metastatic breast cancer
_____6. Patient with abdominal pain following bariatric surgery
_____7. Patient taking acetaminophen regularly for headaches who has a more severe headache this afternoon
_____8. Patient with the onset of chest pain radiating into their shoulder
_____9. Patient whose finger was bent backward playing basketball earlier today
_____10. Patient with ongoing pain following an injury to their neck 9 months ago

## Activity #3

Explain five ways in which you, as the nurse, can minimize bias when assessing the pain of your patients.

1. _____

2. _____

3. _____

4. _____

5. _____

## Activity #4

For each scenario, specify how the nurse will document the type of pain the patient reports.

A. Localized
B. Projected
C. Referred
D. Radiating

_____ 1. Patient with a second-degree burn on the hand
_____ 2. Patient with shoulder pain following a laparoscopic hysterectomy
_____ 3. Patient with a broken ankle whose leg and foot also hurt
_____ 4. Patient with flank pain who also reports abdominal discomfort
_____ 5. Patient with a finger laceration following an accident with a kitchen knife
_____ 6. Patient who reports a tingling sensation from their back down their buttock into the leg
_____ 7. Patient with herpes zoster ("shingles") rash on one side of the body

## Activity #5
List 10 ways that unrelieved pain can affect a patient. Include physiological, quality-of-life, and financial impacts that may occur.

1. _____
2. _____
3. _____
4. _____
5. _____
6. _____
7. _____
8. _____
9. _____
10. _____

## Activity #6
Explain how the nurse interprets findings according to the **Pasero Opioid-Induced Sedation Scale (POSS) with Interventions**. First, explain what the finding listed means, and then list appropriate interventions that match that finding. The first finding is done for you.

1. **S**
   a. Finding: _Sleep, easy to arouse_____
   b. Interventions: _____
   _____

2. **1**
   a. Finding: _____
   b. Interventions: _____
   _____

3. **2**
   a. Finding: _____
   b. Interventions: _____
   _____

4. **3**
   a. Finding: _____
   b. Interventions: _____
   _____

5. **4**
   a. Finding: _____
   b. Interventions: _____
   _____

**Learning Assessment**

**NCLEX Examination Challenge #1**

The nurse is caring for a client with ongoing low back pain for 6 years who just underwent surgery for appendicitis. When the client reports continuing back pain and incisional pain, which kind of pain does the nurse document? **Select all that apply.**

A. Somatic
B. Visceral
C. Radiating
D. Nociceptive
E. Neuropathic

**NCLEX Examination Challenge #2**

The emergency nurse is caring for a client who fell 7 feet from a ladder and is reporting severe back and hip pain. The client has been seen repeatedly for unrelieved back pain over the past year and takes oxycodone regularly. Which nursing action is appropriate? **Select all that apply.**

A. Advocate for adequate pain control for the client.
B. Assume the client is reporting more pain than is truly experienced.
C. Ask the client to describe the pain and rate the intensity on a 0 to 10 scale.
D. Assess how the client's current pain is the same or different as existing pain.
E. Collaborate with the health care provider to convey that they client is overreacting to pain.

**NCLEX Examination Challenge #3**

The nurse is caring for a client residing in a skilled nursing facility who is nonverbal. Which action will the nurse take to assess for pain? **Select all that apply.**

A. Assume there is no pain unless the client cries or attempts to vocalize.
B. Use an evidence-based pain assessment tool when examining the client.
C. Review the electronic health record to assess for potential causes of pain.
D. Collaborate with other nursing staff who have recently cared for the client.
E. Observe trended client behaviors, looking for grimacing, moaning, or guarding.

# 7

# Concepts of Rehabilitation for Chronic and Disabling Health Conditions

## LEARNING OUTCOMES

1. Plan collaborative care with the interprofessional rehabilitation team for patients with chronic and disabling health problems.
2. Explain how to use safe patient-handling practices based on current evidence to prevent self-injury.
3. Plan care coordination and transition management for patients with chronic and disabling health problems.
4. Teach patients with chronic and disabling health problems how to prevent complications associated with decreased mobility.
5. Plan patient and family-centered nursing interventions to decrease the psychosocial impact of living with a chronic and disabling health problem.
6. Interpret health assessment findings associated with conditions that require acute or long-term rehabilitation.
7. Use clinical judgment to plan nursing care to promote health and function in patients in rehabilitative care settings.
8. Incorporate factors that affect health equity into the plan of care for patients with chronic and disabling health problems.

## Preliminary Reading

Read and review Chapter 7, pp. 120–139.

## Chapter Review

### Activity #1

Identify five conditions that can contribute to the need for rehabilitation care.

1. _____

2. _____

3. _____

4. _____

5. _____

### Activity #2

For each statement, specify if the statement is **true (T)** or **false (F)**.

___1. Cognitive therapists diagnose mental health/behavioral health disorders.

___2. Physical assessment data should be collected on residents at least daily.

___3. Acute confusion may be the only sign of a urinary tract infection in an older adult.

_____4. Residents in wheelchairs should be repositioned at least every 1 to 2 hours.
_____5. Pressure-reducing devices should only be used at the first sign of a pressure injury.
_____6. Residents should be toileted every 4 hours during the day and every 6 to 8 hours at night.
_____7. A person who needs mild support with ADLs is best served by being in a skilled nursing facility.
_____8. The Valsalva and Credé maneuvers are used when a patient has bowel problems.
_____9. Telehealth can be used to assist with care coordination in the home setting.
____10. Bisacodyl is only available in suppository form.

## Activity #3
Briefly explain the role of each type of therapist who works in the rehabilitation setting.

1. Physical therapist _____

   _____

2. Occupational therapist _____

   _____

3. Recreational therapist _____

   _____

4. Cognitive therapist _____

   _____

## Activity #4
Match the glossary term with its definition/description.

### Glossary Term
____1. Aphasia
____2. Credé maneuver
____3. Dysphasia
____4. Paresis
____5. Physiatrist
____6. Rehabilitation assistant
____7. Rehabilitation therapists
____8. Resident

### Definition/Description of Glossary Terms
A. Weakness
B. Slurred speech
C. Technique used to assist in urination
D. A person who assists the rehabilitation therapist
E. A physician who specializes in rehabilitative medicine
F. Person living in an inpatient facility with rights of anyone living in their home
G. Inability to use or comprehend spoken or written language because of brain injury or disease
H. Collective group of physical therapists, occupational therapists, and speech-language pathologists

**Activity #5**
List five rights a resident has while living in an assisted-living facility.

1. _____

2. _____

3. _____

4. _____

5. _____

**Activity #6**
List 10 people who are part of the interprofessional health care team in a rehabilitation setting.

1. _____

2. _____

3. _____

4. _____

5. _____

6. _____

7. _____

8. _____

9. _____

10. _____

**Learning Assessment**

**NCLEX Examination Challenge #1**

The nurse is planning care for a client in a rehabilitation setting. To avoid patient constipation, which dietary choices will the nurse include in the plan of care? **Select all that apply.**

A. Apples
B. Green peas
C. Baked beans
D. Bran muffins
E. Whole grain bread

**NCLEX Examination Challenge #2**

The nurse is caring for a client in a rehabilitation setting who has a urinary tract infection with burning and urgency. Which drug does the nurse anticipate will be prescribed?

A. Oxybutynin
B. Solifenacin
C. Tolterodine
D. Trimethoprim

**NCLEX Examination Challenge #3**

The nurse is assessing a new resident in a rehabilitation setting. When the client's Functional Independence Measure (FIM) is 6, which action will the nurse take? **Select all that apply.**

A. Raise all bed rails at night to prevent falls.

B. Encourage dressing self as much as possible.

C. Assign assistive personnel (AP) to provide bathing.

D. Assure there is a clear path from the bed to bathroom.

E. Coordinate full-time care among nursing staff each shift.

# 8 CHAPTER

# *Concepts of Care for Patients at End-of-Life*

## LEARNING OUTCOMES

1. Collaborate within the interprofessional health care team to promote high-quality care for the patient at the end-of-life, including family or other caregivers.
2. Discuss the ethical and legal obligations of the nurse regarding end-of-life care.
3. Explain the purpose of and procedures for advance directives to patients and their families.
4. Assess the ability of the patient and family to cope with the dying process.
5. Incorporate the patient's cultural and spiritual practices and beliefs when providing care during the dying process and death.
6. Assess patients for signs and symptoms related to the end-of-life.
7. Plan evidence-based end-of-life nursing care for the dying patient.

## Preliminary Reading

Read and review Chapter 8, pp. 140–155.

## Chapter Review

### Activity #1

Match the Key Term in Column A with its definition in Column B.

| Column A | Column B |
|---|---|
| ___1. Advance care planning | A. Process of reflecting on life's memories |
| ___2. Advance directive (AD) | B. Care management approach to decrease patient suffering by administration of medications that lower consciousness |
| ___3. Bereavement | C. Legal document in which a person has appointed another person to make health care decisions for them if incapacitated |
| ___4. Do-not-resuscitate (DNR) | |
| ___5. Durable power of attorney for health care (DPOAHC) | D. Compassionate and supportive approach to caring for patients and families living with life-threatening conditions |
| ___6. Living will | E. Written document prepared by a competent person to specify which actions are to be taken or avoided if the patient cannot make personal decisions |
| ___7. Palliative care | |
| ___8. Palliative sedation | F. Legal document instructing health care providers and others about which life-sustaining treatment is wanted or is to be avoided if the patient cannot make decisions for themselves |
| ___9. Reminiscence | |
| | G. Grief and mourning of survivors before and after a death |
| | H. Process in which patients and families discuss end-of-life care |
| | I. Order from physician or authorized health care provider instructing that CPR not be performed in the event of cardiac or respiratory arrest |

### Activity #2

For each statement below, specify if the statement is **true (T)** or **false (F)** regarding the nature of death of people living in the United States.

_____1. Most deaths of patients occur suddenly and unexpectedly.

_____2. Most people die after a long period of chronic illness.

_____3. Most people die after the age of 65 years.

_____4. The most common cause of death is heart disease.

_____5. Medicare covers hospice care for recipients with a prognosis of 6 months or less to live.

_____6. Cheyne-Stokes respirations are one symptom that death is near.

_____7. The nurse must contact a spiritual representative to meet with each patient who is dying.

_____8. Patient needs at the end-of-life can vary based on cultural and spiritual beliefs.

_____9. Family members should be encouraged to refrain from saying "goodbye" when speaking with a dying loved one.

___10. Cannabinoid-based medications can be used in some states for end-of-life care.

### Activity #3

List 10 signs and symptoms that may be noted or that a patient may experience when they are near death.

1. _____

2. _____

3. _____

4. _____

5. _____

6. _____

7. _____

8. _____

9. _____

10. _____

## Activity #4
Briefly explain the how the nurse intervenes to contribute to a patient's "good death."

_____

_____

_____

_____

_____

_____

## Activity #5
Explain how each of the complementary and integrative interventions below can help with pain management of a patient who is dying.

1. Massage _____

   _____

2. Music therapy _____

   _____

3. Guided imagery _____

   _____

4. Aromatherapy/use of essential oils _____

   _____

## Activity #6
List several ways in which hospice care differs from palliative care.

1. _____

2. _____

3. _____

## Learning Assessment

### NCLEX Examination Challenge #1

The hospice nurse is planning care for a client who has been given 3 months to live. Which intervention will the nurse include in the plan of care? **Select all that apply.**

A. Apply oxygen via nasal cannula if dyspnea occurs.

B. Involve family in the caring process if the client and family desire.

C. Discourage friends and family from using the terms "death" and "dying".

D. Withhold opioid drugs so the patient with pain does not develop tolerance.

E. Explain each nursing action to the client and family before they occur.

### NCLEX Examination Challenge #2

The nurse is talking with a family member of a dying client who states, "I am afraid to say goodbye to my mother." Which nursing response is appropriate?

A. "Why do you think it is hard for you to say goodbye?"

B. "It is important that you say goodbye before your mother dies."

C. "Your mother may not die with peace unless she hears you say it."

D. "You can choose to express other thoughts, such as 'I love you.'"

### NCLEX Examination Challenge #3

The nurse is preparing to assess the spirituality of a client who is dying. Which component will the nurse plan to consider? **Select all that apply.**

A. Client's sources of strength and hope

B. Whether the client subscribes to an organized religion

C. The degree to which religion (if any) is important to the client

D. Personal practices the client engages in that are personally meaningful

E. The effect of spirituality and religion on the client's end-of-life decisions

### NCLEX Examination Challenge #4

The nurse has assessed a client who is dying. Which action will the nurse take when cool extremities that are mottled and cyanotic are noted?

A. Administer warmed IV fluids.

B. Place a warm blanket over the client.

C. Gently rub the client's extremities to stimulate circulation.

D. Reposition the client so that the lower extremities are dependent.

# 9 CHAPTER

# Concepts of Care for Perioperative Patients

## LEARNING OUTCOMES

1. Plan collaborative care with the interprofessional team to promote favorable outcomes in perioperative patients.
2. Teach the patient and caregiver(s) about preoperative preparations and how to decrease the risk for postoperative complications.
3. Plan patient- and family-centered nursing interventions to decrease the psychosocial impact of surgery.

4. Use clinical judgment to plan evidence-based nursing care to minimize pain, protect patients from injury and infection, and prevent complications of surgery during the postoperative phase.

## Preliminary Reading

Read and review Chapter 9, pp. 156–193.

## Chapter Review

### Activity #1

Provide a brief definition of each of the following terms.

1. Autologous donation _____

2. Carboxyhemoglobin _____

3. Dehiscence _____

4. Evisceration _____

5. Malignant hyperthermia _____

6. Morbidity _____

7. Myoglobinuria _____

8. Perioperative _____  _____

9. Pulse deficit _____  _____

10. Sanguineous _____  _____

11. Serosanguineous _____  _____

12. Serous _____  _____

## Activity #2

For each statement, specify if the statement is **true (T)** or **false (F).**

_____1. In the case of evisceration, use clean gloves to provide immediate care.

_____2. The intranasal route of naloxone administration has the most rapid onset.

_____3. Music and breathing exercises are examples of nonpharmacologic pain management.

_____4. Acute cholecystitis is an example of surgery that needs to be performed urgently.

_____5. Use of herbal preparations does not have an effect on surgical procedures or outcomes.

_____6. A patient identified as ASA I under the American Society of Anesthesiologists Physical Status Classification System is a normal, healthy, nonsmoking person.

_____7. Loss of lung elasticity and decreased cardiac output are age-related surgical risk factors.

_____8. Following surgery with general anesthesia, the sense of pain is the first conscious function to return.

_____9. Constipation is a common side effect of opioid drug therapy used to manage pain after surgery.

____10. Patients who do not want blood transfusions during surgery have no other options.

## Activity #3

Place the steps in order that the nurse will take when caring for a client with respirations of 8 breaths/min and is suspected of experiencing a benzodiazepine overdose.

A. Apply oxygen.

B. Obtain IV access.

C. Administer flumazenil.

D. Assess IV site every shift.

E. Repeat administration of flumazenil.

F. Do not leave the client unattended until fully responsive.

Order: _____

## Activity #4

Identify which phase the nursing actions below are most likely to occur within.

| Phase |
|---|
| A. Preoperative |
| B. Postoperative |
| C. Both preoperative and postoperative |

___1. Determine if bloodless surgery is preferred.

___2. Assess respiratory effort, rate, rhythm, and depth.

___3. Ask if there is a personal or family history of malignant hyperthermia.

___4. Determine if feeling has returned as anesthesia clears the body.

_____5.   Apply antiembolism stockings.
_____6.   Collect vital signs.
_____7.   Continually monitor pulse oximetry.
_____8.   Assess for sanguineous, serosanguineous, or serous drainage.
_____9.   Provide teaching about how to care for self at home.
____10.   Teach and encourage deep breathing exercises.

**Activity #5**
Identify things the nurse will assess for when collecting a health history and performing a general review of systems.

1.   General (constitutional)_____

_____

2.   Eyes _____

_____

3.   Ears, nose, mouth, and throat_____

_____

4.   Cardiovascular_____

_____

5.   Respiratory _____

_____

6.   Gastrointestinal_____

_____

7.   Genitourinary_____

_____

8.   Musculoskeletal_____

_____

9.   Integumentary (including skin and breasts) _____

_____

10.  Neurologic_____

_____

11. Psychiatric_____

_____

12. Endocrine_____

_____

13. Hematologic and lymphatic_____

_____

14. Allergic and immunologic_____

_____

**Activity #6**

Match the purpose of surgery in Column A with the most likely example of this type of procedure in Column B.

**Column A**

___1. Cosmetic
___2. Curative
___3. Diagnostic
___4. Palliative
___5. Preventive
___6. Reconstructive
___7. Transplantation

**Column B**

A. Total hip replacement
B. Facelift
C. Knee arthroscopy
D. Prophylactic mastectomy
E. Removal of malignant tumor on lung
F. Pancreas transplant
G. Stent placement following vessel blockage

## Learning Assessment

### NCLEX Examination Challenge #1

A client with Crohn's disease who will have a colectomy is having which type of surgical procedure?

A. Curative
B. Diagnostic
C. Preventative (preventive)
D. Transplantation

### NCLEX Examination Challenge #2

Which statement describes the role of the nurse in the process of a client's informed consent for surgery?

A. The nurse provides the client with the benefits and risks associated with surgery.
B. The nurse serves as witness that the surgeon fully informed the client before surgery.
C. The nurse collects informed consent after the surgical procedure has been successful.
D. The nurse's only duty is to ensure that signed informed consent is in the health record.

### NCLEX Examination Challenge #3

The caregiver of a usually healthy 77-year-old client who had a knee replacement this morning states that they are concerned. The client knows the caregiver's name and that they have had surgery but does not know the day or time. Which nursing response is appropriate?

A. Notify the surgeon and request a consultation with a geriatrician.
B. Go to the client's bedside and perform a full mental status assessment.
C. Explain that drugs and anesthesia used in surgery take time to exit the body.
D. Ask the caregiver if there is a family history of dementia or Alzheimer's disease.

## NCLEX Examination Challenge #4

How will the nurse interpret laboratory results of a postoperative client when an increase in band cells is noted?

A. It is likely that infection is present.
B. This result is normal following surgery.
C. Anemia is present, so a transfusion may be needed.
D. Clotting factors are impaired, so the risk for bleeding increases.

# 10 CHAPTER

# Concepts of Emergency and Trauma Nursing

## LEARNING OUTCOMES

1. Describe the emergency department (ED) environment, including vulnerable populations served.
2. Engage in teamwork and collaboration with interprofessional team members to maintain staff and patient safety.
3. Explain selected core competencies required of ED nurses.
4. Prioritize order of ED care delivery via triage and assessment of the injured patient.
5. Implement nursing interventions to support survivors after the death of a loved one.
6. Describe the expected sequence of events from admission through disposition of a patient treated in the ED with trauma or emergent needs.

## Preliminary Reading

Read and review Chapter 10, pp. 194–212.

## Chapter Review

### Activity #1

Match the Key Term in Column A with its definition in Column B.

| Column A | Column B |
|----------|----------|
| ____1. Acceleration-deceleration | A. Category of patients who can wait several hours |
| ____2. Blast effect | B. Comprehensive head-to-toe assessment |
| ____3. Blunt trauma | C. Force involving rapid movement forward then backward |
| ____4. Mechanism of injury | D. Type of trauma resulting from explosive force |
| ____5. Nonurgent triage | E. Category of patients who need treatment quickly |
| ____6. Penetrating trauma | F. System used to sort or classify patients for care |
| ____7. Primary survey | G. Priorities of care based on the *ABCDE* mnemonic |
| ____8. Secondary survey | H. Injuries caused by piercing |
| ____9. Triage | I. Method by which a traumatic event occurred |
| ___10. Urgent triage | J. Type of trauma resulting from impact forces |

### Activity #2

For each statement below, specify if the statement is **true (T)** or **false (F)** regarding emergency care in the United States.

___1. Older adults are considered a vulnerable population.

___2. Contact precautions are required when caring for all patients.

___3. A sexual assault nurse examiner is a type of forensic nurse.

___4. Emergency medical technicians (EMTs) are a type of prehospital care provider.

_____5.   SBAR communication is only used if a patient has a life-threatening condition.
_____6.   Family members are preferred translators instead of telephone language lines.
_____7.   A patient who fell ice skating and has a suspected arm fracture is triaged as urgent.
_____8.   Skin is not cleaned on a patient whose death is under forensic investigation if it could damage evidence.
_____9.   Trauma nursing encompasses a continuum of care from prevention to reintegration.
____10.   Practicing trauma-informed care is a method of ensuring patient safety.

### Activity #3

List ways the nurse can intervene when receiving a patient in the ED who is unconscious and cannot provide their identity or a health history.

1. _____
2. _____
3. _____
4. _____
5. _____
6. _____
7. _____
8. _____
9. _____
10. _____

### Activity #4

Identify which trauma center is most likely represented by the descriptions here.

| Trauma Center Level |
| --- |
| Level I |
| Level II |
| Level III |
| Level IV |

_____1.   Focuses on initial injury stabilization and transfer if necessary
_____2.   Provides total collaborative care to a dense population
_____3.   Offers life support care in a rural area where other access is unavailable
_____4.   Meets needs of most patients, excluding complex or multisystem injury management

## Activity #5

A family arrives and wants to see the body of a client who died in the ED following a motor vehicle crash in which no forensic investigation is required. Describe specific actions the nurse will take before the family enters the room.

1. _____

2. _____

3. _____

4. _____

5. _____

## Activity #6

List signs associated with human trafficking that require the nurse to assess further.

1. _____

2. _____

3. _____

4. _____

5. _____

6. _____

## Learning Assessment

### NCLEX Examination Challenge #1

In which situation would the triage ED nurse, who is working alone, activate the panic button? **Select all that apply.**

A. The line for clients waiting to be triaged becomes overwhelmingly long.

B. A hospital overhead announcement says someone has abducted an infant.

C. A person walks in and starts threatening the registration staff with a weapon.

D. Emergency medical services call on their way to the ED with a client in full arrest.

E. Several clients who have been in the waiting room for a long time begin to complain.

### NCLEX Examination Challenge #2

Which statement would the nurse use **first** when giving a hand-off report to the next shift nurse using the SBAR method?

A. "You will need to contact the hospitalist on call for admission."

B. "The client is a 65-year-old who came to the ED for a severe headache."

C. "Vital signs are T 98.6°F (37°C), HR 98 beats/min, RR 22 breaths/min, BP 190/100 mm Hg."

D. "Medical history includes hypertension; the client stopped taking medications 3 months ago."

**NCLEX Examination Challenge #3**

Five clients enter the emergency department at 0600. Which client will the triage nurse classify as emergent? **Select all that apply.**

A. Client from a long-term care facility with ongoing dysuria
B. Client with potential internal injuries following a motor vehicle crash
C. Client with a dislocated shoulder sustained while playing football
D. Client with back pain and hematuria with a history of kidney stones
E. Client with a generalized skin rash who had shellfish for breakfast two days ago

# 11
## CHAPTER

# Concepts of Care for Patients with Common Environmental Emergencies

## LEARNING OUTCOMES

1. Plan collaborative care with the interprofessional team to promote perfusion and tissue integrity in patients with environmental emergencies.
2. Teach adults how to decrease the risk for exposure to environmental emergencies.
3. Apply knowledge of anatomy, physiology, and pathophysiology to provide evidence-based care for patients with an environmental emergency affecting perfusion, tissue integrity, and pain.
4. Analyze assessment and diagnostic findings to generate solutions and to prioritize nursing care for patients with an environmental emergency.

5. Organize care coordination and transition management for patients with environmental emergencies.
6. Use clinical judgment to plan evidence-based nursing care to promote perfusion, tissue integrity, and pain management and to prevent complications in patients with environmental emergencies.
7. Describe the expected sequence of events from first aid and prehospital interventions through disposition of a patient following an environmental emergency.

## Preliminary Reading

Read and review Chapter 11, pp. 213–230.

## Chapter Review

### Activity #1
Match the Key Term in Column A with its definition in Column B.

| Column A | Column B |
|---|---|
| _____1. Acclimatization | A. Global phenomenon resulting from burning of fossil fuels |
| _____2. Climate action | B. Medical emergency from failure of heat regulatory mechanisms |
| _____3. Climate change | C. Process of adapting top high altitude |
| _____4. Frostbite | D. Decreased arterial carbon dioxide levels |
| _____5. Frostnip | E. Breakdown of muscle tissue |
| _____6. Heat stroke | F. Marks that appear on the skin after a lightning strike |
| _____7. Hyperemia | G. Increased blood flow to an area |
| _____8. Hypocapnia | H. Cold injury that is a form of superficial frostbite |
| _____9. Lichtenberg figures | I. Taking active measures to mitigate and adapt to circumstances that are a result of climate change |
| ____10. Rhabdomyolysis | J. Cold injury in which tissues freezes |

## Activity #2

For each statement, specify if the statement is **true (T)** or **false (F).**

_____1.	Air and water quality can create or contribute to health concerns.

_____2.	Nonexertional heat stroke occurs suddenly with exposure to a hot environment.

_____3.	Bites from deer ticks can result in Lyme disease.

_____4.	A patient who is struck by lightning is electrically charged following the injury.

_____5.	Core rewarming for patients with moderate hypothermia includes warm IV fluids.

_____6.	Patients diagnosed with frostnip are likely to lose the body part that is affected.

_____7.	Acute mountain sickness may be accompanied by high-altitude cerebral edema.

_____8.	Pulmonary edema can result from aspiration of fresh or salt water.

_____9.	After rescue, any patient who has drowned should undergo spine stabilization.

____10.	Bee stings can result in anaphylaxis or in localized skin reactions.

## Activity #3

List important teaching points the nurse will include when providing education to a community group about avoiding lightning injuries.

1.	_____

2.	_____

3.	_____

4.	_____

5.	_____

6.	_____

7.	_____

## Activity #4

Identify which organism is most likely represented by the descriptions.

| Organism | |
| --- | --- |
| A. | Pit viper |
| B. | Coral snake |
| C. | Brown recluse spider |
| D. | Black widow spider |
| E. | Scorpion |
| F. | Honeybee |

_____1.	Retractable curved fangs

_____2.	Fiddle-shaped mark from eyes down the back

_____3.	Red hourglass pattern on torso of shiny black body

_____4.	Pattern of red bands that touch white or yellow bands

_____5.	Small, fixed maxillary fangs

_____6. Stinger on the tail that falls off after stinging
_____7. Triangular head
_____8. Single row of subcaudal scales
_____9. Stinger must be removed by tweezers
____10. Injects venom from a stinging apparatus on the tail; effects are neurotoxic

## Activity #5
List appropriate actions for the nurse to take when a client with heat stroke has been admitted to the ED.

1. _____

2. _____

3. _____

4. _____

5. _____

## Activity #6
Explain *planetary health* and why the nurse must understand this concept.

_____

_____

_____

_____

_____

_____

## Learning Assessment

### NCLEX Examination Challenge #1
Which task will the nurse assign to AP when the ED team is preparing for the arrival of a client who is a drowning victim?
A. Insert a nasogastric tube and attach to suction.
B. Take, report, and record vital signs every 15 minutes.
C. Advise the victim's family of the resuscitation status.
D. Assist with the bag-valve-mask device during intubation.

### NCLEX Examination Challenge #2
Which nursing action is appropriate when providing care for a client with white, waxy skin on the nose, cheeks, and ears?
A. Administer warmed IV fluids.
B. Massage the body parts briskly.
C. Place warm hands over the affected areas.
D. Apply cool water compresses to the waxy areas.

**NCLEX Examination Challenge #3**

The telehealth nurse receives a call from a client who reports being stung by a bee. Which statement prompts the nurse to refer the client to call 911 right away?

A.  "I was stung multiple times by a swarm of bees."
B.  "I'm a little bit anxious, but I am not short of breath."
C.  "The site where I was stung is red, swollen, and painful."
D.  "The last two times I was stung, my provider gave me cortisone cream."

# 12 CHAPTER

# *Concepts of Disaster Preparedness*

## LEARNING OUTCOMES

1. Identify the roles of the nurse and interprofessional team in disaster preparedness and response.
2. Describe components of facility and personal disaster preparedness and response plans.
3. Apply triage principles to prioritize safety in delivery of care to patients affected by a disaster or mass casualty situation.
4. Plan collaborative care with the interprofessional team to promote safety, teamwork and collaboration and communication when caring for patients affected by a disaster or mass casualty situation.
5. Implement nursing interventions to support people coping with life changes after disaster.

## Preliminary Reading

Read and review Chapter 12, pp. 231–245.

## Chapter Review

### Activity #1

Provide a brief definition of each of the following terms.

1. Community relations officer _____

_____

2. Containment _____

_____

3. Emergency preparedness _____

_____

4. Hospital Incident Command Center _____

_____

5. Hospital incident commander _____

_____

6. Medical command physician _____

_____

7. Personal emergency preparedness plan _____

_____

8. Personal readiness supplies _____

_____

9. Triage _____

_____

10. Triage officer _____

_____

### Activity #2
For each statement, specify if the statement is **true (T)** or **false (F).**

____1.   COVID-19 is categorized as an internal disaster.

____2.   A mass casualty event can be managed by a hospital using local resources.

____3.   Health care staff must routinely engage in disaster preparedness and education.

____4.   Nurses are at risk of developing acute stress disorder just as much as disaster victims.

____5.   Mitigation involves planning ahead for what to do if a disaster occurs.

____6.   Disaster victims who need care soon but can wait for a bit of time are tagged yellow.

____7.   When triaging, the nurse uses age of the victim as the primary benchmark for tagging.

____8.   DMAT teams consist of civilian medical, paraprofessional, and support personnel.

____9.   Nurses should assemble a personal emergency preparedness plan when a disaster occurs.

___10.   Rain gear, sunglasses, a cell phone, a pocket knife, and a flashlight are part of a go bag.

### Activity #3
Place the steps in order that the nursing supervisor, who is acting as the hospital incident commander at 0210 will take when notified that an airplane has crashed several miles from the hospital.

A.   Give the order to stand down.

B.   Activate the emergency management plan.

C.   Name officers to oversee essential functions.

D.   Go to the emergency operations center (EOC).

____   Determine the extent of the situation while personnel arrive.

____   Assign nurses to move patients to be discharged to an area to free up beds.

Order: _____

**Activity #4**

Identify which tag the triage nurse would assign to each client below when responding to a mass casualty event.

| Tag |
| --- |
| A. Red |
| B. Yellow |
| C. Green |
| D. Black |

1. \_\_\_\_\_ 19-year-old with airway obstruction
2. \_\_\_\_\_ 39-year-old with signs and symptoms of shock
3. \_\_\_\_\_ 36-year-old with signs of dehydration and systolic BP of 72
4. \_\_\_\_\_ 33-year-old with head injury in and out of consciousness
5. \_\_\_\_\_ 59-year-old with no major injuries and shortness of breath with oxygen saturation level of 88%
6. \_\_\_\_\_ 66-year-old with open fracture of both legs with distal pulses
7. \_\_\_\_\_ 33-year-old with an abdominal wound with no signs of shock
8. \_\_\_\_\_ 45-year-old with fall and fractured right tibia and fibula
9. \_\_\_\_\_ 27-year-old with head injury and no loss of consciousness
10. \_\_\_\_\_ 18-year-old with facial laceration with bleeding controlled with pressure dressing
11. \_\_\_\_\_ 26-year-old with an amputated left index finger
12. \_\_\_\_\_ 89-year-old with nausea and vomiting
13. \_\_\_\_\_ 45-year-old with a sprained right ankle
14. \_\_\_\_\_ 66-year-old with facial and torso lacerations with no major bleeding
15. \_\_\_\_\_ 72-year-old with dislocated right hip
16. \_\_\_\_\_ 75-year-old patient with massive head trauma
17. \_\_\_\_\_ 45-year-old with extensive full-thickness body burns
18. \_\_\_\_\_ 39-year-old patient with high cervical spinal cord injury requiring mechanical ventilation
19. \_\_\_\_\_ 44-year-old with chest trauma and major hemorrhage
20. \_\_\_\_\_ 55-year-old with lacerated femoral artery and thready carotid pulse

**Activity #5**

List ways in which the nurse who provided care during a mass casualty event can reduce the risk for personally developing posttraumatic stress disorder (PTSD).

1. _____

2. _____

3. _____

4. _____

5. _____

6. _____

7. _____

## Activity #6

Explain the role of the nurse in responding when a fire breaks out in the work setting.

_____

_____

_____

_____

_____

_____

_____

_____

## Learning Assessment

### NCLEX Examination Challenge #1

Which action will the nurse take **first** when a client comes to the ED stating they are concerned about being exposed to an infectious bioterrorism agent?

A. Move the client to a quarantined area.
B. Activate the emergency preparedness plan.
C. Call the local police and Department of Public Health.
D. Collect a comprehensive history and assess for any symptoms.

### NCLEX Examination Challenge #2

Which responsibility will be given to the nurse assigned to assist the medical command physician during a disaster?

A. Assist with the triage of disaster victims.
B. Speak to the media about progress in providing care for victims.
C. Determine if the emergency plan is being implemented effectively.
D. Call nursing units to determine how many beds are available for victims.

### NCLEX Examination Challenge #3

The nurse who is part of an Ohio DMAT team has been notified to deploy to a disaster area in Kentucky to provide care following a tornado. Which action will the nurse take?

A. Notify DMAT that Kentucky does not recognize nursing licenses from Ohio.
B. Recognize that deployed DMAT nurses are federal employees with valid licenses.
C. Call the Ohio State Board of Nursing to ask if an Ohio license is valid in Kentucky.
D. Contact the Kentucky Board of Nursing to apply for an emergency Kentucky nursing license.

### NCLEX Examination Challenge #4

Which event will be classified by a hospital as an external disaster? **Select all that apply.**

A. Violent shooter in a park
B. Terrorist act at a shopping mall
C. An Mpox outbreak in the community
D. Fire in a neighboring long-term care agency
E. Broken hospital generator causing an interruption in power

# 13
## CHAPTER

# Concepts of Fluid and Electrolyte Balance and Imbalance

## LEARNING OUTCOMES

1. Use knowledge of anatomy, physiology, and pathophysiology to perform an evidence-based assessment for the patient with a disturbance of fluid and electrolyte balance.
2. Demonstrate clinical judgment to interpret assessment findings for the patient experiencing a disturbance of fluid and electrolyte balance.
3. Explain how physiologic aging increases the risk for disturbances in fluid and electrolyte balance.
4. Teach adults how to decrease the risk for a disturbance in fluid and electrolyte balance.
5. Use clinical judgment to plan evidence-based nursing care to promote fluid and electrolyte balance and prevent fluid and electrolyte disorders.

## Preliminary Reading

Read and review Chapter 13, pp. 246–270.

## Chapter Review

### Terminology Review
### Activity #1
Match the Key Term in Column A with its definition in Column B.

| Column A | Column B |
|---|---|
| _____1. Anions | A. Fluid with osmolarity less than 270 mOsm/L |
| _____2. Cations | B. Number of milliosmoles in a liter of solution |
| _____3. Electrolytes | C. Particles dissolved in solvent of body fluids |
| _____4. Hydrostatic pressure | D. Fluid with solute concentration of 270–300 mOsm/L |
| _____5. Hypertonic | E. Negatively charged electrolytes |
| _____6. Isotonic | F. Pressure exerted by water molecules against surfaces of a confining space |
| _____7. Hypotonic | |
| _____8. Osmolality | G. Number of milliosmoles in a kilogram of solution |
| _____9. Osmolarity | H. Solute particles that express an overall electric charge |
| ____10. Solute | I. Positively charged electrolytes |
| ____11. Solvent | J. Fluid with osmolarity more than 300 mOsm/L |
| | K. Water portion of body fluids |

## Activity #2

For each statement, specify if the statement is **true (T)** or **false (F).**

____1. Malabsorption syndrome can result in hypocalcemia.

____2. 10% dextrose in water ($D_{10}W$) is a hypertonic solution.

____3. 10% dextrose in water ($D_5W$) is a hypotonic solution.

____4. A serum calcium value of 12 mg/dL indicates hypocalcemia.

____5. A serum chloride value of 102 mEq/L is considered normal.

____6. The nurse anticipates that a patient with fluid overload will have warm skin.

____7. The nurse will assess deep tendon reflexes of a patient receiving IV magnesium sulfate ($MgSO_4$) once per shift.

____8. A positive Chvostek sign indicates hypocalcemia.

____9. Hyperkalemia often occurs in patients with normal kidney function.

___10. Lithium is used as a treatment for hyponatremia caused by inappropriate secretion of antidiuretic hormone (ADH).

## Activity #3

Complete the following sentences with the appropriate word or phrase.

1. Insensible water loss takes place via _____, _____, _____, _____, and _____.

2. Hypocalcemia is defined as a serum calcium level below _____.

3. An elevated level of magnesium could indicate _____, _____, _____, or _____.

4. Normal saline solution is _____% saline.

5. The solution of 5% dextrose in Ringer's lactate is _____tonic. (hyper, hypo, iso)

6. Ringer's lactate is _____tonic. (hyper, hypo, iso)

7. The nurse will gather a bag of ____% saline for a patient who is to receive hypotonic fluids.

8. Transfusions of whole blood or packed cells can induce _____.

9. A patient with lactose intolerance is most likely to have _____ as an electrolyte imbalance.

10. A patient with Crohn's disease is most likely to have _____ and _____ as electrolyte imbalances.

## Activity #4

Identify whether each assessment finding below is characteristic of hypokalemia, a normal potassium level, or hyperkalemia.

| Potassium Indication |
|---|
| A. Hypokalemia |
| B. Normal potassium level |
| C. Hyperkalemia |

1. _____ Feet numbness

2. _____ Heart rate 90 beats/min

3. _____ Potassium value of 2.9 mEq/L

4. _____ Respirations 10 breaths/min

5. _____ Potassium value of 4.2 mEq/L

6. _____ Anxiety followed by lethargy

7. _____ Blood pressure 118/72

8. _____ Hyperactive bowel sounds

9. _____ Muscle twitching
10. _____ ST-segment depression
11. _____ New onset of diarrhea
12. _____ Potassium value of 6.1 mEq/L
13. _____ Thready, weak pulse
14. _____ Respirations 18 breaths/min
15. _____ Absence of peristalsis

*Activity #5*
The nurse is providing teaching for a patient who is to follow a low-sodium diet. List foods that the nurse will teach the patient to avoid.

1. _____
2. _____
3. _____
4. _____
5. _____
6. _____
7. _____

*Activity #6*
Explain how calcium functions within the body.

_____
_____
_____
_____
_____
_____
_____

## Learning Assessment

### NCLEX Examination Challenge #1

The nurse is caring for a client with renal disease. Which assessment finding indicates that the client may have fluid overload? **Select all that apply.**

A. Hepatomegaly
B. Pulse rate 120 beats/min
C. Crackles heard on auscultation
D. Respirations 10 breaths/min
E. Bilateral pitting edema in extremities

### NCLEX Examination Challenge #2

Which serum value prompts the nurse to further asses for hypernatremia?

A. Potassium 3.9 mEq/L (mmol/L)
B. Chloride 103 mEq/L (mmol/L)
C. Sodium 149 mEq/L (mmol/L)
D. Magnesium 1.8 mEq/L (mmol/L)

### NCLEX Examination Challenge #3

The nurse notes that a client's urinary output has been 588 mL over the past 24 hours. Which nursing action is appropriate?

A. Decrease fluid volume intake.
B. Assess for electrolyte imbalances.
C. Document the finding as normal.
D. Contact the Rapid Response Team.

### NCLEX Examination Challenge #4

The nurse is caring for a client who has a magnesium value of 1.1 mEq/L. Which assessment will the nurse perform **first**?

A. Check rhythm strip.
B. Listen for bowel sounds.
C. Determine 24-hour urine output.
D. Assess for strength in hand grips.

# 14 CHAPTER

# Concepts of Acid-Base Balance and Imbalance

## LEARNING OUTCOMES

1. Use knowledge of anatomy, physiology, and pathophysiology to perform a focused assessment for the patient with a disturbance of acid-base balance.
2. Demonstrate clinical judgment to interpret assessment findings in a patient with a disturbance of acid-base balance.
3. Explain how physiologic aging changes the effectiveness of mechanisms that maintain acid-base balance.
4. Use clinical judgment to plan evidence-based nursing care to promote acid-base balance.

## Preliminary Reading

Read and review Chapter 14, pp. 271–284.

## Chapter Review

### Terminology Review

#### Activity #1

Match the Key Term in Column A with its definition in Column B.

**Column A**

____1. Acid-base balance
____2. Acidosis
____3. Acids
____4. Alkalosis
____5. Bases
____6. Buffers
____7. Hyperventilation
____8. Hypoventilation
____9. Kussmaul respiration

**Column B**

A. Rate and depth of breathing above normal
B. Substances that bind free hydrogen ions in solution and lower the amount of free hydrogen
C. Substances that release hydrogen ions when dissolved in water or body fluids, increasing the amount of free hydrogen ions
D. Arterial blood pH above 7.45
E. Substances that can react as an acid or base when dissolved in fluid
F. Arterial blood pH below 7.35
G. Rate and depth of breathing above normal
H. Maintenance of arterial blood pH between 7.35 and 7.45
I. Pattern of breathing associated with acidosis

#### Activity #2

For each statement, specify if the statement is **true (T)** or **false (F)**.
_____1. The central nervous system controls respiratory regulation of acid-base balance.
_____2. Bicarbonate is produced from carbonic acid in the pancreas, kidneys, and inside red blood cells.
_____3. Protein metabolism forms carbon dioxide ($CO_2$), which is exhaled by the lungs during breathing.

_____4.   The most common acid in the human body is bicarbonate.

_____5.   Body fluids with a pH level higher than 7.45 have a higher concentration of acids compared with bases.

_____6.   The kidneys and the lungs can compensate for acid-base imbalances.

_____7.   Acid-base problems are fully compensated when adaptive actions are completely successful and the blood pH returns to normal.

_____8.   In full compensation, the levels of oxygen and bicarbonate may be abnormal.

_____9.   Patients with respiratory acidosis benefit from oxygen and bronchodilator therapy.

___10.   A key intervention for a patient with metabolic alkalosis is having them breathe into a paper bag.

## Activity #3

Identify whether each assessment finding is a key feature of acidosis or alkalosis.

| Potassium Indication |
| --- |
| A. Acidosis |
| B. Alkalosis |

1. _____   Positive Trousseau sign
2. _____   Thready peripheral pulses
3. _____   Hyporeflexia
4. _____   Increased digoxin toxicity
5. _____   Flaccid paralysis
6. _____   Muscle cramping
7. _____   Dry skin
8. _____   Kussmaul respirations
9. _____   Hyperreflexia
10. _____   Paresthesias
11. _____   Coma
12. _____   Positive Chvostek sign
13. _____   Widened QRS complex
14. _____   Prolonged PR interval
15. _____   Increased activity

## Activity #4

Identify key assessment points the nurse will complete to determine whether a patient has acid-base balance.

1. _____

2. _____

3. _____

4. _____

5. _____

6. _____

7. _____

*Activity #5*

Explain how buffers work in the body.

_____

_____

_____

_____

_____

_____

_____

## Learning Assessment

### NCLEX Examination Challenge #1

Which client arterial blood gas results would the nurse interpret as within normal limits?

A.  pH 7.26, $PaCO_2$ 28, bicarbonate 16, $PaO_2$ 95
B.  pH 7.40, $PaCO_2$ 44, bicarbonate 24, $PaO_2$ 98
C.  pH 7.36, $PaCO_2$ 26, bicarbonate 17, $PaO_2$ 88
D.  pH 7.31, $PaCO_2$ 53, bicarbonate 30, $PaO_2$ 77

### NCLEX Examination Challenge #2

Which assessment finding does the nurse anticipate in a client with a pH of 7.29? **Select all that apply.**

A.  Decreased serum potassium levels
B.  Increased effectiveness of drugs
C.  Reduced function of hormones
D.  Increased function of enzymes
E.  Decreased cardiac electrical conduction

### NCLEX Examination Challenge #3

Which client will the nurse observe **most closely** for development of a base excess metabolic alkalosis?

A.  26-year-old who received a massive blood transfusion
B.  36-year-old who has a $PaO_2$ of 84 mm Hg and a $PaCO_2$ of 62 mm Hg
C.  56-year-old who has a serum potassium value of 6.0 mEq/L
D.  76-year-old who had surgery and a respiratory rate of 10 breaths/min

### NCLEX Examination Challenge #4

Which laboratory value will the nurse check **first** for a client with metabolic acidosis who now has tall, peaked T waves on the electrocardiogram (ECG)?

A.  Serum glucose
B.  Serum sodium
C.  Serum potassium
D.  Serum magnesium

# 15 CHAPTER

# *Concepts of Infusion Therapy*

## LEARNING OUTCOMES

1. Describe evidence-based practice to safely administer infusion therapy.
2. Identify the evidence-based guidelines for prevention of IV catheter-related bloodstream infection (CRBSI).
3. Describe the population-specific care for older adults receiving infusion therapy, including careful monitoring of fluid and electrolyte balance.
4. Teach the patient and family about infusion therapy and associated care.

5. Explain the evidence-based process of peripheral and central IV therapy, including site selection, insertion, and maintenance.
6. Use clinical judgment to prevent, assess, manage, and document complications related to infusion therapy and vascular access devices (VADs).
7. Describe nursing care associated with intra-arterial, intraperitoneal, subcutaneous, intraosseous, and intraspinal infusion therapy.

## Preliminary Reading

Read and review Chapter 15, pp. 285–315.

## Chapter Review

### Activity #1
List six activities that infusion nurses may perform.

1. _____

2. _____

3. _____

4. _____

5. _____

6. _____

**Activity #2**

For each statement, specify if the statement is **true (T)** or **false (F).**

_____1. The registered nurse is accountable for all aspects of infusion therapy and delegation of associated tasks.

_____2. Standards of practice for all nurses delivering infusion therapy are published by the American Nurses Association.

_____3. Isotonic parenteral solutions are between 270 and 300 mOsm/L.

_____4. Infiltration of an intravenous line always leads to infection.

_____5. Total parenteral nutrition (TPN) solutions have an osmolarity greater than 2000 mOsm/L.

_____6. The nurse can administer intradermal lidocaine before insertion of an IV device without a health care provider's order.

_____7. A peripheral vascular access device (VAD) can be converted into an intermittent IV lock.

_____8. Midline catheters are used for administration of vesicant medications.

_____9. Qualified registered nurses can insert nontunneled central venous catheters (CVCs).

____10. A short secondary administration set is also known as a piggyback set.

____11. Needleless system connections can only be cleaned vigorously with alcohol swabs.

____12. Blood pressure should be taken in an extremity that does not have a catheter in place.

____13. Tape and gauze dressings used with central lines must be changed every 72 hours.

____14. The back of the hand of an older adult with fragile skin is the preferred site for an initial IV site.

____15. Hypodermoclysis is used for long-term fluid volume replacement.

____16. Compartment syndrome is a rare yet potential complication of intraosseous therapy.

____17. Patients receiving intraperitoneal infusion therapy are placed in Trendelenburg position.

**Activity #3**

Provide at least two nursing interventions that can be used to address each given complication of IV therapy.

1. Infiltration

_____

_____

2. Extravasation

_____

_____

3. Phlebitis

_____

_____

4. Thrombosis

_____

_____

5.   Thrombophlebitis

_____

_____

6.   Ecchymosis and hematoma

_____

_____

7.   Site infection

_____

_____

8.   Venous spasm

_____

_____

**Activity #4**
Match the device with its description. (VAD = venous access device)

**Glossary Term**
___1.   Implanted port
___2.   Hemodialysis catheter
___3.   Midline catheter
___4.   Nontunneled central venous catheter (CVC)
___5.   Peripherally inserted central catheter (PICC)
___6.   Short peripheral intravenous catheter (short PIVC)
___7.   Tunneled central venous catheter (CVC)

**Description**
A.   VAD composed of a plastic cannula, built around a sharp stylet for venipuncture, which extends slightly beyond the cannula and is advanced into the vein
B.   Multilumen VAD inserted percutaneously through the subclavian or jugular vein
C.   Single-or double-lumen device inserted by a physician in radiology or a surgeon in an operating room
D.   VAD that is 3 to 8 inches long and inserted through larger peripheral veins in the mid or upper arm
E.   Catheter with very large lumen used to manage renal failure
F.   Surgically implanted VAD used for long-term infusion therapy in which the catheter lies in a subcutaneous tunnel, separating the points where the catheter enters the vein from where it enters the skin
G.   Long catheter inserted through a vein of the antecubital fossa or middle of the upper arm

**Activity #5**

Provide one indication for the use of each gauge of catheter.

1. 24–26 gauge _____

2. 22 gauge _____

3. 20 gauge _____

4. 18 gauge _____

5. 14–16 gauge _____

**Activity #6**

Fill in the blanks for portions of the Catheter-Related Bloodstream Infection (CRBSI) Prevention Bundle.
1. Use a _____ during insertion to make sure that everything is done correctly.
2. _____ before inserting a central line must be thorough (i.e., no quick scrub).
3. Use a _____ before initiation of insertion, correctly identifying patient, procedure, and site.
4. Maximal barrier precautions during line insertion require that the patient be draped from head to toe with a _____ barrier.
5. The primary health care provider who inserts the VAD wears sterile gloves, a gown, and a mask. Anyone in the room during the procedure must also wear a _____.
6. Traffic in and out of the room must be minimized. Many institutions use a _____ sign on the door of the room to prevent people from coming in and going out during the procedure.
7. _____ is used for skin disinfection because it has the best outcomes for preventing infection.
8. The _____ and _____ are the first choice for PICC placement.

**Learning Assessment**

**NCLEX Examination Challenge #1**

Which reason may require the nurse to obtain vascular access in a client? **Select all that apply.**
A. Administer medications.
B. Correct fluid imbalance.
C. Maintain acid-base balance.
D. Provide chemotherapy for clients with cancer.
E. Maintain an open line in case access is needed.

**NCLEX Examination Challenge #2**

Which volume and solution will the nurse use to flush a client's short peripheral intravenous catheter (PIVC)?
A. 5 mL heparin
B. 3 mL normal saline
C. 5 mL heparinized saline
D. 3 mL bacteriostatic saline

**NCLEX Examination Challenge #3**

Which IV fluid will the nurse plan to infuse for a client prescribed a hypotonic solution?
A. 0.9% saline (NS)
B. 0.45% NaCl (1/2 NS)
C. Ringer's lactate solution
D. 5% dextrose with 0.9% saline

# 16 CHAPTER

# *Concepts of Inflammation and Immunity*

## LEARNING OUTCOMES

1. Explain the parts and responses of the immune system.
2. Describe ways in which immunity is acquired.
3. Explain the impact of immunity and inflammation on the aging process.
4. Describe triggers, cell types, responses, and duration of protection associated with different types of immunity.

5. Interpret laboratory findings to assess the patient's risk for a problem with immunity or an increased risk for infection.

## Preliminary Reading

Read and review Chapter 16, pp. 316–332.

## Chapter Review

### Activity #1

List five ways that leukocytes provide protection via defensive actions.

1. _____

2. _____

3. _____

4. _____

5. _____

### Activity #2

For each statement, specify if the statement is **true (T)** or **false (F)**.

___1.   Immature, undifferentiated cells are called stem cells.

___2.   Circulating T lymphocytes decrease as people get older.

___3.   Macrophages are present in the liver, intestinal tract, and spleen.

___4.   *Antibody-mediated immunity* is also known as *innate immunity*.

___5.   A patient who is immunocompetent has maximum protection against infection.

_____6. Red blood cells are also known as erythrocytes.

_____7. Stem cells are sensitized B lymphocytes that produce specific antibodies on all subsequent exposures to the initial sensitizing agent.

_____8. Older adults are at low risk for infection because they have already encountered many bacteria and viruses during their lifetime.

_____9. The majority of white blood cells (WBCs) are eosinophils.

____10. The complement system is a part of a person's innate immunity.

**Activity #3**
Explain each stage of the inflammatory sequence.

1. Stage I

_____

_____

_____

_____

2. Stage II

_____

_____

_____

_____

_____

3. Stage III

_____

_____

_____

_____

## Activity #4
Match the type of immunity below with its description.

### Immunity Type
___1.   Active immunity
___2.   Artificial active immunity
___3.   Artificial passive immunity
___4.   Natural active immunity
___5.   Natural passive immunity
___6.   Passive immunity

### Description
A.   Occurs when a fetus obtains antibodies through the placenta or a newborn obtains antibodies through the mother's colostrum or breast milk
B.   Takes place when a killed or weakened form of a disease organism is introduced into the body through vaccination
C.   Develops when people are given antibodies to a disease instead of producing them within their own immune system
D.   Occurs when the body is exposed to a disease organism through infection and the immune system produces antibodies to that disease
E.   Takes place when the body is infected with a disease and responds through illness and recovery
F.   Occurs when the body is injected with antibodies that were created in the body of another person or animal (e.g., immune globulin)

## Activity #5
Identify the type of immunity the nurse will document in these situations

| Immunity Type Choices |
| --- |
| Natural active immunity |
| Artificial active immunity |
| Natural passive immunity |
| Artificial passive immunity |
| Innate immunity |

1.   A patient is given an influenza vaccine.

_____

2.   A patient with COVID-19 receives a monoclonal antibody infusion.

_____

3.   A patient contracts a GI virus and recovers 48 hours later.

_____

4.   A patient who is pregnant says, "My newborn will get antibodies when I breastfeed."

_____

5.   A patient gets a chemical on their skin that they can easily wash away.

_____

## Activity #6
List the five cardinal signs of inflammation.

1.   _____

2.   _____

3.   _____

4.   _____

5.   _____

## Learning Assessment

### NCLEX Examination Challenge #1
1.   Which client condition does the nurse identify that may reduce immune function? **Select all that apply.**
     A.   Takes NSAIDs and corticosteroids daily
     B.   Maintains control of type 2 diabetes mellitus
     C.   Is older than age 80 years and lives alone in own home
     D.   Used large public shelters during cold weather
     E.   Eats a restricted diet for several weeks to quickly lose weight

### NCLEX Examination Challenge #2
Which WBC differential laboratory value indicates to the nurse that a client has a serious ongoing bacterial infection?
A.   "Bands" are equal to the "segs".
B.   Lymphocytes outnumber the basophils.
C.   Monocyte count is 600/mm$^3$ (0.6 $\times$ 10$^9$/L).
D.   Total WBC count is 9000/mm$^3$ (9 $\times$ 10$^9$/L).

### NCLEX Examination Challenge #3
The nurse is caring for a client who asks, "What kind of health problems might develop because I have decreased regulator T-cells?" Which nursing response is appropriate?
A.   "You will need extra vaccinations because your ability to make antibodies is reduced."
B.   "You are much more susceptible to bacterial and viral infections than other people."
C.   "You may have an increased number of allergic reactions when exposed to allergens."
D.   "Your risk for cancer development is increased because your cells aren't functioning."

# 17 CHAPTER

# *Concepts of Care for Patients with Allergy and Immunity Conditions*

## Preliminary Reading

Read and review Chapter 17, pp. 333–374.

## Chapter Review

### Pathophysiology Review

#1. For each symptom or condition, identify the type of hypersensitivity reaction from the choices listed.

| Hypersensitivity Reaction Choices |
| --- |
| Type I |
| Type II |
| Type III |
| Type IV |

\_\_\_\_\_1.    Hemolytic transfusion reaction
\_\_\_\_\_2.    Rheumatoid arthritis
\_\_\_\_\_3.    Rash after poison ivy exposure

_____4.    Anaphylaxis
_____5.    Local response to a bee sting
_____6.    Allergy to penicillin
_____7.    Peanut allergy
_____8.    Sarcoidosis
_____9.    Systemic lupus erythematosus
____10.   Drug-induced hemolytic anemia

#2.  Fill in the chart to include the onset after exposure and at least three signs and symptoms of the given type of allergic reaction. In some instances, areas have been completed for you.

| Type | Onset After Exposure | Signs and Symptoms |
|---|---|---|
| **Type I**<br>or<br>**Anaphylactic Reaction**<br>or<br>**Immediate Reaction** | Immediate reaction occurs in _____ to _____ minutes<br>Accelerated reaction occurs in ___ to _____ hours | 1. _____<br><br>2. _____<br><br>3. _____ |
| **Type II**<br>or<br>**Cytotoxic-Mediated Response** | Can happen in minutes to hours | Specific symptoms are associated with the causative agent<br>(e.g., difficulty breathing, sense of anxiety, elevated pulse, and increased respiratory rate that arises during blood infusion) |
| **Type III**<br>or Immunocomplex **Reaction** | Can happen in hours to _____ | Dependent on specific disorder(s) |
| **Type IV**<br>or<br>**Delayed Hypersensitivity Reaction** | _____ to _____ hours | 1. _____<br><br>2. _____<br><br>3. _____ |

## Activities

### Activity #1
For each statement, specify if the statement is **true (T)** or **false (F)**.
_____1.    HIV is transmitted only by sexual contact.
_____2.    Fusion occurs when the HIV envelope and CD4 cell membrane join.
_____3.    Stage II of HIV infection is also known as AIDS.
_____4.    Autoimmune conditions are often genetically linked.
_____5.    Bone damage is uncommon in patients with systemic lupus erythematosus.
_____6.    The first-line intervention for anaphylaxis is application of oxygen to the patient.
_____7.    Patients with any type of food allergy should carry an epinephrine autoinjector.
_____8.    Anaphylaxis is a Type I hypersensitivity reaction.
_____9.    Contact dermatitis is a Type IV hypersensitivity reaction.
____10.   Preexposure prophylaxis is the use of HIV antiretroviral drugs by an HIV-uninfected adult to prevent infection after exposure to the HIV virus.

## Activity #2

List at least two signs and symptoms of rejection for each given organ.

| Organ | Signs and Symptoms of Rejection |
|---|---|
| Heart | 1. _____<br>2. _____ |
| Kidney | 1. _____<br>2. _____ |
| Liver | 1. _____<br>2. _____ |
| Lung | 1. _____<br>2. _____ |
| Pancreas | 1. _____<br>2. _____ |

## Activity #3

Match each drug in Column A with its appropriate class in Column B.

**Column A**
___1. Enfuvirtide
___2. Raltegravir
___3. Ritonavir
___4. Ibalizumab-uiyk
___5. Abacavir
___6. Efavirenz
___7. Darunavir

**Column B**
A. PK enhancer
B. Monoclonal antibody
C. Protease inhibitor
D. Integrase inhibitor
E. Entry inhibitor
F. Nucleoside reverse transcriptase inhibitor (NRTI)
G. Nonnucleoside reverse transcriptase inhibitor (NNTRI)

**Activity #4**

For each system, list potential assessment findings the nurse would anticipate in a client with Stage III HIV infection (AIDS).

| System | Potential Assessment Findings |
|---|---|
| **Cardiovascular** | |
| Heart failure | |
| **Endocrine** | |
| Hormonal changes | |
| **Gastrointestinal** | |
| Anorexia, malabsorption, weight loss | |
| Diarrhea (can result in "AIDS wasting syndrome") | |
| Oral and esophageal lesions | |
| **Immune** | |
| *Candida albicans* | |
| Human papillomavirus (HPV) | |
| **Integumentary** | |
| Kaposi's sarcoma (KS) | |
| **Neurologic** | |
| HIV-associated dementia (HAD) | |
| **Renal** | |
| HIV-associated nephropathy (HIVAN) | |
| **Respiratory** | |
| *Pneumocystis jiroveci* pneumonia (PCP) | |
| Tuberculosis (TB) | |

**Activity #5**

List 10 common autoimmune disorders.

1. _____

2. _____

3. _____

4. _____

5. _____

6. _____

7. _____

8. _____

9. _____

10. _____

## Learning Assessments

### NCLEX Examination Challenge #1
The nurse is caring for a client scheduled to undergo testing with contrast dye. Which client statement requires the nurse to intervene?
A. "Diabetes and high blood pressure are part of my family history."
B. "My sister is allergic to the red dye that is used in juice beverages."
C. "I have a lot of seasonal allergies, and they make me pretty miserable."
D. "Last year I had a test with contrast dye, and my face got very swollen."

### NCLEX Examination Challenge #2
The nurse has started IV administration of a newly prescribed drug. Which client symptom prompts the nurse to initiate the Rapid Response Team for possible anaphylaxis? **Select all that apply**.
A. Facial flushing
B. Heart rate 58 beats/min
C. Oxygen saturation of 88%
D. Wheezing on exhalation
E. Increased deep tendon reflexes

### NCLEX Examination Challenge #3
The nurse is caring for a client who went camping and hiking 1 month prior. Which new symptom does the nurse associate with the possibility of Stage I of Lyme disease?
A. Acute confusion
B. Cardiac dysrhythmias
C. Erythema migrans rash
D. Sudden onset of painful, swollen joints

**NGN Challenge #1**

The nurse reviews the Nurses Notes for a 29-year-old female client who has come to the primary health care provider with flu-like symptoms.

| Nurses Notes | Health Care Provider's Orders | Diagnostic Testing Results |
|---|---|---|

**1232:** Client here to see the health care provider to establish care. She has moved here recently after living in three states previously over the past 4 years. Reports having seen numerous health care providers who have diagnosed her with recurrent viral infections. She states that over the past few years she has experienced intermittent low-grade fevers that do not respond to acetaminophen or ibuprofen. She states she also has rashes that come and go over the body and facial redness that seems to have increased over the past year. They do resolve on their own but recur frequently. States that she has ongoing fatigue and consistent pain in her joints yet says, "I am too young for arthritis." Rates joint pain as a 4 or 5 on a 0 to 10 scale. Denies any changes in bowel or bladder habits. Other than these ongoing symptoms, her medical history is unremarkable. Family history positive for type 2 diabetes, rheumatoid arthritis, and hypertension. Current on immunizations.
Current VS: T 99.9°F (37.7°C); HR 62 beats/min and regular; RR 14 breaths/min; BP 110/70 mm Hg; SpO$_2$ 97%. Alert and oriented × 4. Slight redness on face noted across bridge of nose. Breath sounds clear in all lung fields. No wheezes, crackles, or dyspnea. S$_1$ and S$_2$ present; no murmurs. Bowel sounds present × 4; no abdominal tenderness noted on palpation. Joints in hands and knees appear slightly swollen.

Complete the diagram by selecting from the choices to specify what **one** potential condition the client may be experiencing, **two** actions the nurse would take to address that condition, and **two** parameters the nurse would monitor to assess the client's progress.

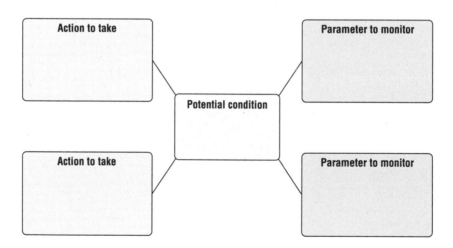

| Actions to Take | Potential Condition | Parameters to Monitor |
|---|---|---|
| Remind to have laboratory work performed for CBC and ANA | Lyme disease | Confusion as disease stages progress |
| Conduct further pain assessment for patterns | Stage I HIV infection | Formation of scaled lesions |
| Arrange for family member to drive her to appointment to receive HIV testing results | Systemic lupus erythematosus | Development of opportunistic infections |
| Encourage use of ice packs over joints | Psoriasis | Bone density |
| Teach how to apply topical antibiotic to rash on face | ///////////////////////////// | Cardiac changes |

**NGN Challenge #2**

The nurse reviews the Nurses Notes for a 21-year-old client who is seeing the primary health care provider for flu-like symptoms.

| Nurses Notes | Health Care Provider's Orders | Diagnostic Testing Results |
|---|---|---|

**1030:** Client here to see provider for flu-like symptoms. Reports that he attended a large party 2 weeks ago and, following that event, had ongoing symptoms such as sore throat, chills, fever, night sweats, headache, fatigue, and muscle aches. States, "I have felt better since yesterday but I had already made this appointment so I thought I would still come in. When I made this appointment, I was worried that I had COVID-19." Acknowledges that at the party, he was drinking heavily and engaging in unprotected sexual activity with two other males in attendance. Medical history unremarkable. Social history positive for occasional use of marijuana. Family history positive for hypertension and glaucoma. Current VS: T 98.9°F (37.2°C); HR 74 beats/min and regular; RR 18 breaths/min; BP 118/74 mm Hg; SpO$_2$ 98%. Alert and oriented × 4. Throat slightly red. Breath sounds clear in all lung fields. No wheezes, crackles, or dyspnea noted. S$_1$ and S$_2$ present; no murmurs. Bowel sounds present × 4; no abdominal tenderness noted on palpation.

Complete the diagram by selecting from the choices to specify what **one** potential condition the client may be experiencing, **two** actions the nurse would take to address that condition, and **two** parameters the nurse would monitor to assess the client's progress.

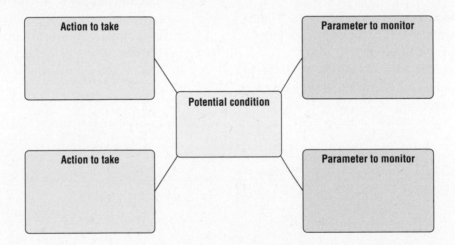

| Actions to Take | Potential Condition | Parameters to Monitor |
|---|---|---|
| Offer PrEP therapy | COVID-19, resolving | Observation of bedrest |
| Teach about Epstein-Barr virus | Mononucleosis | Viral load |
| Prepare to administer monoclonal antibodies | Influenza, resolving | Finishing full course of antibiotics |
| Encourage regular use of condoms during sexual encounters | Stage I HIV infection | Maintenance of quarantine |
| Explain stages of disease and associated symptomology | //////////////////////////////// | Adherence to antiretroviral therapy |

# 18
CHAPTER

# *Concepts of Care for Patients with Cancer*

## LEARNING OUTCOMES

1. Apply knowledge of anatomy, physiology, and pathophysiology to provide evidence-based care for patients with cancer affecting cellular regulation.
2. Teach adults behaviors that reduce the risk for cancer development.
3. Teach the patient and caregiver(s) about common drugs and other management strategies used for cancer.
4. Plan patient- and family-centered nursing interventions to decrease the psychosocial impact caused by living with cancer.
5. Analyze assessment and diagnostic findings to generate solutions and prioritize nursing care for patients with cancer.
6. Plan collaborative care with the interprofessional team to coordinate high-quality care to patients with cancer.
7. Organize care coordination and transition management for patients with cancer.
8. Protect yourself and others from cytotoxic agents and radiation.
9. Use clinical judgment to plan evidence-based nursing care to promote cellular regulation and prevent complications in patients with cancer.
10. Incorporate factors that affect health equity into the plan of care for patients with cancer.

## Preliminary Reading

Read and review Chapter 18, pp. 375–405.

## Chapter Review

### Pathophysiology Review

#1. Match the Key Term in Column A with its description in Column B.

| Column A | Column B |
|---|---|
| \_\_\_\_1. Carcinogenesis | A. Invasion and spreading of cancer cells from the primary tumor to other locations |
| \_\_\_\_2. Carcinogen | B. Substance that can induce nausea and vomiting |
| \_\_\_\_3. Emetogenic | C. Decreased platelets |
| \_\_\_\_4. Extravasation | D. Drugs designed to activate body's immune system to attack cancer cells |
| \_\_\_\_5. Immunotherapy | E. Change of a normal cell into a cancer cell |
| \_\_\_\_6. Metastasis | F. Vesicant leaking or infiltration into surrounding tissue |
| \_\_\_\_7. Nadir | G. Decreased neutrophils |
| \_\_\_\_8. Neutropenia | H. Drugs that can cause severe tissue damage |
| \_\_\_\_9. Thrombocytopenia | I. Period in which bone marrow suppression is the greatest |
| \_\_\_10. Vesicant | J. Substances that change cell gene activity so cell becomes a cancer cell |

#2. Fill in the chart to describe the actions that take place in each step of carcinogenesis.

| Step | Actions |
|---|---|
| Initiation | |
| Promotion | |
| Progression | |
| Metastasis | |

## Activities

### Activity #1

For each statement, specific if the statement is **true (T)** or **false (F)**.

\_\_\_\_1. Cancers are classified according to the type of tissue from which they arise.

\_\_\_\_2. Pathologic staging assesses tumor size, number, sites, and lymph node spread.

\_\_\_\_3. Cruciferous vegetables should be avoided to minimize the risk for cancer.

\_\_\_\_4. Having mutations of the *APC* gene increases the risk for colon cancer.

\_\_\_\_5. Radiation is a type of systemic treatment for various types of cancer.

\_\_\_\_6. Intravesicular chemotherapy is given directly into the cerebrospinal fluid.

\_\_\_\_7. Patients who are immunosuppressed benefit from being in a private room.

\_\_\_\_8. Patients with a low white blood count should never prepare meals.

\_\_\_\_9. Teach the patient with mucositis to drink at least 3 or more liters of water daily.

\_\_\_10. Endocrine therapy can include the use of antiandrogens and antiestrogens.

### Activity #2

Fill in the chart to include at least two early and two late sides effects (where applicable) of radiation therapy per body location.

| Body Location | Early Effect | Late Effect |
|---|---|---|
| Central nervous system | | |
| Head and neck | | |
| Breast and chest wall | | |

| Body Location | Early Effect | Late Effect |
|---|---|---|
| Chest and lung | | XXXXXXXXXXXXXXXXXXXXXXXXXXX |
| Abdomen and pelvis | | |
| Eye | | XXXXXXXXXXXXXXXXXXXXXXXXXX |

## Activity #3

Fill in the blanks to demonstrate the Seven Warning Signs of Cancer.

| | |
|---|---|
| **C** | C _____ |
| **A** | A _____ |
| **U** | U _____ |
| **T** | T _____ |
| **I** | I _____ |
| **O** | O _____ |
| **N** | N _____ |

## Activity #4

For each cancer type, identify three methods of assessment the nurse would use when examining an older adult for that condition. These methods may include questions the nurse would ask the patient, observations the nurse would make, or hands-on modes of assessment.

| Cancer Type | Assessment Methods |
|---|---|
| Colorectal cancer | 1. _____ <br> _____ <br><br> 2. _____ <br> _____ <br><br> 3. _____ <br> _____ |
| Lung cancer | 1. _____ <br> _____ <br><br> 2. _____ <br> _____ <br><br> 3. _____ <br> _____ |
| Prostate cancer | 1. _____ <br> _____ <br><br> 2. _____ <br> _____ <br><br> 3. _____ <br> _____ |

| Cancer Type | Assessment Methods |
|---|---|
| Skin cancer | 1. _____<br>_____<br>2. _____<br>_____<br>3. _____<br>_____ |
| Leukemia | 1. _____<br>_____<br>2. _____<br>_____<br>3. _____<br>_____ |
| Bladder cancer | 1. _____<br>_____<br>2. _____<br>_____<br>3. _____<br>_____ |

**Activity #5**

Explain characteristics of each type of surgery that can be used to address a cancer diagnosis.

*Prophylactic surgery:*

_____

_____

_____

*Diagnostic surgery:*

_____

_____

_____

*Curative surgery:*

_____

_____

_____

*Debulking surgery:*

_____

_____

_____

*Palliative surgery:*

_____

_____

_____

*Reconstructive or restorative surgery:*

_____

_____

_____

## Learning Assessment

### NCLEX Examination Challenge #1

Which precaution will the nurse teach a client undergoing 6 weeks of daily external beam radiation for breast cancer? **Select all that apply**.
A.   Do not remove the markings.
B.   Avoid direct skin exposure to sunlight for up to a year.
C.   Wash the area with your hand using only mild soap and water.
D.   Apply a heating pad to treated areas to stimulate circulation.
E.   Avoid wearing a tight-fitting bra during treatment and when the area is irritated.

### NCLEX Examination Challenge #2

Which statement by a client taking an oral cancer agent indicates to the nurse that further teaching is required?
A.   "This drug is much more convenient than my old IV drugs."
B.   "I understand that not skipping doses is important in controlling cancer."
C.   "My partner wants to help me, but I told him that only I should touch this drug."
D.   "I have been crushing the drug and putting it in my tea because it is hard to swallow."

## NCLEX Examination Challenge #3

Which intervention will the nurse choose when caring for a client whose platelet count is 18,000/mm³ ($18 \times 10^9$/L) (Reference range: 150,000–400,000/mm³ or $150–400 \times 10^9$/L [SI units])?

A. Apply pressure after blood draws.
B. Assign to a contact isolation room.
C. Use oxygen to reduce dyspnea.
D. Restrict fluids to prevent edema.

## NGN Challenge #1

The nurse documents assessment findings for a 58-year-old client who is seeing the primary health care provider for an annual checkup.

| Health History | Nurses Notes | Vital Signs | Laboratory Results |
|---|---|---|---|

**1010:** Client is here to see primary care provider for an annual health checkup. Electronic health record shows it has been 16 months since his last annual evaluation. Denies any health changes other than a bit of blood in stool recently that he attributes to hemorrhoids. Quantifies that "recently" means that the blood in stool began about 2 months ago and occurs several times a week. States it is not profuse, noting about 1 tablespoon of bright red blood in toilet following some bowel movements. Denies pain with defecation. No changes in urinary habits. Medical history positive for GERD controlled by omeprazole 20 mg, three times daily before meals. Reports that this usually works most of the time, but has been experiencing some abdominal discomfort and reflux following meals over the last few months. States, "a couple of times I took a double dose of omeprazole but it didn't help." Alert and oriented × 4. Breath sounds clear in all lung fields. No wheezes, crackles, or dyspnea. $S_1$ and $S_2$ present; no murmurs. Bowel sounds present × 4. Abdomen nontender upon gentle palpation. Current VS: T 98.4°F (36.9°C); HR 84 beats/min and regular; RR 18 breaths/min; BP 130/90 mm Hg; SpO$_2$ 99%.

**Highlight the client findings in the above note that are abnormal.**

The nurse analyzes the findings to determine the client's condition. **Select two findings that require immediate follow-up by the nurse.**

☐ Blood in stool
☐ Taking double doses of omeprazole
☐ Blood pressure 130/90 mm Hg
☐ Bright red blood in toilet
☐ Has not seen provider in 16 months
☐ Experiencing increased instances of reflux

| Health History | Nurses Notes | Vital Signs | Laboratory Results |
|---|---|---|---|

**1010:** Client is here to see primary care provider for an annual health checkup. Electronic health record shows it has been 16 months since his last annual evaluation. Denies any health changes other than a bit of blood in stool recently that he attributes to hemorrhoids. Quantifies that "recently" means that the blood in stool began about 2 months ago and occurs several times a week. States it is not profuse, noting about 1 tablespoon of bright red blood in toilet following some bowel movements. Denies pain with defecation. No changes in urinary habits. Medical history positive for GERD controlled by omeprazole 20 mg, three times daily before meals. Reports that this usually works most of the time, but has been experiencing some abdominal discomfort and reflux following meals over the last few months. States, "a couple of times I took a double dose of omeprazole but it didn't help." Alert and oriented × 3. Breath sounds clear in all lung fields. No wheezes, crackles, or dyspnea. $S_1$ and $S_2$ present; no murmurs. Bowel sounds present × 4. Abdomen nontender upon gentle palpation. Current VS: T 98.4°F (36.9°C); HR 84 beats/min and regular; RR 18 breaths/min; BP 130/90 mm Hg; SpO$_2$ 99%.

The nurse considers the client data to determine the priority for the plan of care. Choose the **most likely** options for the information missing from the statement below by selecting from the list of options provided.

The client is at highest risk for having _____(1)_____ cancer as evidenced by _____(2)_____ and _____(3)_____.

| Options for 1 | Options for 2 and 3 |
|---|---|
| Stomach | Increased reflux |
| Prostate | Blood in toilet |
| Colon | Taking extra GERD medication |
| Esophageal | Blood in stool |
| Throat | Hypertension |

While the health care provider is reviewing the electronic health record before seeing the patient, the nurse gathers supplies.

Which item will the nurse gather for the examination and remainder of the visit? **Select all that apply.**
A. Hemoccult card
B. Plastic speculum
C. Handout on colonoscopies
D. Information about a low-fat diet
E. Brochure on high-fiber food choices
F. Plate for gonorrhea and chlamydia smears

One week later, the client has had a colonoscopy and his hemoccult results are complete. The client is diagnosed by the health care provider with colon cancer. Surgery and chemotherapy are scheduled. The nurse provides teaching before beginning chemotherapy.

Select three pieces of information the nurse will teach the client about chemotherapy.
A. Chemotherapy can be immunosuppressive.
B. It is normal to have a fever and rash during chemotherapy.
C. Certain chemotherapy side effects can be life-threatening.
D. If oral chemotherapy drugs expire, flush them down the toilet.
E. Oral chemotherapy drugs are less toxic than intravenous chemotherapy.
F. Chemotherapeutic agents kill only the cancer cells that are present in the body.
G. If children are desired in the future, a sperm bank representative can provide options.

At the last chemotherapy appointment, the nurse conducts an assessment. For each client finding, use an X to indicate whether the initial nursing interventions implemented during chemotherapy were **Effective** (helped to meet expected outcomes) or **Not Effective** (did not help to meet expected outcomes).

| Previous Client Finding | Current Client Finding | Effective | Not Effective |
|---|---|---|---|
| Blood in stool | No further blood in stool reported | | |
| Blood in toilet | States no blood has been found in the toilet since surgery and chemotherapy | | |
| Platelet count 225,000/mm$^3$ (225 $\times$ 10$^9$/L) (Reference range 150,000–400,000/mm$^3$ or 150–400 $\times$ 10$^9$/L [SI units]) | Platelet count 176,000/mm$^3$ (176 $\times$ 10$^9$/L) | | |
| White blood cell count 6500/mm$^3$ (6.5 $\times$ 10$^9$/L) (Reference range 5000–10,000/mm$^3$ or 5–10 $\times$ 10$^9$/L [SI units]) | White blood cell count 5300/mm$^3$ (5.3 $\times$ 10$^9$/L) | | |

# 19 CHAPTER

# Concepts of Care for Patients with Infection

## LEARNING OUTCOMES

1. Use clinical judgment to determine infection control measures based on the infection transmission method.
2. List factors that increase the risk for infection in older adults.
3. Describe evidence-based infection control measures used in hospitals and other inpatient health care facilities.
4. Summarize infection control issues that were recognized as a result of the COVID-19 pandemic.
5. Recognize relevant assessment findings associated with local and systemic infections.
6. Identify nursing implications associated with common multidrug-resistant organisms.
7. Plan actions to manage fever in the patient with systemic infection.

## Preliminary Reading

Read and review Chapter 19, pp. 406–421.

## Chapter Review

### Activity #1

Name two major normal physiologic defenses the body has against infection.

1. _____

2. _____

### Activity #2

Match the term in Column A with its definition in Column B.

**Column A**

____1. Communicability
____2. Microbiome
____3. Endemic
____4. Virulence
____5. Immunity
____6. Sepsis
____7. Colonization
____8. Cohorting

**Column B**

A. A disease with a relatively high and predictable rate of infection in a particular population or region
B. A life-threatening clinical syndrome caused by an infection and resulting in organ dysfunction
C. The protection from illness or disease that is maintained by the body's defenses
D. The ability of pathogens to spread from one person to another and cause disease
E. Genomes of all the microorganisms that coexist in and on a person
F. The practice of grouping patients who are colonized or infected with the same pathogen
G. The ability of a pathogen to cause severe disease or infection
H. The presence of pathogens in host tissues that do not cause symptomatic disease because of normal flora

## Activity #3
Older adults are more at risk for infection than their younger counterparts. List at least four physiologic changes of aging or other factors that contribute to this increased risk.

1. _____

2. _____

3. _____

4. _____

## Activity #4
Match the transmission precaution type in Column A with the client condition in Column B.

**Column A**
___1.   Standard precautions
___2.   Contact precautions
___3.   Droplet precautions
___4.   Airborne precautions

**Column B**
A.   Pneumonia
B.   Disseminated varicella zoster
C.   Peritonitis
D.   Scabies

## Activity #5
List three nursing interventions that are appropriate to manage a fever for clients who have systemic infection.

1. _____

2. _____

3. _____

## Activity #6
For each statement, specify if the statement is **true (T)** or **false (F).**
___1.   Indwelling urinary catheters are the primary cause of urinary tract infections.
___2.   One of the results of the COVID-19 pandemic was an increase in other hospital infections.
___3.   Hand hygiene refers only to handwashing for at least 15 to 30 seconds.
___4.   Infections caused by multidrug-resistant organisms have a higher mortality than other infection types.
___5.   When administering delafloxacin, give the drug with meals or immediately before eating.
___6.   To prevent acquiring an infection, nurses should change their clothes from scrubs to personal clothes before leaving work.

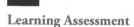 

## Learning Assessment

### NCLEX Examination Challenge #1

1. The nurse is reviewing regulations related to infection control and injury prevention for the workplace. Which U.S. federal organization oversees worker protection from injury and illness?
   A. Centers for Disease Control and Prevention (CDC)
   B. Occupational Safety and Health Administration (OSHA)
   C. Food and Drug Administration (FDA)
   D. National Institutes of Health (NIH)

### NCLEX Examination Challenge #2

The nurse is caring for a client with a chronic respiratory condition that was likely caused by particulate matter exposure. When conducting a client history, which questions would the nurse include? **Select all that apply.**
A. "What activities do you engage in at your current workplace?"
B. "What activities did you engage in at your previous places of employment?"
C. "What health concerns do you have about your current work environment?"
D. "Is your workplace part of a corporate chain or a private company?"
E. "If you live in a house or apartment, when was it built?"

### NCLEX Examination Challenge #3

The nurse is caring for a client with a systemic infection as a result of a gunshot wound (GSW). Which laboratory finding would the nurse expect?
A. Increased WBC count
B. Decreased erythrocyte sedimentation rate (ESR)
C. Decreased neutrophil count
D. Negative wound culture

# 20
CHAPTER

# *Assessment of Skin, Hair, and Nails*

## LEARNING OUTCOMES

1. Use knowledge of anatomy and physiology to perform a focused assessment of the skin, hair, and nails.
2. Teach evidence-based health promotion activities to help prevent skin, hair, and nail health problems or trauma.
3. Identify factors that affect health equity for patients with skin, hair, or nail health problems.
4. Explain how genetic implications and physiologic aging of the skin, hair, and nails affect tissue integrity.
5. Interpret assessment findings for patients with a suspected or actual skin, hair, or nail problem.
6. Plan evidence-based care and support for patients undergoing diagnostic testing of the skin or nails.

## Preliminary Reading

Read and review Chapter 20, pp. 422–441.

## Chapter Review

### Anatomy & Physiology Review

#1. Label the parts skin using the Anatomy Labels provided on the following page.

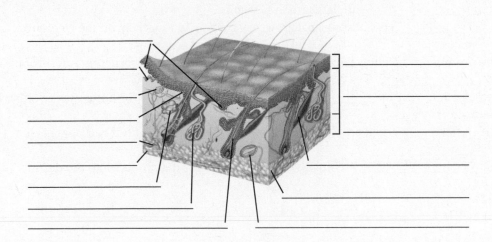

| Anatomy Labels |
|---|
| Rete pegs |
| Dermal papillae |
| Meissner corpuscle |
| Melanocytes |
| Artery |
| Vein |
| Sebaceous gland |
| Sweat gland |
| Hair shaft |
| Pacinian corpuscle |
| Fat |
| Arrector pili muscle |
| Epidermis |
| Dermis |
| Subcutaneous layer |

#2. Complete the sentences by filling in the blanks with terms or phrases listed. Not all terms will be used.

1. The _____ is the outermost layer of skin.
2. Purple patches on the skin that may be caused by blood disorders, trauma, or vascular abnormalities are called _____.
3. The function of _____ is to lubricate the skin and to reduce water loss from the surface of the skin.
4. Lice eggs are called _____.
5. _____ are larger than petechiae.
6. _____ is the abnormal growth of body hair, especially on the face, chest, and abdomen of females.
7. The protein produced by keratinocytes that makes the stratum corneum waterproof is called _____.
8. Some people develop _____, an accumulation of patchy or diffuse white or gray scales on the scalp's surface.
9. The initial reaction to a problem altering one of the skin's structural components is a _____.
10. The _____ are fingers of epidermal tissue that project into the dermis.

## Choices for Sentence Completion

| |
|---|
| Bioburden |
| Dandruff |
| Dermal papillae |
| Dystrophic |
| Ecchymoses |
| Ground substance |
| Hirsutism |
| Keratin |
| Lunula |
| Macular |
| Nits |
| Papular |
| Petechiae |
| Primary lesion |
| Purpura |
| Sebum |
| Secondary lesion |
| Stratum corneum |

## Activities

### Activity #1
List five common skin changes associated with aging.

1. _____

2. _____

3. _____

4. _____

5. _____

**Activity #2**

Complete the sentences with the correct term or phrase.

1.  Intact skin helps regulate _____ and maintain _____.
2.  The _____ and _____ in the dermis serve to exchange oxygen and heat.
3.  A person's hair color is determined by their rate of _____.
4.  The nurse teaches patients to avoid exposure to _____ and _____ to minimize the chance of developing skin cancer.
5.  _____ can develop as the result of a patient's activities.
6.  The term used describe a skin lesion with wavy borders is _____.
7.  Red discoloration of the lunula can indicate _____.
8.  Early clubbing can be a sign of _____ or _____.
9.  The procedure of cutting and removing a small plug of tissue is called a _____.
10. A _____ lamp can be used to determine if a skin infection is present.

**Activity #3**

For each statement, specify if the statement is **true (T)** or **false (F)**.

_____1.  Shave biopsies remove only the part of the skin that rises above the surrounding tissue when injected with a local anesthetic.
_____2.  Dandruff flaking occurs when a patient's scalp is very dry.
_____3.  Inspect the mucous membranes of a patient with dark skin to assess for pallor.
_____4.  Hirsutism can be a sign of a hormonal imbalance or a side effect of drug therapy.
_____5.  Sterile gloves are necessary when collecting samples from the skin for laboratory testing.
_____6.  Informed consent is not needed for a skin biopsy because it is a minor procedure.
_____7.  The nurse teaches patients who had a skin biopsy to remove dried blood or crusting with tap water or saline.
_____8.  The patient who will have diascopy performed must give informed consent.
_____9.  The ABCDE method is used to assess for melanoma.
_____10.  A lesion with border irregularity, symmetrical shape, and less than 1/4" does not require further assessment.

**Activity #4**

List pertinent questions the nurse will ask about the current concerns of a patient with a skin condition.

1.  _____

2.  _____

3.  _____

4.  _____

5.  _____

6.  _____

7.  _____

## Learning Assessments

### NCLEX Examination Challenge #1

The nurse has used the ABCDE method to assess a client for melanoma. Which assessment finding requires the nurse to notify the health care provider? **Select all that apply.**

A. Border regularity of a lesion
B. Asymmetry of a lesion's shape
C. Small amount of bleeding from a lesion
D. Diameter of one lesion approximately 7 mm
E. Change in the color of a lesion since the last visit

### NCLEX Examination Challenge #2

Which laboratory test will the nurse check as the **priority** when caring for a client with a large amount of ecchymoses?

A. Platelet count
B. Hemoglobin level
C. White blood cell count
D. International normalized ratio (INR)

### NCLEX Examination Challenge #3

How will the nurse document a client's rash that is red, raised, and itching over much of the body?

A. Red, macular, lichenified
B. Cyanotic, annular, circinate
C. Linear, universal, nummular
D. Erythematous, diffuse, pruritic

# 21 CHAPTER

# Concepts of Care for Patients with Conditions of the Skin, Hair, and Nails

## LEARNING OUTCOMES

1. Plan collaborative care with the interprofessional team to promote tissue integrity in patients with skin disorders.
2. Teach adults how to decrease the risk for skin disorders.
3. Teach the patient and caregiver(s) about common drugs and other management strategies used for skin disorders.
4. Plan patient- and family-centered nursing interventions to decrease the psychosocial impact caused by living with skin disorders.
5. Apply knowledge of anatomy, physiology, and pathophysiology to provide evidence-based care for patients with skin disorders affecting tissue integrity.
6. Analyze assessment and diagnostic findings to generate solutions and prioritize nursing care for patients with skin disorders.
7. Organize care coordination and transition management for patients with skin disorders.
8. Use clinical judgment to plan evidence-based nursing care to promote tissue integrity and fluid and electrolyte balance and prevent complications in patients with skin disorders.
9. Incorporate factors that affect health equity into the plan of care for patients with skin disorders.

## Preliminary Reading

Read and review Chapter 21, pp. 442–493.

## Chapter Review

### Pathophysiology Review

#1. Match the Key Term in Column A with its description in Column B.

| Column A | | Column B | |
|---|---|---|---|
| _____1. | Allograft | A. | Cutting layers to release pressure or tension |
| _____2. | Autograft | B. | Mechanical entrapment and detachment of dead tissue |
| _____3. | Contraction | C. | Skin replacement using another person's tissue |
| _____4. | Escharotomy | D. | Release of eschar when burns compromise circulation or respiration |
| _____5. | Fasciotomy | E. | Regrowth across a wound's open area |
| _____6. | Granulation | F. | Skin replacement using nonhuman tissue |
| _____7. | Mechanical débridement | G. | Hidden wounds extending into surrounding tissues |
| _____8. | Resurfacing | H. | Skin replacement using patient's own tissue |
| _____9. | Tunneling | I. | Formation of scar tissue for wound healing |
| ___10. | Xenograft | J. | Wound closure by new collagen replacing damaged tissue |

#2.  Fill in the chart to describe the given lesion type. Some columns may support more than one word choice.

| Lesion Type | Flat or Raised? | Description | Primary Location |
|---|---|---|---|
| Actinic (solar) keratosis (premalignant) | | | |
| Squamous cell carcinoma | | | |
| Basal cell carcinoma | | | |
| Melanoma | | | |

### Word choices for "flat or raised"

| |
|---|
| Flat |
| Raised |

### Word choices for "description"

| |
|---|
| Central crater |
| Crust |
| Indurated |
| Macule |
| Nodule |
| Papule |
| Pigmented |
| Plaque |

### Word choices for "primary location"

| |
|---|
| Back – upper |
| Burns |
| Cheeks |
| Ears |
| Hands – back |
| Hands – palms |
| Head |
| Forehead |
| Forearms |
| Legs – lower |
| Lip |
| Neck |
| Nevi (nearby) |
| Scars |
| Soles of feet |

#3. Regarding the Burn Resuscitation Phase, indicate in the chart below whether the laboratory test is anticipated to be <u>increased</u> or <u>decreased</u> along with the rationale for why this finding is expected.

| Test | Normal Ranges (SI Units) | Increased or Decreased with Rationale |
|---|---|---|
| **Blood studies** | | |
| Hemoglobin, total | *Females:* 12–16 g/dL (7.4–9.9 mmol/L)<br>*Males:* 14–18 g/dL (8.7–11.2 mmol/L) | Increased or decreased?<br>_____<br>Rationale: |
| Hematocrit | *Females:* 37%–47% (0.37–0.47 volume fraction)<br>*Males:* 40%–52% (0.40–0.52 volume fraction) | Increased or decreased?<br>_____<br>Rationale: |
| Urea nitrogen | *Adult:* 10–20 mg/dL or 3.6–7.1 mmol/L (SI units)<br>*Older adult:* May be slightly higher than adult | Increased or decreased?<br>_____<br>Rationale: |
| Glucose | *Adult:* 74–106 mg/dL or 4.1–5.9 mmol/L<br>*Older adult aged 60–90 years:* 82–115 mg/dL or 4.6–6.4 mmol/L<br>*Older adult aged >90 years:* 75–121 mg/dL or 4.2–6.7 mmol/L | Increased or decreased?<br>_____<br>Rationale: |
| **Electrolytes** | | |
| Sodium | *Adult and older adults:* 136–145 mEq/L or 136–145 mmol/L (SI units) | Increased or decreased?<br>_____<br>Rationale: |
| Potassium | *Adult and older adults:* 3.5–5.0 mEq/L or 3.5–5.0 mmol/L (SI units) | Increased or decreased?<br>_____<br>Rationale: |
| Chloride | *Adult and older adults:* 98–106 mEq/L or 98–106 mmol/L (SI units) | Increased or decreased?<br>_____<br>Rationale: |
| **Arterial blood gases** | | |
| $PO_2$ | 80–100 mm Hg<br>*Older adults:* values may be lower | Increased or decreased?<br>_____<br>Rationale: |

| PCO$_2$ | 35–45 mm Hg | Increased or decreased? _____ Rationale: |
| --- | --- | --- |
| pH | 7.35–7.45 | Increased or decreased? _____ Rationale: |
| Carboxyhemoglobin (COHb, carbon monoxide) | Saturation of hemoglobin<br>Nonsmoker: <3%<br>Smoker: 12% | Increased or decreased? _____ Rationale: |
| **Other** | | |
| Total protein | *Adult/older adult:*<br>6.4–8.3 g/dL or 64–83 g/L (SI units) | Increased or decreased? _____ Rationale: |
| Albumin | 3.5–5 g/dL or 35–50 g/L (SI units) | Increased or decreased? _____ Rationale: |

## Activities

### Activity #1

For each statement below, specify if the statement is **true (T)** or **false (F)**.

_____1.   Collagen dressings can be used in the treatment of stage 3 or 4 pressure injuries.
_____2.   Sterile maggots are an approved treatment to consume necrotic wound tissue.
_____3.   Skin shearing only occurs after patients become older adults.
_____4.   The most common skin cancer worldwide is basal cell carcinoma.
_____5.   Grafting is a procedure that is done to cover burn wounds.
_____6.   Emergency tracheostomy is needed for any patient with smoke inhalation.
_____7.   Patients with pediculosis are usually prescribed lindane for treatment.
_____8.   A herpes zoster outbreak extends from one side of the body across the midline.
_____9.   Topical corticosteroids are contraindicated in the treatment of plaque psoriasis.
_____10.  Teach patients with contact dermatitis to avoid perfumed hygiene products.

**Activity #2**

Indicate whether the finding below is a <u>local indicator</u> or <u>systemic indicator</u> of infection.

| | Finding | Local Indicator | Systemic Indicator |
|---|---|---|---|
| 1 | Excessive burn wound drainage | | |
| 2 | Oliguria | | |
| 3 | Hypoxemia | | |
| 4 | Graft sloughing | | |
| 5 | Wound odor | | |
| 6 | Heart rate 122 beats/min | | |
| 7 | Crusting of granulation tissue | | |
| 8 | Edema arising around burn wound | | |
| 9 | Glucose 362 mg/dL | | |
| 10 | Body temperature instability | | |
| 11 | Eruption of vesicular lesions in healed skin | | |
| 12 | Blood pressure 90/60 mm Hg | | |
| 13 | Change in level of consciousness | | |
| 14 | Ulceration of skin surrounding burn site | | |
| 15 | Respiratory rate 32 breaths/min | | |

**Activity #3**

Provide two expected findings that the nurse would anticipate in a client with <u>no</u>, <u>mild</u>, <u>moderate</u>, or <u>severe</u> carbon monoxide poisoning.

1. 1% to 10% (no carbon monoxide poisoning)

    a. _____

    b. _____

2. 11% to 20% (mild carbon monoxide poisoning)

    a. _____

    b. _____

3. 21% to 40% (moderate carbon monoxide poisoning)

    a. _____

    b. _____

4. 41% to 60% (severe carbon monoxide poisoning)

    a. _____

    b. _____

## Activity #4
Identify the burn depth based on each description.

| Burn Description | Burn Depth |
|---|---|
| 1. Extends to dermis<br>2. Moderate edema<br>3. Pain rated at 8 on 0–10 scale<br>4. No eschar | |
| 1. Extends to tendon<br>2. Black in color<br>3. No blistering<br>4. Eschar present | |
| 1. Yellow in color<br>2. Severe edema<br>3. No pain<br>4. Inelastic eschar | |
| 1. Dry appearance<br>2. No edema<br>3. Pain rated 4 on 0–10 scale<br>4. New epidermis noted | |
| 1. Extends into dermis<br>2. Moderate edema<br>3. No blistering<br>4. Soft eschar | |

## Activity #5
List at least three unique characteristics of each type of pressure injury.

Stage 1:

    1. _____

    2. _____

    3. _____

Stage 2:

    1. _____

    2. _____

    3. _____

Stage 3:

1. _____

2. _____

3. _____

Stage 4:

1. _____

2. _____

3. _____

Unstageable:

1. _____

2. _____

3. _____

Deep tissue pressure injury:

1. _____

2. _____

3. _____

## Learning Assessment

### NCLEX Examination Challenge #1

Which client does the nurse identify that is at risk for pressure injuries? **Select all that apply.**

A. Middle-aged client with quadriplegia who is alert and conversant

B. Ambulatory client who has occasional urinary incontinence

C. Client who sits for long periods in a chair and refuses meals

D. Client with obesity who must be assisted to move and turn in the bed

E. Older adult who is bedridden and in a late stage of Alzheimer's disease

### NCLEX Examination Challenge #2

Which assessment finding does the emergency department (ED) nurse anticipate may be present when a client has a smoke-related inhalation injury? **Select all that apply.**

A. Cough

B. Cherry red skin

C. Shortness of breath

D. Speech hoarseness

E. Singed nasal hairs

## NCLEX Examination Challenge #3

Which preventive strategies for skin cancer does the nurse teach to an adult client? **Select all that apply.**

A.  Avoid sun exposure when the sun is at its brightest point.
B.  Wear a hat and sunglasses when you are outside in the sun.
C.  Use tanning beds no more than 30 to 60 minutes twice weekly.
D.  Take pictures of lesions and compare them monthly for changes.
E.  Use sunscreen if you will be outside in the sun for more than an hour.

## NGN Challenge #1

The nurse documents assessment findings for a 32-year-old client brought to the emergency department with multiple first- and second-degree burns.

| Health History | Nurses Notes | Vital Signs | Laboratory Results |
| --- | --- | --- | --- |

**1644:** Brought to emergency department by squad after experiencing first- and second-degree burns. Client was at work when a fire broke out; client returned to primary work station to obtain sketches of a building that was being worked on and was burned in the process when attempting to escape. Client has obesity. Other health history unremarkable. Multiple first- and second-degree burns noted on arms. Height: 74 in (188 cm); weight: 298 lb (135.2 kg). VS: T 99.0°F (37.2°C); HR 110 beats/min; RR 22 breaths/min; BP180/98 mm Hg. SpO$_2$ 96% on RA. Reports pain of 4 on 0 to 10 scale.

**Highlight the client findings in the above note that are abnormal.**

The nurse documents further interventions that have been implemented at 1305.

| Health History | Nurses Notes | Vital Signs | Laboratory Results |
| --- | --- | --- | --- |

**1644:** Brought to emergency department by squad after experiencing first- and second-degree burns. Client was at work when a fire broke out; client returned to primary work station to obtain sketches of a building that was being worked on and was burned in the process when attempting to escape. Client has obesity. Other health history unremarkable. Multiple first- and second-degree burns noted on arms. Height: 74 in (188 cm); weight: 298 lb (135.2 kg). VS: T 99.0°F (37.2°C); HR 110 beats/min; RR 22 breaths/min; BP 180/98 mm Hg. SpO$_2$ 96% on RA. Reports pain of 4 on 0 to 10 scale.

**1700:** Removed shirt and pants. No burns noted on legs. Burns on arms assessed and noted:
• Anterior and posterior right arm and hands – first and second degree (both sides)
  Estimated percent of body burned: 18% per Rule of Nines

The nurse analyzes the findings to determine the client's condition. Choose the *most likely* options for the information missing from the statement by selecting from the lists of options provided.

The client is at high risk for _____ [1]_[Select]_____ as evidenced by _____ [2] [Select]_____.

| Options for 1 | Options for 2 |
| --- | --- |
| Shock | Respiratory rate 22 breaths/min |
| Hyperosmolar hyperglycemic state | Blood pressure 180/98 mm Hg |
| Fluid volume deficit | Temperature 99.0°F (37.2°C) |
| Infection | 18% TBSA burned |

| Health History | Nurses Notes | Vital Signs | Laboratory Results | |
|---|---|---|---|---|

**1644:** Brought to emergency department by squad after experiencing first- and second-degree burns. Client was at work when a fire broke out; client returned to primary work station to obtain sketches of a building that was being worked on and was burned in the process when attempting to escape. Client has obesity. Other health history unremarkable. Multiple first- and second-degree burns noted on arms. Height: 74 in (188 cm); weight: 298 lb (135.2 kg). VS: T 99.0°F (37.2°C); HR 110 beats/min; RR 22 breaths/min; BP 180/98 mm Hg. SpO$_2$ 96% on RA. Reports pain of 4 on 0 to 10 scale.

**1700:** Removed shirt and pants. No burns noted on legs. Burns on arms assessed and noted:
- Anterior and posterior right arm and hands – first and second degree (both sides)
  Estimated percent of body burned: 18% per Rule of Nines

The nurse considers the client data to determine the priority for the plan of care. Choose the **most likely** options for the information missing from the statement by selecting from the list of options provided.

The *priority* for the client at this time is to manage_____ to prevent _____.

| Options |
|---|
| Fever |
| Fluid balance |
| Open wounds |
| Infection |
| Disfigurement |

The nurse is preparing to gather supplies to manage the client's wounds. **Select three items the nurse will take into the client's room.**
A.   Gauze
B.   Foam sheets
C.   Cotton 4 × 4s
D.   Normal saline
E.   Sterile maggots
F.   Hydrogel sheets
G.   Alginate dressing
H.   Sharp instrument for débridement
I.   3M Tegaderm superabsorbent dressing

After dressing the more significant second-degree wounds, the nurse provides teaching about how to care for the burns. Which information will the nurse include? **Select all that apply.**
A.   Change dressings at least twice daily
B.   Use acetaminophen or ibuprofen to manage pain
C.   Apply ice packs directly to the skin to cool the wounds
D.   Take antiviral medication to minimize the chance for infection
E.   Clean wounds with normal saline each time dressings are changed
F.   An over-the-counter topical triple antibiotic can be used on the burns
G.   If any purulent or odorous drainage arises, report this to the health care provider

One week later, the client sees their primary health care provider to follow up on their burn injuries. For each client finding, use an X to indicate whether the initial nursing interventions implemented in the emergency department were **Effective** (helped to meet expected outcomes) or **Not Effective** (did not help to meet expected outcomes).

| Previous Client Finding | Current Client Finding | Effective | Not Effective |
|---|---|---|---|
| Multiple first-degree burns noted | Several first-degree burns appear to be healed over | | |
| Multiple second-degree burns noted | Greenish-yellow drainage is noted from two second-degree burns | | |
| Reported pain of 4 on 0 to 10 scale | Reports that pain is 2 on 0 to 10 scale and some areas are "itchy" | | |
| Temperature = 99.0°F (37.2°C) | Temperature = 101.0°F (38.3°C) | | |

# 22 CHAPTER

# *Assessment of the Respiratory System*

## LEARNING OUTCOMES

1. Use knowledge of anatomy and physiology to perform a focused assessment of the respiratory system.
2. Teach evidence-based health promotion activities to prevent respiratory system health problems or trauma.
3. Demonstrate clinical judgment to interpret assessment findings for the patient with a respiratory health problem.
4. Identify factors that affect health equity for patients with respiratory system health problems.
5. Explain how genetic implications and physiologic aging of the respiratory system affect gas exchange and perfusion.
6. Interpret assessment findings for patients with a suspected or actual respiratory system problem.
7. Plan evidence-based care and support for patients undergoing diagnostic testing of the system.

## Preliminary Reading

Read and review Chapter 22, pp. 494–520.

## Chapter Review

### Anatomy & Physiology Review

#1. Label the parts of the upper respiratory tract using the Anatomy Labels provided on the following page.

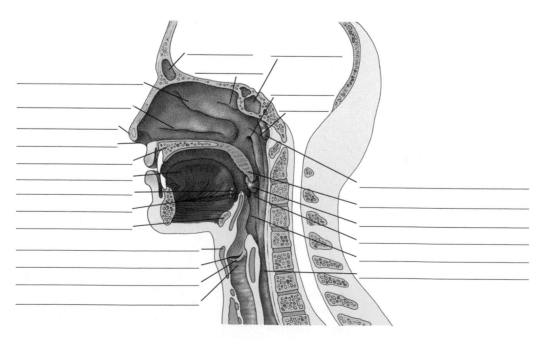

## Anatomy Labels

| Frontal sinus |
| --- |
| Nares |
| Hard palate |
| Tongue |
| Lingual tonsils |
| Epiglottis |
| Hyoid bone |
| Glottis |
| Thyroid cartilage |
| Vocal cord |
| Adenoids |
| Soft palate |
| Oropharynx |
| Laryngopharynx |
| Esophagus |

#2. Complete the sentences by filling in the blanks with terms or phrases listed. Not all terms will be used.

1. _____ is the vibration of the chest wall felt on the surface by palpation when the patient speaks.
2. Blood in the sputum is referred to as _____.
3. The fatty protein that line alveoli and reduces alveolar surface tension is _____.
4. _____ is air trapped in and under the skin that is felt as a crackling sensation beneath the fingertips.
5. A _____ is performed by a needle aspiration of pleural fluid or air from the pleural space.
6. The number of packs per day multiplied by the number of years a patient has smoked is referred as _____.
7. During a _____, a tube is inserted into the airways to the secondary bronchi to view airway structures.
8. The nurse documents that a patient has _____ when they must sit up to decrease shortness of breath.

## Choices for Sentence Completion

| Atelectasis |
| --- |
| Bronchoscopy |
| Crepitus |
| Fremitus |
| Gas exchange |
| Hemoptysis |

| Choices for Sentence Completion |
|---|
| Mediastinal shift |
| Orthopnea |
| Pack-years |
| Perfusion |
| Respiratory diffusion |
| Surfactant |
| Thoracentesis |
| Ventilation |

## Activities

### Activity #1
Describe the characteristics of these adventitious breath sounds.
1. Fine rales _____
2. Coarse crackles _____
3. Rhonchi _____
4. Pleural friction rub _____

### Activity #2
Complete the sentences with the correct term or phrase.
1. When the nurse hears squeaky, musical continuous sounds on auscultation of the lung, _____ will be documented.
2. A patient smoked a pack of cigarettes daily for 10 years, quit for 4 years, then resumed smoking 2 packs per day for 25 years. The nurse documents the pack-year smoking history as _____ years.
3. The nurse recommends that a patient at risk for osteoporosis begin taking the mineral _____.
4. The "Adam's apple" refers to the anatomic structure of the _____.
5. Various ways of smoking include use of _____, _____, _____, and _____.

### Activity #3
For each statement, specify if the statement is **true (T)** or **false (F)**.
_____1. The Joint Commission states tobacco cessation measures must be offered to patients.
_____2. Nicotine replacement therapies are available over the counter in the form of transdermal patches, gums, and lozenges.
_____3. Bupropion is one of the safest treatments for young adults who wish to stop smoking.
_____4. A person who has worked as a painter for many years should be screened by the nurse for complications associated with particulate matter.
_____5. Pulse oximetry readings should be trended over time to accurately assess oxygenation of a patient with dark skin.
_____6. The nurse will assess a patient from the southwestern portion of the United States for *histoplasmosis*.
_____7. The lungs can produce up to 190 mL of sputum daily.
_____8. Ideal normal pulse oximetry values are between 90% and 100%.
_____9. Cellular metabolism is increased by fever, acidosis, and heavy exercise.
_____10. The nurse will monitor a patient for respiratory depression following bronchoscopy.

## Activity #4
List 10 age-related changes that affect the respiratory system.

1. _____
2. _____
3. _____
4. _____
5. _____
6. _____
7. _____
8. _____
9. _____
10. _____

## Activity #5
List five interventions the nurse will provide to address changes in the respiratory system of an older adult.

1. _____
2. _____
3. _____
4. _____
5. _____

## Learning Assessments
### NCLEX Examination Challenge #1
The nurse has provided teaching about smoking cessation. Which client statement requires the nurse to intervene by providing further education? **Select all that apply.**
A. "I won't have lung problems because I only smoke occasionally."
B. "I heard that cigarette smoking can cause lung and heart problems."
C. "I plan to change to 'vaping' because it is safer than smoking cigarettes."
D. "I know I have a problem because I ask friends for cigarettes when I'm socializing."
E. "I started using a hookah, but I'm quitting because it's bad for my health."

**NCLEX Examination Challenge #2**

The nurse is assessing a client who began taking varenicline as prescribed. Which client statement demonstrates to the nurse that drug therapy is effective?
A. "I don't gain much pleasure from smoking now."
B. "I am not craving cigarettes as much as I used to."
C. "I've cut back on smoking because the taste now makes me sick."
D. "I get nicotine from the drug when I chew it so I don't need cigarettes."

**NCLEX Examination Challenge #3**

The nurse is caring for a client in the emergency department reporting difficulty breathing. Which assessment finding does the nurse report to the health care provider? **Select all that apply.**
A. Moveable trachea
B. Use of pursed-lip breathing
C. Breath sounds absent below the diaphragm
D. Flat percussive sound in the upper center chest
E. Rough scratching sounds over the right lower lobe

# 23
## CHAPTER

# Concepts of Care for Patients with Noninfectious Upper Respiratory Conditions

## LEARNING OUTCOMES

1. Plan collaborative care with the interprofessional team to promote gas exchange for patients with upper respiratory problems.
2. Teach adults how to decrease the risk for upper respiratory problems.
3. Teach the patient and caregiver(s) about common drugs and other management strategies used for upper respiratory problems.
4. Plan patient- and family-centered nursing interventions to decrease the psychosocial impact caused by living with upper respiratory problems.
5. Apply knowledge of anatomy, physiology, and pathophysiology to provide evidence-based care for patients with upper respiratory problems affecting gas exchange.
6. Analyze assessment and diagnostic findings to generate solutions and prioritize nursing care for patients with upper respiratory problems.
7. Organize care coordination and transition management for patients with upper respiratory problems.
8. Use clinical judgment to plan evidence-based nursing care to promote gas exchange and prevent complications in patients with upper respiratory problems.
9. Incorporate factors that affect health equity into the plan of care for patients with upper respiratory problems.

## Preliminary Reading

Read and review Chapter 23, pp. 521–538.

## Chapter Review
### Pathophysiology Review

#1. Identify four warning signs of head and neck cancer.

1. _____

2. _____

3. _____

4. _____

#2. For each statement listed, specify if the statement is **true (T)** or **false (F).**

_____1.   Partial airway obstruction produces general symptoms such as diaphoresis, tachycardia, anxiety, and elevated blood pressure.

_____2.   Obstructive sleep apnea syndrome is associated with increased risk for hypertension and other cardiovascular disorders, insulin resistance, stroke, and cognitive impairment such as dementia.

_____3.   Nasal fractures are the most common type of facial trauma.

_____4.   The Le Fort classification of facial fractures is widely used.

_____5.   Head and neck cancers are usually slow-growing squamous cell carcinomas that are curable when diagnosed and treated at an early stage.

_____6.   Head and neck cancer is more common in men, and diagnosis is greater among adults over the age of 30.

_____7.   Surgery for head and neck cancer increases the risk for aspiration because of changes in the upper respiratory tract and altered swallowing mechanisms.

## Activities

### Activity #1
List four risk factors for head and neck cancer that the nurse would include in health teaching.

1.   _____

2.   _____

3.   _____

4.   _____

### Activity #2
For each statement listed, specify if the statement is **true (T)** or **false (F).**

_____1.   Abdominal thrust maneuver is performed on an unconscious patient instead of chest compressions *only* when a known obstruction is present and the patient has a palpable pulse.

_____2.   Patients receiving mechanical ventilation for upper airway obstruction or respiratory failure may require a tracheostomy after 7 or more days of continuous endotracheal intubation.

_____3.   Symptoms of obstructive sleep apnea syndrome include fatigue, daytime sleepiness, headaches, waking with gasping or choking sensation, difficulty concentrating, irritability, depression, and memory problems.

_____4.   A polysomnography (PSG) is a sleep study testing for wakefulness and sleepiness.

_____5.   Noninvasive positive-pressure ventilation via continuous positive airway pressure (CPAP) to hold open the upper airways is the most commonly used form of nonsurgical management for obstructive sleep apnea.

_____6.   Relieving pain after surgery for obstructive sleep apnea is the highest priority because the oropharynx has a rich nerve supply and is extremely sensitive.

_____7.   Assessing how often the patient swallows after nasal surgery is a priority because repeated swallowing may indicate posterior nasal bleeding.

_____8.   Laryngectomy is a surgical reconstruction of the nose performed to repair a fractured nose or to change the shape of the nose for improved function or appearance.

_____9.   The priority action when caring for a patient with facial trauma is airway assessment for gas exchange.

_____10.   Most patients have hoarseness, sore throat, dysphagia, skin problems, impaired taste, and dry mouth for weeks after radiation after head and neck surgery for cancer.

**Activity #3**

Identify three actions the nurse would implement as part of emergency care for a client who has an anterior nosebleed.

1. _____

2. _____

3. _____

**Activity #4**

List three discharge teaching points the nurse would include about home laryngectomy care.

1. _____

2. _____

3. _____

## Learning Assessments

### NCLEX Examination Challenge #1

The nurse is caring for a client who had reconstructive surgery for obstructive sleep apnea syndrome. When planning care, which expected outcome will the nurse determine is the **priority** for the client?

A. Client will maintain a patent airway.

B. Client will state pain is reduced to acceptable level.

C. Client will remain free from infection.

D. Client will not experience excessive bleeding.

### NCLEX Examination Challenge #2

The nurse is planning discharge teaching for a client who had an inner maxillary fixation (IMF) to treat a fractured jaw. What is the **most important** statement the nurse would include in the teaching?

A. "Be sure to use the irrigating device to clean your teeth often."

B. "Try to drink protein shakes and other high nutrient liquids."

C. "Expect that you will have your jaws wired for several weeks."

D. "Keep wire cutters with you to prevent aspiration if you vomit."

### NCLEX Examination Challenge #3

The nurse is caring for a client preparing to begin external radiation therapy for head and neck cancer following surgery. Which instruction(s) will the nurse provide to the client about skin care related to radiation? **Select all that apply.**

A. "Avoid exposing the radiated area to sun, heat, and cold."

B. "Avoid abrasive actions such as shaving."

C. "Wear protective clothing made of soft cotton."

D. "Remove the dead skin where it was radiated."

E. "Wash the radiated area gently with a mild soap."

## NGN Challenge #1

The nurse reviews the postoperative Nurses Note for a 55-year-old client admitted following reconstructive surgery for obstructive sleep apnea syndrome (OSAS).

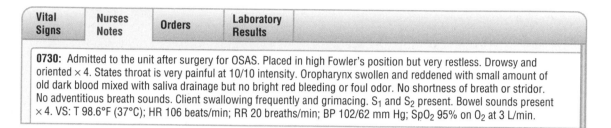

| Vital Signs | Nurses Notes | Orders | Laboratory Results |
|---|---|---|---|

**0730:** Admitted to the unit after surgery for OSAS. Placed in high Fowler's position but very restless. Drowsy and oriented × 4. States throat is very painful at 10/10 intensity. Oropharynx swollen and reddened with small amount of old dark blood mixed with saliva drainage but no bright red bleeding or foul odor. No shortness of breath or stridor. No adventitious breath sounds. Client swallowing frequently and grimacing. $S_1$ and $S_2$ present. Bowel sounds present × 4. VS: T 98.6°F (37°C); HR 106 beats/min; RR 20 breaths/min; BP 102/62 mm Hg; $SpO_2$ 95% on $O_2$ at 3 L/min.

Complete the diagram by selecting from the choices to specify what **one** potential condition the client may be experiencing, **two** actions the nurse would take to address that condition, and **two** parameters the nurse would monitor to assess the client's progress.

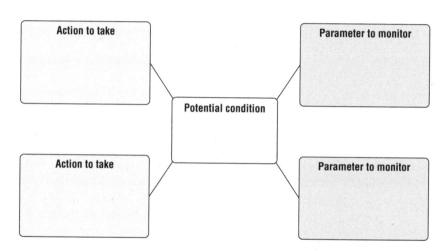

| Actions to Take | Potential Condition | Parameters to Monitor |
|---|---|---|
| Administer analgesic medication | Partial airway obstruction | Vital signs |
| Monitor surgical site frequently | Bleeding | $SpO_2$ levels |
| Administer IV antibiotic therapy | Infection | Pain intensity level |
| Notify surgeon | Hypoxia | Frequency of swallowing |
| Increase oxygen flow rate | ///////////////////////////////// | Respiratory effort |

# 24 CHAPTER

# Concepts of Care for Patients with Noninfectious Lower Respiratory Conditions

## LEARNING OUTCOMES

1. Plan collaborative care with the interprofessional team to promote gas exchange in patients with chronic lower respiratory problems.
2. Teach adults how to decrease the risk for lower respiratory problems.
3. Teach the patient and caregiver(s) about common drugs and other management strategies used for lower respiratory problems.
4. Plan patient- and family-centered nursing interventions to decrease the psychosocial impact caused by living with lower respiratory problems.
5. Apply knowledge of anatomy, physiology, and pathophysiology to provide evidence-based care to patients with lower respiratory problems affecting gas exchange or perfusion.
6. Analyze assessment and diagnostic findings to generate solutions and prioritize nursing care for patients with lower respiratory problems.
7. Organize care coordination and transition management for patients with lower respiratory problems.
8. Use clinical judgment to plan evidence-based nursing care to promote gas exchange and prevent complications in patients with lower respiratory problems.
9. Incorporate factors that affect health equity into the plan of care for patients with lower respiratory disorders.

## Preliminary Reading

Read and review Chapter 24, pp. 539–572.

## Chapter Review

### Pathophysiology Review

#1. Match the Key Term in Column A with its definition in Column B.

**Column A**

1. Asthma
2. Chronic bronchitis
3. Chronic obstructive pulmonary disease
4. Cor pulmonale
5. Cystic fibrosis
6. Emphysema
7. Hypercapnia
8. Hypoxemia
9. Orthopnea

**Column B**

A. Right-sided heart failure caused by pulmonary disease
B. Breathlessness worse in a supine position
C. Destructive problem of lung elastic tissue leading to lung hyperinflation
D. Chronic disease in which acute reversible airway obstruction occurs intermittently
E. Low blood oxygen level
F. Inflammation of the bronchi and bronchioles caused by irritants such as smoking
G. Autosomal recessive genetic disease affecting mostly the lungs and pancreas
H. Group of lower airway disorders that impairs airflow and gas exchange
I. High blood carbon dioxide level

#2. For each statement, specify if the statement is **true (T)** or **false (F)**.

_____1. Airway inflammation and sensitivity can trigger bronchiolar constriction, and many adults with asthma have both problems.

_____2. The major mediator that activates eosinophils and increases inflammation leading to asthma attacks is interleukin 5 (IL-5).

_____3. Bronchospasm is narrowing of the bronchial tubes by constriction of the smooth muscle around and within the bronchial walls.

_____4. Individuals who have long-term COPD often develop respiratory alkalosis.

_____5. Cigarette smoking is the greatest risk factor for COPD.

_____6. The underlying problem of cystic fibrosis is blocked sodium transport in the cell membranes.

_____7. The pulmonary problems of cystic fibrosis result from the constant presence of thick, sticky mucus and are the most serious complications of the disease.

_____8. Pulmonary artery hypertension progresses and leads to left-sided heart failure with reduced perfusion and gas exchange.

_____9. Lung cancers occur as a result of repeated exposure to inhaled substances that cause chronic tissue irritation or inflammation interfering with cellular regulation of cell growth.

_____10. Idiopathic pulmonary fibrosis is a restrictive lung disease with no known cause.

## Activities

### Activity #1

List three nursing considerations when caring for an older adult who has a respiratory condition.

1. _____

2. _____

3. _____

**Activity #2**

For each statement, specify if the statement is **true (T)** or **false (F)**.

_____1.  Nurses should teach patients with asthma to keep a symptom and intervention diary to learn specific triggers, early cues for impending attacks, and personal response to drugs.

_____2.  If status asthmaticus is not reversed, the patient may develop pneumothorax and cardiac or respiratory arrest.

_____3.  The patient with COPD often sits in a forward-bending posture with the arms held forward, a position known as the orthopneic or tripod position.

_____4.  The chronically hypoxic patient is usually anemic as evidenced by decreased red blood cell production.

_____5.  The patient with chronic bronchitis often has a cyanotic, or blue-tinged, dusky appearance and has excessive sputum production.

_____6.  Diaphragmatic or abdominal and pursed-lip breathing may be helpful for managing dyspneic episodes in the client with chronic lung disease.

_____7.  All hypoxic patients, even those with COPD and hypercarbia, should receive oxygen therapy at rates appropriate to reduce hypoxia and bring $SpO_2$ levels up between 88% and 92%.

_____8.  The most common respiratory infection for patients with cystic fibrosis is _Pseudomonas aeruginosa_.

_____9.  The nurse assesses for complications of lung transplantation, which includes bleeding, infection, and transplant rejection.

____10.  Postoperative nursing care after a pneumonectomy includes managing one or more chest tubes.

**Activity #3**

Match the drug in Column A with its classification in Column B.

**Column A**

_____1.  Albuterol
_____2.  Salmeterol
_____3.  Aclidinium
_____4.  Fluticasone
_____5.  Nedocromil
_____6.  Montelukast
_____7.  Reslizumab
_____8.  Omalizumab
_____9.  Guaifenesin
____10.  Ivacaftor
____11.  Bosentan
____12.  Epoprostenol

**Column B**

A.  Mucolytic
B.  Endothelin-receptor antagonists
C.  Leukotriene modifier
D.  Cholinergic antagonist
E.  Prostacyclin agonist
F.  IgE antagonist
G.  Long-acting beta$_2$ agonist
H.  Interleukin antagonist
I.  CFTR modulator
J.  Corticosteroid
K.  Cromolyn
L.  Bronchodilator

**Activity #4**

Identify four assessments or actions a home health nurse would consider for the patient who has COPD.

1.  _____

2.  _____

3.  _____

4.  _____

### Activity #5

Complete each sentence with the appropriate word(s).

1. Patients who have long-term chronic lung disease often have a change in their physical appearance referred to as a _____ chest.
2. The most accurate tests for measuring airflow in asthma are the _____ using spirometry.
3. _____ therapy drugs help to prevent asthma attacks from occurring.
4. _____ deliver drugs as a fine liquid spray.
5. Patients who have COPD need to consume foods high in _____ and _____.
6. _____ is a common complication of COPD, especially among older adults.
7. For patients who have a closed chest drainage system for chest tubes, the nurse keeps the drainage system _____ the level of the patient's chest.
8. _____ is a procedure performed when pleural effusion is a problem for the patient with lung cancer.

### Learning Assessments

#### NCLEX Examination Challenge #1

The nurse is evaluating the effectiveness of discharge teaching for a client newly diagnosed with asthma. Which statement by the client indicates a **need for further teaching**?

A. "I plan to get a gas insert to replace my old wood-burning fireplace."
B. "I plan to avoid any food that has been prepared with monosodium glutamate (MSG) or metabisulfite."
C. "When I exercise, I will use my bronchodilator 15 minutes after I start with my workout."
D. "I'll wash my bed linens with hot water to kill any dust mites that could cause an attack."

#### NCLEX Examination Challenge #2

The nurse is planning care for a client who has anorexia and weight loss because of severe, advanced COPD. Which action(s) would the nurse select as part of the care plan? **Select all that apply.**

A. Consult with the registered dietitian nutritionist.
B. Teach the client to eat small, frequent meals.
C. Select foods that are easy to chew and not gas-forming.
D. Remind the client to drink extra fluids before meals to thin secretions.
E. Instruct the client to avoid dry foods and caffeine-containing food or fluids.

#### NCLEX Examination Challenge #3

The nurse is preparing to provide health teaching about bosentan to manage pulmonary arterial hypertension. What is the **priority** statement for the nurse to include for a female client?

A. "Take the drug with a full glass of water."
B. "Follow up with laboratory tests to evaluate your liver function."
C. "Swallow the tablets whole and do not chew or break them."
D. "Use two types of contraception to avoid pregnancy while taking this drug."

## NGN Challenge #1

The nurse reviews the Nurses Notes for a 61-year-old client admitted with long-term COPD on continuous oxygen therapy.

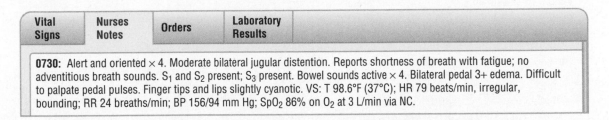

| Vital Signs | Nurses Notes | Orders | Laboratory Results |
|---|---|---|---|

**0730:** Alert and oriented × 4. Moderate bilateral jugular distention. Reports shortness of breath with fatigue; no adventitious breath sounds. $S_1$ and $S_2$ present; $S_3$ present. Bowel sounds active × 4. Bilateral pedal 3+ edema. Difficult to palpate pedal pulses. Finger tips and lips slightly cyanotic. VS: T 98.6°F (37°C); HR 79 beats/min, irregular, bounding; RR 24 breaths/min; BP 156/94 mm Hg; $SpO_2$ 86% on $O_2$ at 3 L/min via NC.

Complete the diagram by selecting from the choices to specify what **one** potential condition the client may be experiencing, **two** actions the nurse would take to address that condition, and **two** parameters the nurse would monitor to assess the client's progress.

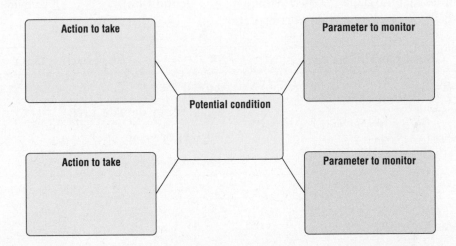

| Actions to Take | Potential Condition | Parameters to Monitor |
|---|---|---|
| Administer analgesic medication | Pulmonary arterial hypertension | Cardiac rhythm |
| Initiate continuous cardiac monitoring | Respiratory failure | $SpO_2$ levels |
| Administer IV antibiotic therapy | Cor pulmonale | Body temperature |
| Prepare client for intubation | Chronic bronchitis | Pulmonary function tests |
| Increase oxygen flow rate | ///////////////////////////////// | Respiratory effort |

**NGN Challenge #2**

The nurse reviews recent laboratory results for a client with long-term chronic obstructive pulmonary disease.

| Vital Signs | Laboratory Results | Orders | Nurses Notes | |
|---|---|---|---|---|

| Lab Test | Today | Two Days Ago | Normal Range* |
|---|---|---|---|
| Arterial pH | 7.33 | 7.28 | 7.35–7.45 |
| $PaCO_2$ | 65 mm Hg | 57 mm Hg | 35–45 mm Hg |
| $HCO_3$ | 52 mEq/L | 39 mEq/L | 21–28 mEq/L |
| $PaO_2$ | 69 mm Hg | 71 mm Hg | 80–100 mm Hg |

*Normal range for U.S. and international measures.

Based on an analysis of the client's laboratory results and condition, complete the following sentence from the lists of options provided.

The nurse determines that the client is experiencing _____[**condition**]_____ as evidenced by _____ [**supporting data**]_____ and _____[**supporting data**]_____.

| Client Condition | Supporting Data |
|---|---|
| Respiratory failure | Low arterial pH |
| Metabolic alkalosis | High carbon dioxide level |
| Respiratory acidosis | High bicarbonate level |
| Hypocarbia | Low oxygen level |

# 25 CHAPTER

# *Concepts of Care for Patients with Infectious Respiratory Conditions*

## LEARNING OUTCOMES

1. Plan collaborative care with the interprofessional team to promote gas exchange in patients with infectious respiratory problems.
2. Teach adults how to decrease the risk for of respiratory infection.
3. Teach the patient and caregiver(s) about common drugs and other management strategies used for infectious respiratory problems.
4. Plan patient- and family-centered nursing interventions to decrease the psychosocial impact caused by living with an infectious respiratory problem.
5. Apply knowledge of anatomy, physiology, and pathophysiology to provide evidence-based care for patients with respiratory infections that affect gas exchange.

6. Analyze assessment and diagnostic findings to generate solutions and prioritize nursing care for patients with infectious respiratory problems.
7. Organize care coordination and transition management for patients with infectious respiratory problems.
8. Use clinical judgment to plan evidence-based nursing care to promote gas exchange and prevent complications in patients with infectious respiratory problems.
9. Incorporate factors that affect health equity into the plan of care for patients with infectious respiratory problems.

## Preliminary Reading

Read and review Chapter 25, pp. 573–595.

## Chapter Review

### Pathophysiology Review

#1. Match the Key Term in Column A with its definition in Column B.

**Column A**

_____1. Anergy
_____2. Ageusia
_____3. Anosmia
_____4. Consolidation
_____5. COVID-19
_____6. Empyema
_____7. Endemic infection
_____8. Induration
_____9. Pandemic infection
_____10. Tuberculosis

**Column B**

A. Collection of pus in the pleural cavity
B. Highly communicable disease caused by infection with *Mycobacterium tuberculosis*
C. Localized swelling with hardness of soft tissue
D. Loss of taste
E. Abnormal solidification in the lung
F. Infection with an organism to which most humans have no immunity and spreads globally
G. Failure to have a skin response to TB skin testing because of reduced immunity
H. Severe acute respiratory syndrome coronavirus-2 (SARS-CoV-2)
I. Infection caused by an organism that is common but the incidence is low
J. Loss of smell

#2. For each statement, specify if the statement is **true (T)** or **false (F)**.

_____1. Adults with influenza are not contagious until symptoms occur but can be contagious up to 10 days after the symptoms begin.
_____2. The patient with influenza often has a rapid onset of severe headache, muscle aches, fever, chills, fatigue, and weakness.
_____3. SARS-CoV-2 enters the host cell by binding to the angiotensin-converting enzyme 2 (ACE 2) receptors, which are found in vascular endothelial cells, lungs, heart, brain, kidneys, intestine, liver, pharynx, and other tissue.
_____4. Effects of SARS-CoV-2 (COVID-19) include inflammation, vasoconstriction, hypercoagulability, endothelial dysfunction, and edema.
_____5. Pneumonia from respiratory infection is associated with the formation of thick exudate containing proteins and other particles that seriously reduce gas exchange.
_____6. Pneumonia may occur as lobar pneumonia with consolidation in a segment or in an entire lobe of the lung or as bronchopneumonia with diffusely scattered patches around the bronchi.
_____7. Pulmonary tuberculosis is spread by skin-to-skin contact.
_____8. Complications of rhinosinusitis include cellulitis, abscess, and meningitis.
_____9. Anything that blocks the flow of secretions from the sinuses can result in rhinosinusitis.
_____10. Pneumonia is most common in young and middle-aged adults.

## Activities

### Activity #1

List four activities or lifestyle habits that nurses would include in health teaching about how to prevent respiratory infection in the community.

1. _____

2. _____

3. _____

4. _____

### Activity #2

For each statement, specify if the statement is **true (T)** or **false (F)**.

_____1.   Antivirals to treat influenza should be taken within 72 to 96 hours after symptoms begin.

_____2.   Whenever possible, the patient with COVID-19 is managed at home to limit the potential for transmission of infection to others.

_____3.   Nursing priorities for patients who have COVID-19 infection include teaching about symptom management, warning signs of disease progression, and preventing the spread of the infection to others.

_____4.   COVID-19 vaccinations are available for individuals 6 months and older.

_____5.   In the older adult, the chest x-ray is essential for early diagnosis because other pneumonia symptoms are often vague.

_____6.   The older adult with pneumonia typically has weakness, fatigue (which can lead to falls), lethargy, confusion, and poor appetite.

_____7.   The most common symptom of pneumonia in the older-adult patient is a change in cognition with acute confusion from hypoxia.

_____8.   The nurse encourages the alert patient to drink at least 4 L of fluid daily to prevent dehydration and to thin secretions caused by pneumonia unless another health problem requires fluid restriction.

_____9.   Nursing priorities to increase gas exchange in patients who have pneumonia include delivery of oxygen therapy and assisting with bronchial hygiene.

_____10.   Tuberculosis can be effectively managed; however, it requires a long period of treatment and care.

### Activity #3

Match the drug in Column A with the respiratory infection for which it is used in Column B. Some infections in Column B may be used more than once.

**Column A**

_____1.   Isoniazid

_____2.   Nirmatrelvir-ritonavir

_____3.   Zanamivir

_____4.   Rifapentine

_____5.   Remdesivir

_____6.   Moxifloxacin

_____7.   Oseltamivir

_____8.   Pyrazinamide

**Column B**

A.   Influenza

B.   Tuberculosis

C.   COVID-19

**Activity #4**

Identify four nursing interventions that can help prevent transmission of COVID-19 in an inpatient setting.

1. _____

2. _____

3. _____

4. _____

## Learning Assessments

### NCLEX Examination Challenge #1

The nurse is assessing risk factors for a client who is concerned about contracting COVID-19 infection. Which comorbidities would the nurse include in the risk assessment? **Select all that apply.**
A. Diabetes mellitus
B. Obesity
C. Cancer
D. Physical disabilities
E. Age younger than 60 years of age

### NCLEX Examination Challenge #2

The nurse is assigned to caring for a client diagnosed with COVID-19 in an acute care respiratory unit. Which **essential** personal protective equipment would the nurse wear? **Select all that apply.**
A. Shoe covering
B. Isolation gown
C. N95 mask
D. Hair covering
E. Nonsterile gloves
F. Protective eyewear

### NCLEX Examination Challenge #3

The nurse is caring for a client who does not adhere to a complex drug regimen prescribed to manage pulmonary tuberculosis. Which action would be the best for the client at this time?
A. Change to a less complex drug regimen.
B. Admit the client to acute care.
C. Initiate directly observed therapy.
D. Determine why the client does not adhere to therapy.

**NGN Challenge #1**

The nurse reviews the Nurses Notes for a 78-year-old client admitted to the medical unit from home with a history of chronic obstructive lung disease.

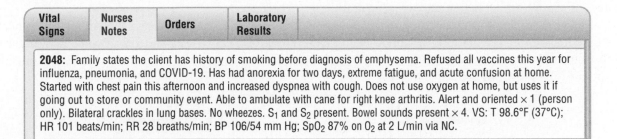

| Vital Signs | Nurses Notes | Orders | Laboratory Results |

**2048:** Family states the client has history of smoking before diagnosis of emphysema. Refused all vaccines this year for influenza, pneumonia, and COVID-19. Has had anorexia for two days, extreme fatigue, and acute confusion at home. Started with chest pain this afternoon and increased dyspnea with cough. Does not use oxygen at home, but uses it if going out to store or community event. Able to ambulate with cane for right knee arthritis. Alert and oriented × 1 (person only). Bilateral crackles in lung bases. No wheezes. $S_1$ and $S_2$ present. Bowel sounds present × 4. VS: T 98.6°F (37°C); HR 101 beats/min; RR 28 breaths/min; BP 106/54 mm Hg; $SpO_2$ 87% on $O_2$ at 2 L/min via NC.

Complete the diagram by selecting from the choices to specify what **one** potential condition the client may be experiencing, **two** actions the nurse would take to address that condition, and **two** parameters the nurse would monitor to assess the client's progress.

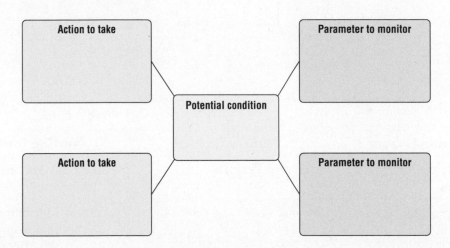

| Actions to Take | Potential Condition | Parameters to Monitor |
|---|---|---|
| Consult with respiratory therapist | Pneumonia | Cardiac rhythm |
| Initiate continuous cardiac monitoring | Tuberculosis | $SpO_2$ levels |
| Administer IV antibiotic therapy | COVID-19 | Body temperature |
| Prepare client for intubation | Acute bronchitis | Pulmonary function tests |
| Increase oxygen flow rate | /////////////////////////////// | Respiratory rate and effort |

**NGN Challenge #2**

The nurse reviews the history of an obese Hispanic client who is concerned about obtaining the COVID-19 vaccine series because of its adverse effects. The nurse recognizes that people of color are more at risk for life-threatening complications of COVID-19 when compared with Whites, and therefore, need the vaccine for protection from hospitalization and possible death.

Complete the diagram by selecting from the choices to specify what **one** primary problem related to health care outcomes across populations became evident as a result of the COVID-19 pandemic, **two** factors (determinants of health) that contribute to this problem for people of color, and **two** <u>priority</u> nursing interventions that can help address this problem.

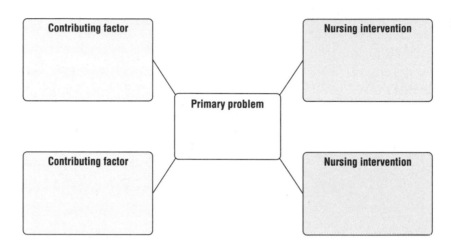

| **Contributing Factors** | **Primary Problem** | **Nursing Interventions** |
|---|---|---|
| Lack of trust and misinformation about vaccines | Cultural differences | Take a class on culture and inclusivity |
| Higher formal educational level | Personal biases and values | Acknowledge differences related to health outcomes |
| More comorbidities that are not always diagnosed or well-managed | Health inequity | Take a cultural screening test to determine implicit bias |
| Poorly designed research studies | Poor quality of rural health care | Refer clients to Social Services to ensure quality care |
| Differences in the quality of health care | ///////////////////////////// | Establish trusting relationships and provide accurate health information |

# 26 CHAPTER

# *Critical Care of Patients with Respiratory Emergencies*

## LEARNING OUTCOMES

1. Plan collaborative care with the interprofessional team to promote gas exchange in critically ill patients with a respiratory emergency, including tracheostomy.
2. Teach adults how to decrease the risk for severe respiratory damage or disease.
3. Teach the patient and caregiver(s) about common drugs and management strategies used for critically ill patients with respiratory problems.
4. Plan patient- and family-centered nursing interventions to decrease the psychosocial impact caused by respiratory emergencies.
5. Apply knowledge of anatomy, physiology, and pathophysiology to provide evidence-based care for critically ill patients with respiratory problems affecting gas exchange or perfusion.
6. Analyze assessment and diagnostic findings to generate solutions and prioritize nursing care for critically ill patients with respiratory emergencies.
7. Organize care coordination and transition management for critically ill patients with respiratory problems.
8. Use clinical judgment to plan evidence-based nursing care to promote gas exchange and perfusion in critically ill patients with respiratory emergencies.
9. Incorporate factors that affect health equity into the plan of care for critically ill patients with respiratory emergencies.

## Preliminary Reading

Read and review Chapter 26, pp. 596–635.

## Chapter Review

### Pathophysiology Review

#1. Match the Key Term in Column A with its definition in Column B.

**Column A**

_____1. Barotrauma
_____2. Biotrauma
_____3. Embolism
_____4. Extubation
_____5. Hemoptysis
_____6. Hemothorax
_____7. Hypoventilation
_____8. Hypoxemia
_____9. Hypoxia
_____10. Lung compliance
_____11. Pneumothorax
_____12. Weaning

**Column B**

A. Decreased tissue oxygenation
B. Bloody sputum
C. Process of going from ventilatory dependence to spontaneous breathing
D. Inflammatory response-mediated damage to alveoli
E. Elasticity and recoil of lung tissue
F. Poor respiratory movements
G. Ventilator-induced damage to the lungs from positive pressure
H. Air in the pleural space, which can lead to lung collapse
I. Low arterial blood oxygen level
J. Blood clot or other object (e.g., air bubble) that dislodges and travels in the blood stream to another area of the body
K. Bleeding into the chest cavity
L. Removal of an endotracheal (ET) tube

#2. For each statement, specify if the statement is **true (T)** or **false (F)**.

_____1. Most often, pulmonary embolism develops because of a deep vein thrombosis.
_____2. Major risk factors for pulmonary embolism include anything that promotes abnormal blood flow in veins (venous stasis), increases the tendency to clot (hypercoagulable state), or a vessel wall injury.
_____3. Venous thromboembolism (VTE) includes deep vein thrombosis and pulmonary embolism.
_____4. Age is one of the most important risk factors for VTE because VTE risk decreases with age.
_____5. A complication of pulmonary embolism is acute respiratory failure.
_____6. Acute respiratory failure occurs over 1 or more weeks before physiological compensatory mechanisms are activated.
_____7. Acute respiratory failure can be ventilatory failure, oxygenation failure, or a combination of ventilatory and oxygenation failure and is classified by abnormal blood gas values.
_____8. Lungs can be injured during sepsis, pulmonary embolism, shock, aspiration, severe inflammation from COVID-19 infection, or pneumonia.
_____9. Sepsis is the most common cause of acute respiratory distress syndrome (ARDS).
_____10. The trigger for ARDS is an alveolar injury leading to a systemic inflammatory response that activates a variety of proinflammatory cytokines.

## Activities

### Activity #1

List four risk factors for the development of venous thromboembolism that can lead to pulmonary embolism.

1. _____

2. _____

3. _____

4. _____

## Activity #2

For each statement, specify if the statement is **true (T)** or **false (F)**.

_____1.   Computed tomography pulmonary angiography (CTPA) is the standard for diagnosing a pulmonary embolism (PE).

_____2.   When a patient has a sudden onset of dyspnea and chest pain or other symptoms of respiratory impairment, the nurse would immediately initiate the Rapid Response Team.

_____3.   To treat PE, low-molecular-weight heparin and fondaparinux are preferred over unfractionated heparin because they are less likely to cause major bleeding or heparin-induced thrombocytopenia.

_____4.   Patients who receive fibrinolytic therapy for PE are hemodynamically unstable and are at a high risk for bleeding; therefore, these patients require monitoring in an ICU setting.

_____5.   The purpose of anticoagulant therapy for PE management is to dissolve the clot to relieve symptoms.

_____6.   Most patients are started on an oral anticoagulant such as warfarin on day 1 or 2 of heparin therapy.

_____7.   Direct-acting oral anticoagulants have a rapid onset of action and require laboratory monitoring unlike warfarin.

_____8.   Oxygen therapy is appropriate for any patient with acute hypoxemia.

_____9.   The nursing priority in the prevention of ARDS is early recognition of patients at high risk for the syndrome.

_____10.   The nursing priorities in caring for the patient during mechanical ventilation are monitoring and evaluating patient responses, managing the ventilator system safely, and preventing complications.

## Activity #3

Complete the following sentences with the appropriate word or phrase.

1.   Using the Wells Criteria/Modified Wells Criteria scoring tool, if a client has a total score of _____, the client likely has a pulmonary embolism.

2.   The antidote for heparin is _____; the antidote for warfarin is _____.

3.   The symptoms of acute respiratory failure are related to the systemic effects of hypoxemia, hypercapnia, and/or _____, an acid-base imbalance.

4.   Oxygen therapy is used in acute respiratory failure (ARF) to keep the arterial oxygen ($PaO_2$) level above _____ mm Hg while treating the cause of ARF.

5.   A cardinal pathologic change that occurs in clients with ARDS is hypoxemia even when _____.

6.   Because one of the side effects of positive end-expiratory pressure (PEEP) is _____, the nurse needs to assess lung sounds hourly and suction as often as needed to maintain a patent airway.

7.   Similar to ARDS, _____ positioning has been found to improve oxygenation in COVID-19 patients.

8.   The most common type of airway for short-term mechanical ventilation is the _____.

9.   Patients often receive a _____ drug before intubation to facilitate tube placement into the airway and to minimize risk of aspiration.

10.   Immediately after an ET tube is inserted, placement is verified by checking _____ levels and by chest x-ray.

11.   The priority nursing action when caring for an intubated patient is maintaining a _____.

12.   Frequent oral care for clients who are mechanically ventilated is essential to help prevent ventilator-associated _____.

## Activity #4

Match the drug in Column A with its classification in Column B.

**Column A**

___1. Alteplase
___2. Dalteparin
___3. Apixaban
___4. Dabigatran
___5. Dopamine
___6. Baricitinib
___7. Tocilizumab

**Column B**

A. Vasopressor
B. IL-6 pathway inhibitor
C. Fibrinolytic agent
D. Direct-acting oral anticoagulant
E. Janus kinase (JAK) inhibitor
F. Xa inhibitor
G. Low-molecular-weight heparin

## Activity #5

Identify four potential postoperative complications of tracheostomy and at least one appropriate nursing intervention:

| Potential Postoperative Complications | Nursing Interventions |
|---|---|
| | |
| | |
| | |
| | |

## Learning Assessment

### NCLEX Examination Challenge #1

The nurse is planning care for a postoperative client to help prevent the development of venous thromboembolism. Which action(s) would the nurse include in the client's collaborative plan of care? **Select all that apply.**

A. Start passive and active range-of-motion exercises for the client's extremities.
B. Place one or two pillows under the client's knees while in bed to promote venous return.
C. Reposition the client at least every 2 hours, or ambulate as tolerated.
D. Instruct the client not to cross the legs because it can obstruct venous return.
E. Remind assistive personnel not to massage the client's legs.

### NCLEX Examination Challenge #2

The nurse is caring for a client with acute respiratory failure who is mechanically ventilated when the high-pressure alarm sounds. The nurse determines that the client's endotracheal tube is secure in the correct position. Which action would be the most appropriate for the nurse to take next?

A. Call the Rapid Response Team.
B. Check all tubing connections for leaks.
C. Request a bedside chest x-ray.
D. Suction the client for excess secretions or mucous plugs.

### NCLEX Examination Challenge #3

The nurse is reviewing laboratory results of a client who is hospitalized with severe COVID-19 infection. Which laboratory finding(s) would the nurse expect for this client? **Select all that apply.**

A. Increased D-dimer
B. Increased C-reactive protein
C. Decreased platelet count
D. Decreased creatine phosphokinase
E. Increased prothrombin time

## NGN Challenge
### Item #1
The nurse reviews the initial Nurses Notes for a 67-year-old client admitted to the ED.

| Vital Signs | Nurses Notes | Orders | Laboratory Results | |
|---|---|---|---|---|

**0545:** Family brought client to ED because of increasingly worsening shortness of breath, frequent cough, fatigue, and low-grade fever. Tested positive for COVID-19 using a rapid test at home yesterday. History of hypertension controlled by medication; no other significant medical history. Alert and oriented ×4. Bilateral crackles throughout lung fields. No wheezes. $S_1$ and $S_2$ present. Bowel sounds present ×4. VS: T 100.6°F (38.1°C); HR 98 beats/min; RR 32 breaths/min; BP 126/70 mm Hg; $SpO_2$ 90% on RA. BMI 25.8. Oxygen started at 4 L/min via NC. $SpO_2$ increased to 94%.

**0720:** Awaiting stat labs. Chest x-ray shows 50% of lung fields with diffuse infiltrates. Peripheral IV with NS started in left forearm. $SpO_2$ 94% on $O_2$ at 4 L/min via NC.

Which client findings are of immediate concern to the nurse? **Select all that apply.**
A. Fever
B. Frequent cough
C. BMI 25.8
D. $SpO_2$ 92% of RA
E. History of hypertension
F. Worsening shortness of breath
G. 50% of lung fields with infiltrates
H. Bilateral crackles throughout lung fields

### Item #2
The nurse reviews the Nurses Notes for a 67-year-old client admitted to the ED.

| Vital Signs | Nurses Notes | Orders | Laboratory Results | |
|---|---|---|---|---|

**0545:** Family brought client to ED because of increasingly worsening shortness of breath, frequent cough, fatigue, and low-grade fever. Tested positive for COVID-19 using a rapid test at home yesterday. History of hypertension controlled by medication; no other significant medical history. Alert and oriented × 4. Bilateral crackles throughout lung fields. No wheezes. $S_1$ and $S_2$ present. Bowel sounds present × 4. VS: T 100.6°F (38.1°C); HR 98 beats/min; RR 32 breaths/min; BP 126/70 mm Hg; $SpO_2$ 90% on RA. BMI 25.8. Oxygen started at 4 L/min via NC. $SpO_2$ increased to 94%.

**0720:** Awaiting stat labs. Chest x-ray shows 50% of lung fields with diffuse infiltrates. Peripheral IV with NS started in left forearm. $SpO_2$ 94% on $O_2$ at 4 L/min via NC.

Complete the following sentence by selecting from the list of options listed.
Based on analysis of relevant client findings, the nurse determines that the client has _____ as a result of COVID-19 infection.

| Options |
|---|
| Acute respiratory failure |
| Acute respiratory distress syndrome |
| Viral pneumonia |
| Pulmonary embolism |

*Item #3*

The nurse reviews the Nurses Notes, including the 0815 entry, for a 67-year-old client admitted to COVID unit from the ED.

| Vital Signs | Nurses Notes | Orders | Laboratory Results | |
|---|---|---|---|---|

**0545:** Family brought client to ED because of increasingly worsening shortness of breath, frequent cough, fatigue, and low-grade fever. Tested positive for COVID-19 using a rapid test at home yesterday. History of hypertension controlled by medication; no other significant medical history. Alert and oriented × 4. Bilateral crackles throughout lung fields. No wheezes. $S_1$ and $S_2$ present. Bowel sounds present × 4. VS: T 100.6°F (38.1°C); HR 98 beats/min; RR 32 breaths/min; BP 126/70 mm Hg; $SpO_2$ 90% on RA. BMI 25.8. Oxygen started at 4 L/min via NC.

**0720:** Awaiting stat labs. Chest x-ray shows 50% of lung fields with diffuse infiltrates. Peripheral IV with NS started in left forearm. $SpO_2$ 94% on $O_2$ at 4 L/min via NC.

**0815:** Admitted to the COVID unit with oxygen at 4 L/min via NC. Started on drug therapy for pneumonia. Consult requested for respiratory therapy. Alert and oriented × 4. Bilateral crackles throughout lung fields. No wheezes. Reports continued shortness of breath. VS: T 100.6°F (37°C); HR 102 beats/min; RR 28 breaths/min; BP 122/66 mm Hg; $SpO_2$ 90% on $O_2$ at 4 L/min. Increased to 6 L/min; $SpO_2$ now 86%. ABGs drawn.

Complete the following sentence using the lists of options listed.

The nurse's ***priority*** for the client's care would be to implement interventions to prevent _____ _____**1 [Select]**_____ which could result because of _____**2 [Select]**_____ caused by COVID-19 pneumonia.

| Option 1 | Option 2 |
|---|---|
| Acute lung injury | Consolidation |
| Asthma | Pneumothorax |
| Atelectasis | Emboli |
| Pulmonary embolism | Inflammation |

*Item #4*

The nurse caring for a 67-year-old client admitted to a COVID unit reviews the Nurses Notes and recent ABG results.

| Vital Signs | Nurses Notes | Orders | Laboratory Results | |
|---|---|---|---|---|

**0545:** Family brought client to ED because of increasingly worsening shortness of breath, frequent cough, fatigue, and low-grade fever. Tested positive for COVID-19 using a rapid test at home yesterday. History of hypertension controlled by medication; no other significant medical history. Alert and oriented × 3. Bilateral crackles throughout lung fields. No wheezes. $S_1$ and $S_2$ present. Bowel sounds present × 4. VS: T 100.6°F (38.1°C); HR 98 beats/min; RR 32 breaths/min; BP 126/70 mm Hg; $SpO_2$ 90% on RA. BMI 25.8. Oxygen started at 4 L/min via NC.

**0720:** Awaiting stat labs. Chest x-ray shows 50% of lung fields with diffuse infiltrates. Peripheral IV with NS started in left forearm. $SpO_2$ 94% on $O_2$ at 4 L/min via NC.

**0815:** Admitted to the COVID unit with oxygen at 4 L/min via NC. Started on drug therapy for pneumonia. Consult requested for respiratory therapy. Alert and oriented × 4. Bilateral crackles throughout lung fields. No wheezes. Reports continued shortness of breath. VS: T 100.6°F (38.1°C); HR 102 beats/min; RR 28 breaths/min; BP 122/66 mm Hg; $SpO_2$ 90% on $O_2$ at 4 L/min. Increased to 6 L/min; $SpO_2$ now 86%. ABGs drawn.

| Vital Signs | Laboratory Results | Orders | Nurses Notes | |
|---|---|---|---|---|

| ABG Lab Test | Today at 0815 | Normal Range |
|---|---|---|
| Arterial pH | 7.33 | 7.35–7.45 |
| $PaCO_2$ | 52 mm Hg | 35–45 mm Hg |
| $HCO_3$ | 31 mEq/L | 21–28 mEq/L |
| $PaO_2$ | 74 mm Hg | 80–100 mm Hg |
| Base excess | 2 mEq/L | $0 \pm 2$ mEq/L |

Based on the client findings, the nurse communicates with the primary health care provider using an SBAR report. Indicate which of these actions would be **Appropriate** or **Not Appropriate** for the nurse to request at this time.

| Potential Nursing Action | Appropriate | Not Appropriate |
|---|---|---|
| Initiate high-flow nasal cannula oxygen at 60 L/min | | |
| Assess respiratory status every 4 hours | | |
| Schedule awake pronation periods | | |
| Prepare for possible intubation and mechanical ventilation | | |

*Item #5*

The nurse caring for a 67-year-old client admitted to a COVID unit reviews the Nurses Notes and recent ABG results.

| Vital Signs | Nurses Notes | Orders | Laboratory Results | |
|---|---|---|---|---|

**0545:** Family brought client to ED because of increasingly worsening shortness of breath, frequent cough, fatigue, and low-grade fever. Tested positive for COVID-19 using a rapid test at home yesterday. History of hypertension controlled by medication; no other significant medical history. Alert and oriented × 4. Bilateral crackles throughout lung fields. No wheezes. $S_1$ and $S_2$ present. Bowel sounds present × 4. VS: T 100.6°F (38.1°C); HR 98 beats/min; RR 32 breaths/min; BP 126/70 mm Hg; $SpO_2$ 90% on RA. BMI 25.8. Oxygen started at 4 L/min via NC.

**0720:** Awaiting stat labs. Chest x-ray shows 50% of lung fields with diffuse infiltrates. Peripheral IV with NS started in left forearm. $SpO_2$ 94% on $O_2$ at 4 L/min via NC.

**0815:** Admitted to the COVID unit with oxygen at 4 L/min via NC. Started on drug therapy for pneumonia. Consult requested for respiratory therapy. Alert and oriented × 4. Bilateral crackles throughout lung fields. No wheezes. Reports continued shortness of breath. VS: T 100.6°F (38.1°C); HR 102 beats/min; RR 28 breaths/min; BP 122/66 mm Hg; $SpO_2$ 90% on $O_2$ at 4 L/min. Increased to 6 L/min; $SpO_2$ now 86%. ABGs drawn.

| Vital Signs | Laboratory Results | Orders | Nurses Notes | |
|---|---|---|---|---|

| ABG Lab Test | Today at 0815 | Normal Range |
|---|---|---|
| Arterial pH | 7.33 | 7.35–7.45 |
| $PaCO_2$ | 52 mm Hg | 35–45 mm Hg |
| $HCO_3$ | 31 mEq/L | 21–28 mEq/L |
| $PaO_2$ | 74 mm Hg | 80–100 mm Hg |
| Base excess | 2 mEq/L | 0 ± 2 mEq/L |

After consulting with respiratory therapy, the nurse plans care appropriate for the client. Select **four actions** that the nurse would take at this time?

A. Assess and document respiratory status every hour.

B. Schedule at least 6 hours of awake pronation as tolerated.

C. Prepare for intubation and mechanical ventilation.

D. Draw arterial blood gases every 6 hours.

E. Administer IV antibiotic therapy.

F. Administer IV corticosteroids per protocol.

*Item #6*

A 67-year-old client hospitalized with severe COVID-19 is being discharged tomorrow after a week. The nurse assesses the client and compares findings with client findings on admission. Indicate whether nursing and collaborative actions were effective or not effective for the client.

| Current Client Findings | Client Findings on Admission | Effective | Not Effective |
|---|---|---|---|
| Bilateral crackles in both lung bases | Bilateral crackles throughout lung fields | | |
| Respiratory rate 20 breaths/min | Respiratory rate 32 breaths/min | | |
| SpO$_2$ 90% on RA | SpO$_2$ 96% on RA | | |
| Heart rate 98 beats/min | Heart rate 96 beats/min | | |
| Chest x-ray shows 50% of lung fields with diffuse infiltrates | Chest x-ray shows 20% of lung fields with few infiltrates | | |

# *Assessment of the Cardiovascular System*

## LEARNING OUTCOMES

1. Use knowledge of anatomy and physiology to perform a focused assessment of the cardiovascular system.
2. Teach evidence-based health promotion activities to help prevent cardiovascular health problems or trauma.
3. Demonstrate clinical judgment to interpret assessment findings in a patient with a cardiovascular health problem.
4. Identify factors that affect health equity for patients with cardiovascular health problems.
5. Explain how genetic implications and physiologic aging of the cardiovascular system affect perfusion.
6. Plan evidence-based care and support for patients undergoing diagnostic testing of the cardiovascular system.

## Preliminary Reading

Read and review Chapter 27, pp. 636–658.

## Chapter Review

### Anatomy & Physiology Review

#1. Label the parts of the heart and large vessels using the Anatomy Labels provided on the following page.

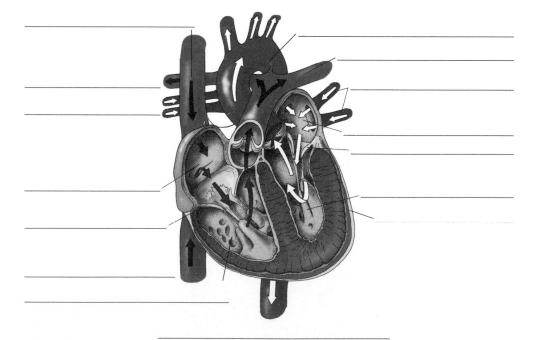

| **Anatomy Labels** |
|---|
| Right atrium |
| Left atrium |
| Right ventricle |
| Left ventricle |
| Aortic arch |
| Descending aorta |
| Right pulmonary artery |
| Left pulmonary artery |
| Right pulmonary vein |
| Left pulmonary vein |
| Tricuspid valve |
| Mitral valve |
| Myocardium |
| Superior vena cava |
| Inferior vena cava |

#2. Complete the sentences by filling in the blanks with terms or phrases listed. Not all terms will be used.

1. _____ is the volume of blood ejected by the heart each minute.
2. The right atrium (RA) receives deoxygenated _____ blood, which is returned from the body through the superior and inferior venae cavae.
3. Blood moves from the _____ throughout the systemic circulation to the various tissues of the body.
4. A mean arterial pressure between _____ mm Hg is necessary to maintain perfusion of major body organs, such as the kidneys and brain.
5. _____ is the amount of blood ejected by the left ventricle during each contraction.
6. _____ in the aortic arch and the internal carotid arteries are stimulated when the arterial walls are stretched by an increased BP.
7. The primary function of the _____ system is to deliver oxygen and nutrients to various tissues in the body.
8. _____ is the pressure or resistance that the ventricles must overcome to eject blood through the semilunar valves and into the peripheral blood vessels.

| **Choices for Sentence Completion** |
|---|
| Afterload |
| Aorta |
| Arterial |
| Baroreceptors |
| Cardiac output |

| Choices for Sentence Completion |
|---|
| Chemoreceptors |
| Deoxygenated |
| Preload |
| Stroke volume |
| Vena cava |
| Venous |
| 60 to 70 |
| 90 to 100 |

## Activities

### Activity #1
List at least four common physiologic cardiovascular system changes associated with aging.

1. _____

2. _____

3. _____

4. _____

### Activity #2
Complete the sentences with the correct term or phrase.
1. _____ is the leading cause of diabetes-related death for both men and women.
2. The nurse documents a client's smoking history in _____, which is the number of packs per day multiplied by the number of years the patient has smoked.
3. A feeling of fluttering or an unpleasant feeling in the chest caused by an irregular heartbeat is referred to as _____.
4. _____ refers to a brief loss of consciousness.
5. _____ occurs when the BP is not adequately maintained while moving from a lying to a sitting or standing position.
6. The difference between systolic and diastolic blood pressure values is referred to as _____.
7. _____ are detected by placing the bell of the stethoscope on the neck over the carotid artery while the patient holds a breath.
8. The desired range of total cholesterol is less than _____ mg/dL.
9. The most definitive but most invasive test in the diagnosis of heart disease is _____ _____.
10. _____ uses ultrasound waves to assess cardiac structure and mobility, particularly of the valves.

## Activity #3

For each statement, specify if the statement is **true (T)** or **false (F)**.

_____1. Cigarette smoking is a major risk factor for CVD, specifically coronary artery disease (CAD) and peripheral vascular disease (PVD).

_____2. About two-thirds of American adults are overweight as defined by a body mass index (BMI) of 25 to 30.

_____3. Females typically have mid-sternal chest pain when there is impaired perfusion to the heart muscle.

_____4. Syncope refers to a brief loss of consciousness and is often caused by decreased perfusion to the brain.

_____5. The ankle-brachial index (ABI) can be used to assess the vascular status of the lower extremities; the normal value is 1.00 or higher.

_____6. The second heart sound ($S_2$) is created by the closure of the mitral and tricuspid valves (atrioventricular valves).

_____7. After a cardiac catheterization, the patient remains in bed for 2 to 6 hours depending on the type of vascular closure device used.

_____8. The stress test helps determine the functional capacity of the heart and screens for asymptomatic coronary artery disease.

_____9. Cardiac CT imaging is a noninvasive option to evaluate calcium formation in the coronary arteries.

_____10. Although not common, stroke or myocardial infarction may occur after a right-sided cardiac catheterization.

## Activity #4

Match the Key Term in Column A with its definition in Column B.

| Column A | Column B |
|---|---|
| _____1. Apical impulse | A. Abnormal heart sound that reflects turbulent blood flow through heart valves |
| _____2. Blood pressure | B. Point of maximal impulse (PMI) |
| _____3. Bruit | C. Myocardial muscle protein released into the bloodstream with injury to the myocardium |
| _____4. Highly sensitive C-reactive protein | D. Swishing sound resulting from turbulent blood flow in a narrowed artery |
| _____5. Homocysteine | E. Abnormal sound that originates from the pericardial sac with movements of the heart |
| _____6. Murmur | F. Amino acid, which can be a risk factor for cardiovascular disease when elevated |
| _____7. Paradoxical blood pressure | G. Force of blood exerted against vessel walls |
| _____8. Pericardial friction rub | H. Serum lipid profile that includes the measurement of cholesterol and lipoproteins |
| _____9. Triglycerides | I. Exaggerated decrease in systolic pressure by more than 10 mm Hg during the inspiratory phase |
| _____10. Troponin | J. Serum marker of inflammation |

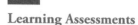 

## Learning Assessments

### NCLEX Examination Challenge #1

The nurse auscultates a loud swishing sound over a client's left neck. How will the nurse document this client finding?

A. Murmur auscultated over left carotid artery
B. Murmur auscultated over left jugular vein
C. Bruit auscultated over left carotid artery
D. Bruit auscultated over left jugular vein

### NCLEX Examination Challenge #2

The nurse is reviewing the laboratory profile of an older adult who has diabetes mellitus. Which laboratory test result would the nurse recognize as being desirable?

A. Elevated high-density lipoproteins
B. Elevated low-density lipoproteins
C. Elevated triglycerides
D. Elevated total cholesterol

### NCLEX Examination Challenge #3

The nurse is caring for a client following a left-sided cardiac catheterization. What is the nurse's **priority** assessment after this procedure?

A. Fluid and electrolyte balance
B. Neurologic status
C. Pain intensity
D. Vital signs

# 28

CHAPTER

# Concepts of Care for Patients with Dysrhythmias

## LEARNING OUTCOMES

1. Plan collaborative care with the interprofessional team to promote perfusion in patients with dysrhythmias.
2. Teach adults how to decrease the risk for dysrhythmias.
3. Provide a safe environment for patients and staff when using a cardiac defibrillator.
4. Teach the patient and caregiver(s) about common drugs and other management strategies used for common dysrhythmias.
5. Plan patient- and family-centered nursing interventions to decrease the psychosocial impact caused by life-threatening dysrhythmias and emergency care procedures.
6. Apply knowledge of anatomy, physiology, and pathophysiology to provide evidence-based care for patients with common dysrhythmias.
7. Analyze assessment and diagnostic findings to generate solutions and prioritize nursing care for patients with dysrhythmias.
8. Organize care coordination and transition management for patients with dysrhythmias.
9. Use clinical judgment to plan evidence-based nursing care to promote perfusion and prevent complications in patients experiencing common dysrhythmias.
10. Incorporate factors that affect health equity into the plan of care for patients with dysrhythmias.

## Preliminary Reading

Read and review Chapter 28, pp. 659–688.

## Chapter Review

### Pathophysiology Review

#1.  Match the Key Term in Column A with its definition in Column B.

**Column A**

_____1.   Atrial fibrillation
_____2.   Contractility
_____3.   Dysrhythmia
_____4.   Normal sinus rhythm
_____5.   Premature ventricular complex
_____6.   Sinus bradycardia
_____7.   Sinus tachycardia
_____8.   Torsades de pointes
_____9.   Ventricular fibrillation
_____10.  Ventricular tachycardia

**Column B**

A.  Life-threatening type of ventricular tachycardia related to prolonged QT interval
B.  Cardiac dysrhythmia in which multiple rapid impulses from many atrial foci depolarize in a disorganized manner
C.  Ventricular contractions resulting from ventricular irritability followed by a pause
D.  Dysrhythmia caused by electrical chaos in the ventricles
E.  Disturbance in cardiac rhythm; irregular pulse
F.  Dysrhythmia caused by decreased sinus node discharge with a heart rate less than 60 beats/min
G.  Ability of atrial and ventricular muscle to push blood through the heart
H.  Dysrhythmia caused by firing of an irritable ventricular ectopic focus
I.  Cardiac rhythm originated from sinoatrial node with a heart rate between 60 and 100 beats/min
J.  Dysrhythmia caused by an increased sinus node discharge with a heart rate more than 100 beats/min

#2.  For each statement, specify if the statement is **true (T)** or **false (F).**

_____1.   Bigeminy occurs when normal and premature complexes occur in pairs.
_____2.   Coronary perfusion pressure may decrease if the heart rate is too slow to provide adequate cardiac output and blood pressure.
_____3.   Increased sympathetic nervous system stimulation causes a decrease in heart rate.
_____4.   Atrial fibrillation (AF) is the most common dysrhythmia, and its incidence increases with age.
_____5.   Atrial fibrillation causes serious problems in older people, leading to stroke and/or heart failure.
_____6.   For patients experiencing ventricular fibrillation (VF), there is no cardiac output or pulse and, therefore, no cerebral, myocardial, or systemic perfusion.
_____7.   Patients who have a myocardial infarction (heart attack) are at great risk for atrial fibrillation.
_____8.   Ventricular asystole, sometimes called ventricular standstill, is the complete absence of any ventricular rhythm.

## Activities

### Activity #1
List four risk factors for the development of atrial fibrillation.

1.  _____

2.  _____

3.  _____

4.  _____

## Activity #2
For each statement, specify if the statement is **true (T)** or **false (F)**.

_____1.  Artifact is interference seen on the monitor or rhythm strip that can be caused by patient movement, lose or defective electrodes, improper grounding, or faulty equipment.

_____2.  The ECG provides a graphic representation, or picture, of cardiac electrical activity.

_____3.  The first step in analyzing an ECG strip is to determine the heart rate.

_____4.  Temporary pacing is used to treat conduction disorders such as complete heart block.

_____5.  Permanent pacemaker checks are done on an ambulatory-care basis at regular intervals.

_____6.  Teach patients who have permanent pacemakers to avoid sources of strong electromagnetic fields, such as magnets and telecommunications transmitters.

_____7.  When administering adenosine, be sure to have emergency equipment readily available.

_____8.  Electrical cardioversion is a synchronized countershock that may be performed to restore normal conduction in a hospitalized patient with new-onset atrial fibrillation.

_____9.  Radiofrequency catheter ablation is an invasive procedure that may be used to destroy an irritable focus in atrial or ventricular conduction.

_____10.  For the unstable patient with sustained ventricular tachycardia (SVT), the nurse administers oxygen and confirms the rhythm via a 12-lead ECG.

_____11.  Magnesium sulfate is an electrolyte administered to treat refractory VT or VF because these patients may be hypomagnesemic, with increased ventricular irritability.

## Activity #3
Complete the following sentences with the appropriate word or phrase.

1.  CPR, also known as Basic Cardiac Life Support (BCLS), must be initiated immediately when _____ occurs.
2.  The loss of coordinated atrial contractions in AF can lead to pooling of blood, causing patients to be at high risk for _____.
3.  _____ is an asynchronous countershock that allows the sinus node to regain control of the heart.
4.  The _____ procedure is an open chest surgical technique performed with coronary artery bypass grafting for patients in atrial fibrillation with decompensation.
5.  _____ is the use of a battery-powered transmitter system for continuous cardiac rhythm monitoring.
6.  In the United States the FDA approved _____ as the reversal agent for rivaroxaban and apixaban.
7.  Dronedarone is a potassium channel blocker that is contraindicated in patients who have _____.
8.  Beta blockers such as sotalol can cause _____ and decreased blood pressure.

## Activity #4
Match the drug in Column A with its classification in Column B. Classifications in Column B may be used more than once.

**Column A**
___1.  Flecainide
___2.  Propranolol
___3.  Amiodarone
___4.  Ibutilide
___5.  Verapamil
___6.  Dabigatran
___7.  Esmolol
___8.  Diltiazem

**Column B**
A.  Calcium channel blocker
B.  Sodium channel blocker
C.  Beta adrenergic blocker
D.  Potassium channel blocker
E.  Direct oral anticoagulant

## Learning Assessments

### NCLEX Examination Challenge #1

The nurse is caring for a client who just had a cardioversion for AF. What actions will the nurse include in this client's care? **Select all that apply.**

A. Maintain a patent airway.
B. Administer supplemental oxygen therapy.
C. Assess vital signs and the level of consciousness.
D. Assess surgical wound for integrity.
E. Monitor for dysrhythmias.
F. Assess for chest burns from electrodes.

### NCLEX Examination Challenge #2

The nurse is caring for an older adult who was prescribed verapamil for newly diagnosed AF. Which statement would the nurse include as a **priority** for health teaching?

A. "Do not take the drug with grapefruit or grapefruit juice."
B. "Be aware that chest pain is a common side effect."
C. "Change position from sitting or lying to standing slowly."
D. "Report bleeding or excessive bruising to the provider."

### NCLEX Examination Challenge #3

The nurse is caring for a client who has a history of asthma and tachydysrhythmias. Which drug would be contraindicated for this client?

A. Propranolol
B. Diltiazem
C. Digoxin
D. Amiodarone

### NCLEX Examination Challenge #4

The nurse is caring for a client on continuous cardiac monitoring. When the nurse walks into the room, the client seems nonresponsive. The client's ECG strip is shown.

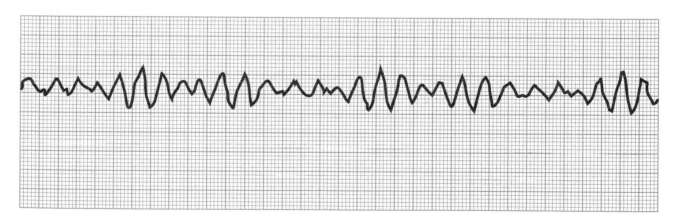

What is the appropriate action by the nurse?

A. Initiate cardiopulmonary resuscitation.
B. Give the client an IV beta blocker.
C. Start oxygen therapy via nonrebreathing mask.
D. Prepare to defibrillate client.

**NGN Challenge**

The nurse reviews the Nurses Notes for a 40-year-old client admitted to the urgent care center.

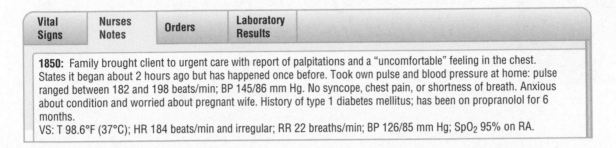

| Vital Signs | Nurses Notes | Orders | Laboratory Results |
| --- | --- | --- | --- |

**1850:** Family brought client to urgent care with report of palpitations and a "uncomfortable" feeling in the chest. States it began about 2 hours ago but has happened once before. Took own pulse and blood pressure at home: pulse ranged between 182 and 198 beats/min; BP 145/86 mm Hg. No syncope, chest pain, or shortness of breath. Anxious about condition and worried about pregnant wife. History of type 1 diabetes mellitus; has been on propranolol for 6 months.
VS: T 98.6°F (37°C); HR 184 beats/min and irregular; RR 22 breaths/min; BP 126/85 mm Hg; SpO$_2$ 95% on RA.

Complete the diagram by selecting from the choices to specify what **one** potential condition the client may be experiencing, **two** actions the nurse would take to address that condition, and **two** parameters the nurse would monitor to assess the client's progress.

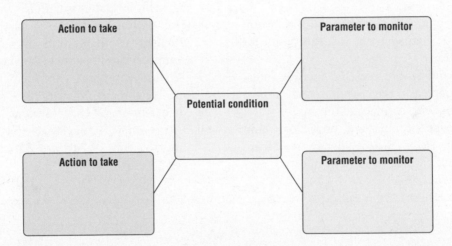

| Actions to Take | Potential Condition | Parameters to Monitor |
| --- | --- | --- |
| Give antihypertensive drug per protocol | Premature ventricular contractions | Cardiac rate and rhythm |
| Initiate continuous cardiac monitoring | Sinus tachycardia | SpO$_2$ levels |
| Prepare client for temporary pacing | Ventricular fibrillation | Blood pressure |
| Prepare client for cardioversion if antidysrhythmic drug is not effective | Atrial fibrillation | Pain intensity |
| Administer supplemental oxygen | ///////////////////////////////// | Respiratory rate and effort |

# 29
## CHAPTER

# Concepts of Care for Patients with Cardiac Conditions

## LEARNING OUTCOMES

1. Plan collaborative care with the interprofessional team to promote perfusion and gas exchange in patients with cardiac conditions.
2. Teach adults how to decrease the risk of cardiac conditions.
3. Teach the patient and caregiver(s) about common drugs and other management strategies used for cardiac conditions.
4. Plan patient- and family-centered nursing interventions to decrease the psychosocial impact caused by living with cardiac conditions.
5. Apply knowledge of anatomy, physiology, and pathophysiology to provide evidence-based care for patients with cardiac conditions affecting perfusion and gas exchange.
6. Analyze assessment and diagnostic findings to generate solutions and prioritize nursing care for patients with cardiac conditions.
7. Organize care coordination and transition management for patients with cardiac conditions.
8. Use clinical judgment to plan evidence-based nursing care to promote perfusion and prevent complications in patients with cardiac conditions.
9. Provide emergency care for patients experiencing life-threatening complications, such as cardiac tamponade and pulmonary edema.
10. Incorporate factors that affect health equity into the plan of care for patients with cardiac conditions.

## Preliminary Reading

Read and review Chapter 29, pp. 689–724.

## Chapter Review

## Pathophysiology Review

#1. Match the Key Term in Column A with its definition in Column B.

**Column A**

_____1.  Acute pericarditis
_____2.  Aortic stenosis
_____3.  Cardiac tamponade
_____4.  Cardiomegaly
_____5.  Heart failure
_____6.  Infective endocarditis
_____7.  Mitral valve prolapse
_____8.  Myocardial hypertrophy
_____9.  Pericardial effusion
____10.  Petechiae
____11.  Pulse alternans
____12.  Splinter hemorrhage

**Column B**

A.  Pinpoint red or purple spots on the mucous membranes or skin caused by bleeding
B.  Enlargement of the heart
C.  Black, longitudinal line or small red streak on the distal nail bed
D.  Microbial infection of the endocardium
E.  Inflammation of the pericardium
F.  Fluid accumulation in the pericardium
G.  Inadequacy of the heart to pump blood through the body
H.  Compression of the myocardium by fluid that has accumulated around the heart
I.  Enlargement of the cardiac muscle
J.  Type of pulse in which a weak pulse alternates with a strong pulse
K.  Narrowing of the aortic valve orifice and obstruction of left ventricular outflow during systole
L.  Dysfunction of the mitral valve that occurs when valvular leaflets slip into the left atrium during systole

#2. For each statement, specify if the statement is **true (T)** or **false (F).**

_____1.  Most heart failure begins with failure of the right ventricle and progresses to failure of both ventricles.
_____2.  In patients who have systolic heart failure, the ejection fraction drops from a normal level of 50% to 70% to below 40% with ventricular dilation.
_____3.  In heart failure, stimulation of the sympathetic nervous system (i.e., increasing catecholamines) as a result of tissue hypoxia represents the most immediate compensatory mechanism.
_____4.  The B-type natriuretic peptide (BNP) is produced and released by the ventricles as they stretch in response to fluid overload from HF.
_____5.  HF is caused by systemic hypertension in most cases.
_____6.  HF is the most common reason for hospital admission for people older than 65 years.
_____7.  With right ventricular systolic dysfunction, cardiac output (CO) is diminished, leading to impaired tissue *perfusion,* anaerobic metabolism, and unusual fatigue.
_____8.  An $S_3$ gallop is often the first sign of HF.
_____9.  Rheumatic fever is the most common cause of mitral stenosis.
____10.  Aortic stenosis is the most common cardiac valve dysfunction in the United States and is often considered a condition of "wear and tear."
____11.  Infective endocarditis occurs primarily in patients with injection drug use (IDU) and those who have had valve replacements, have experienced systemic alterations in immunity, or have structural cardiac defects.
____12.  Rheumatic carditis, also called rheumatic endocarditis, is a sensitivity response that develops after an upper respiratory tract infection with group A beta-hemolytic streptococci.

## Activities

### Activity #1

One standardized and commonly used self-management plan is called MAWDS. Complete the table with the components of this plan and one health teaching statement for each component.

| Component | Health Teaching Associated with Component |
|---|---|
|  |  |
|  |  |
|  |  |
|  |  |
|  |  |

### Activity #2

For each statement, specify if the statement is **true (T)** or **false (F)**.

_____1. Patients with HF, especially those with advanced disease, are at high risk for depression.

_____2. B-type natriuretic peptide (BNP) is used for diagnosing HF (in particular, diastolic HF) in patients with acute dyspnea.

_____3. Electrocardiography is considered the best tool in diagnosing heart failure.

_____4. Cardiac resynchronization therapy (CRT), also called biventricular pacing, uses a permanent pacemaker alone or is combined with an implantable cardioverter/defibrillator.

_____5. Having a ventricular assistive device (VAD) is considered destination therapy, meaning that patients will have the device for the rest of their lives.

_____6. The patient diagnosed with pulmonary edema is admitted to the acute care hospital, often in a critical care unit.

_____7. Transesophageal echocardiography (TEE) or transthoracic echocardiography (TTE) is performed to assess most valve problems.

_____8. Nurses need to teach patients with valve disease the importance of prophylactic antibiotic therapy before any invasive dental or oral procedure.

_____9. For valvular heart disease and chronic atrial fibrillation, anticoagulation with heparin is usually part of the plan of care.

___10. After valvuloplasty, the nurse observes the patient closely for bleeding from the catheter insertion site and institutes postangiogram precautions.

### Activity #3

Match the drug in Column A with its classification in Column B.

**Column A**

_____1. Enalapril

_____2. Valsartan

_____3. Furosemide

_____4. Spironolactone

_____5. Nitroglycerin

_____6. Digoxin

_____7. Dobutamine

_____8. Milrinone

_____9. Carvedilol

___10. Ivabradine

**Column B**

A. Beta-adrenergic blocker

B. Aldosterone antagonist

C. Angiotensin-converting enzyme inhibitor

D. Beta-adrenergic agonist

E. HCN channel blocker

F. Loop diuretic

G. Phosphodiesterase inhibitor

H. Angiotensin-receptor blocker

I. Cardiac glycoside

J. Nitrate

## Activity #4

Match the drug classification in Column A with one of its side effects in Column B.

**Column A**

1. Angiotensin-converting enzyme inhibitors
2. Angiotensin-receptor blockers
3. Loop diuretics
4. Nitrates
5. Cardiac glycosides
6. HCN channel blockers
7. Anticoagulants

**Column B**

A. Cardiac dysrhythmias
B. Bleeding
C. Dry cough and orthostatic hypotension
D. Dehydration and hypokalemia
E. Bradycardia and hypertension
F. Angioedema and orthostatic hypotension
G. Headache

## Activity #5

List four symptoms that patients with a history of heart failure should report to the primary health care provider because they could indicate worsening or recurrent heart failure.

1. _____

2. _____

3. _____

4. _____

## Learning Assessments

### NCLEX Examination Challenge #1

The nurse is caring for a client who has an exacerbation of heart failure and fluid and electrolyte imbalance. What is the best assessment to determine if the client is retaining fluid?

A. Assess for pitting ankle and foot edema.
B. Check the quality of the client's pulse.
C. Monitor intake and output amounts.
D. Weigh the client on the same scale every morning.

### NCLEX Examination Challenge #2

The nurse is caring for a client with heart failure who has dyspnea, especially on exertion. Which nursing action(s) are appropriate for the client to manage the dyspnea? **Select all that apply.**

A. Administer oxygen to maintain the $SpO_2$ at 100% or higher.
B. Position the client in a sitting position rather than lying flat.
C. Encourage deep breathing and coughing every 2 hours.
D. Monitor the client's respiratory status and breath sounds frequently.
E. Consult with the respiratory therapist to plan client care.

### NCLEX Examination Challenge #3

The nurse evaluates an older client who had an initial dose of losartan for management of heart failure. The client's current BP is 88/50 mm Hg. What is the nurse's **priority** action?

A. Retake the BP in 30 minutes.
B. Initiate continuous cardiac monitoring.
C. Lie the client flat and elevate the client's legs.
D. Prepare for transfer to the critical care unit.

### NCLEX Examination Challenge #4

The most recent laboratory findings for an older client who has been on digoxin for chronic heart failure show hypokalemia and hyponatremia. What is the nurse's **priority** concern for the client?

A. Potential for fluid imbalance
B. Potential for digoxin toxicity
C. Potential for mental status changes
D. Potential for falls

## NGN Challenge #1

The nurse reviews the Nurses Notes for a 77-year-old client admitted to the ED from home with acute confusion and worsening dyspnea.

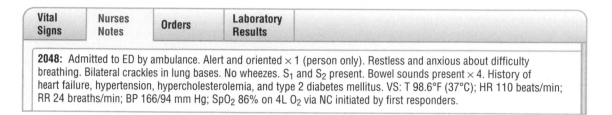

**2048:** Admitted to ED by ambulance. Alert and oriented × 1 (person only). Restless and anxious about difficulty breathing. Bilateral crackles in lung bases. No wheezes. $S_1$ and $S_2$ present. Bowel sounds present × 4. History of heart failure, hypertension, hypercholesterolemia, and type 2 diabetes mellitus. VS: T 98.6°F (37°C); HR 110 beats/min; RR 24 breaths/min; BP 166/94 mm Hg; $SpO_2$ 86% on 4L $O_2$ via NC initiated by first responders.

Complete the diagram below by selecting from the choices to specify what **one** potential condition the client may be experiencing, **two** priority actions the nurse would take to address that condition, and **two** parameters the nurse would monitor to assess the client's progress.

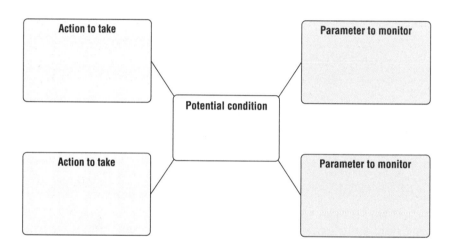

| Priority Actions to Take | Potential Condition | Parameters to Monitor |
|---|---|---|
| Administer IV diuretic drugs per protocol | Cor pulmonale | Cardiac rhythm |
| Initiate continuous cardiac monitoring | Acute pulmonary edema | $SpO_2$ levels |
| Administer oxygen therapy at 5 to 12 L/min by simple facemask or at 6 to 10 L/min by nonrebreathing mask with reservoir | Pulmonary embolism | Renal function |
| Prepare client for intubation and mechanical ventilation | Left-sided heart failure | Pulmonary function tests |
| Give IV antihypertensive drug per protocol | ///////////////////////////// | Respiratory rate and effort |

**NGN Challenge #2**

The nurse reviews the Nurses Notes for a 55-year-old client admitted to the Emergency Department with chest pain.

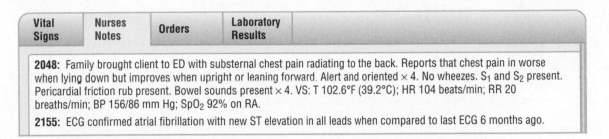

| Vital Signs | Nurses Notes | Orders | Laboratory Results |
|---|---|---|---|

**2048:** Family brought client to ED with substernal chest pain radiating to the back. Reports that chest pain in worse when lying down but improves when upright or leaning forward. Alert and oriented × 4. No wheezes. $S_1$ and $S_2$ present. Pericardial friction rub present. Bowel sounds present × 4. VS: T 102.6°F (39.2°C); HR 104 beats/min; RR 20 breaths/min; BP 156/86 mm Hg; $SpO_2$ 92% on RA.

**2155:** ECG confirmed atrial fibrillation with new ST elevation in all leads when compared to last ECG 6 months ago.

Complete the diagram by selecting from the choices to specify what **one** potential condition the client may be experiencing, **two** actions the nurse would take to address that condition, and **two** parameters the nurse would monitor to assess the client's progress.

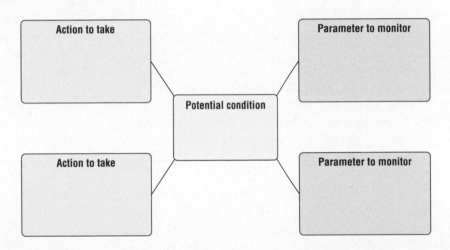

| Actions to Take | Potential Condition | Parameters to Monitor |
|---|---|---|
| Administer antiinflammatory drug for pain | Infective endocarditis | Body temperature |
| Initiate supplemental oxygen therapy | Rheumatic carditis | $SpO_2$ levels |
| Administer antibiotic therapy per protocol | Acute pericarditis | Chest pain intensity |
| Administer anticoagulant to prevent emboli | Myocardial infarction | Pulmonary function tests |
| Give IV antihypertensive drug per protocol | /////////////////////////////// | Respiratory rate and effort |

# 30 CHAPTER

# *Concepts of Care for Patients with Vascular Conditions*

## LEARNING OUTCOMES

1. Plan collaborative care with the interprofessional team to promote perfusion in patients with vascular conditions.
2. Teach adults how to decrease the risk for vascular conditions.
3. Teach the patient and caregiver(s) about common drugs and other management strategies used for vascular conditions.
4. Plan patient- and family-centered nursing interventions to decrease the psychosocial impact caused by living with vascular conditions.
5. Apply knowledge of anatomy, physiology, and pathophysiology to provide evidence-based care for patients with vascular conditions affecting perfusion and clotting.
6. Analyze assessment and diagnostic findings to generate solutions and prioritize nursing care for patients with vascular conditions.
7. Organize care coordination and transition management for patients with vascular conditions.
8. Use clinical judgment to plan evidence-based nursing care to promote perfusion and prevent complications in patients with vascular conditions.
9. Incorporate factors that affect health equity into the plan of care for patients with vascular conditions.

## Preliminary Reading

Read and review Chapter 30, pp. 725–759.

## Chapter Review
## Pathophysiology Review

#1. Match the Key Term in Column A with its definition in Column B.

| Column A | Column B |
|---|---|
| ____1. Acute arterial occlusion | A. Inflammation of a vein |
| ____2. Aneurysm | B. Thickening or hardening of the arterial wall |
| ____3. Arterial ulcers | C. Distended, protruding, and tortuous veins |
| ____4. Arteriosclerosis | D. Obstructions in the distal end of the aorta and the iliac arteries |
| ____5. Atherosclerosis | E. Ulcer resulting from long-term venous insufficiency, usually on malleolus |
| ____6. Deep vein thrombosis | F. Sudden blockage of an artery, usually in the lower extremities |
| ____7. Hypertensive crisis | G. Disorders that change the peripheral flow of blood in veins and arteries |
| ____8. Inflow disease | H. Blood clot in one or more deep veins, usually in the legs |
| ____9. Intermittent claudication | I. Three factors that contribute to thrombosis: stasis of blood flow, endothelial injury, and hypercoagulability |
| ___10. Outflow disease | J. Painful ulcers caused by diminished blood flow through an artery, usually on the toes |
| ___11. Peripheral vascular disease | K. Dusky red discoloration of the skin |
| ___12. Phlebitis | L. Vascular lesions with a red center and radiating branches |
| ___13. Rubor | M. Permanent localized dilation of an artery |
| ___14. Stasis ulcers | N. Severe elevation in blood pressure that can cause major organ damage |
| ___15. Telangiectasias | O. Leg pain experienced by patients who have peripheral arterial disease |
| ___16. Varicose veins | P. Refers to both deep vein thrombosis and pulmonary embolism |
| ___17. Venous thromboembolism | Q. Arteriosclerosis with plaque on vessel walls |
| ___18. Virchow triad | R. Obstructions in the femoral, popliteal, and tibial arteries |

#2. For each statement, specify if the statement is **true (T)** or **false (F).**

_____1. Kidney disease is one of the most common causes of primary hypertension.

_____2. The exact pathophysiology of atherosclerosis is not known, but the condition is thought to occur from blood vessel damage that causes inflammation in response to cellular injury.

_____3. Adult patients of any age with severe diabetes mellitus frequently have premature and severe atherosclerosis from microvascular damage.

_____4. Emboli originating from the heart are the most common cause of acute arterial occlusions.

_____5. An aneurysm forms when the middle layer (media) of the artery is weakened, producing a stretching effect in the inner layer (intima) and outer layers of the artery.

_____6. Aortic dissection is thought to be caused by a sudden tear in the aortic intima, allowing blood to enter the aortic wall.

_____7. The highest incidence of clot formation occurs in patients who have undergone hip surgery, total knee replacement, or open prostate surgery.

_____8. In people with long-term venous insufficiency, arterial ulcers often form.

_____9. The classic signs and symptoms of deep vein thrombosis are calf or groin tenderness and pain and sudden onset of unilateral swelling of the leg.

____10. Rupture is the most frequent complication of an aneurysm and is life threatening because abrupt and massive hemorrhagic shock results.

## Activities

### Activity #1

List four risk factors associated with the development of primary hypertension.

1. _____

2. _____

3. _____

4. _____

### Activity #2

For each statement, specify if the statement is **true (T)** or **false (F)**.

_____1.   Diuretics are the first type of drugs for managing primary hypertension.

_____2.   Thiazide diuretics should be used with caution in patients with diabetes mellitus because they can interfere with serum glucose control.

_____3.   The most frequent side effect associated with thiazide and loop diuretics is hyponatremia.

_____4.   Patients in hypertensive crisis are admitted to critical care units where they receive IV antihypertensive therapy such as nitroprusside, clevidipine, fenoldopam, or labetalol.

_____5.   Patients with atherosclerosis often have elevated lipids, including cholesterol and triglycerides.

_____6.   All patients with peripheral vascular disease need to avoid crossing their legs and avoid wearing restrictive clothing because these actions interfere with blood flow.

_____7.   For patients with chronic PAD, prescribed drugs usually include antiplatelet agents such as aspirin and heparin.

_____8.   Graft occlusion (blockage) is a postoperative emergency that can occur within the first 24 hours after arterial revascularization.

_____9.   The repair of abdominal aortic aneurysms with endovascular stent grafts is the procedure of choice for almost all patients on an elective or emergent basis.

___10.   Checking a Homans sign is not advised because it is an unreliable tool to detect deep vein thrombosis.

___11.   The health care provider discontinues heparin administration if severe heparin-induced thrombocytopenia (HIT) occurs.

___12.   According to the National Patient Safety Goals, therapeutic levels of warfarin must be monitored by measuring the international normalized ratio at frequent intervals.

### Activity #3

Match the drug in Column A with its classification in Column B.

| **Column A** | **Column B** |
|---|---|
| _____1.   Bumetanide | A.   Angiotensin II-receptor blocker |
| _____2.   Metoprolol | B.   Low-molecular-weight heparin |
| _____3.   Amlodipine | C.   Beta-adrenergic blocker |
| _____4.   Lisinopril | D.   Antiplatelet agent |
| _____5.   Valsartan | E.   Loop diuretic |
| _____6.   Simvastatin | F.   Direct oral anticoagulant |
| _____7.   Clopidogrel | G.   Calcium channel blocker |
| _____8.   Dabigatran | H.   HMG-CoA reductase inhibitor |
| _____9.   Enoxaparin | I.   Angiotensin-converting enzyme inhibitor |
| ___10.   Alirocumab | J.   PCSK9 inhibitor |

## Activity #4
Match the drug classification in Column A with a corresponding nursing implication in Column B.

**Column A**

___1.  Furosemide
___2.  Atenolol
___3.  Diltiazem
___4.  Captopril
___5.  Valsartan
___6.  Lovastatin
___7.  Rivaroxaban

**Column B**

A.  Report to provider if muscle cramping occurs on a regular basis.
B.  Assess HR and BP before giving drug; hold drug if systolic BP is less than 90 mm Hg.
C.  Report bleeding or excessive bruising to the provider.
D.  Teach to avoid grapefruit and grapefruit juice.
E.  Teach to avoid foods high in potassium.
F.  Teach to eat foods high in potassium.
G.  Report dry, hacking cough to provider.

## Activity #5
Identify four areas of health teaching that the nurse would provide to help clients who have hypertension manage their care.

1. _____

2. _____

3. _____

4. _____

## Learning Assessments

### NCLEX Examination Challenge #1
The nurse is caring for a client who returned from having percutaneous vascular intervention for peripheral arterial disease. What is the nurse's **priority** for postprocedure assessment?
A.  Monitor the client's level of consciousness.
B.  Observe for bleeding at the arterial puncture site.
C.  Monitor the client's hematocrit values.
D.  Assess the client's femoral pulses.

### NCLEX Examination Challenge #2
The nurse is providing health teaching for a client who is starting diuretic therapy with hydrochlorothiazide (HCTZ). What statement(s) will the nurse **include** in the teaching? **Select all that apply.**
A.  "If you have a history of gout, you should not take this medication."
B.  "Follow up for lab testing to determine if you have too much potassium."
C.  "You may experience decreased libido (desire for sex) when taking this drug."
D.  "Report severe weakness or irregular heartbeat to your provider."
E.  "Expect that you will void more often and in larger amounts."

### NCLEX Examination Challenge #3
The nurse is caring for a client following a femorotibial bypass. Which nursing action is the **priority** for the postoperative care of the client?
A.  Perform frequent neurologic assessments.
B.  Monitor postoperative pain intensity.
C.  Assess operative leg circulation frequently.
D.  Observe for bleeding at the venous puncture site.

**NGN Challenge #1**

The nurse reviews the Nurses Notes for an 87-year-old client residing in an assisted living facility.

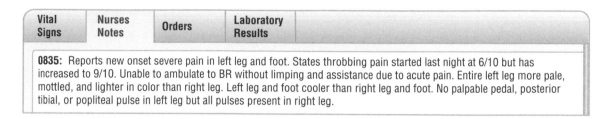

| Vital Signs | Nurses Notes | Orders | Laboratory Results |
|---|---|---|---|

**0835:** Reports new onset severe pain in left leg and foot. States throbbing pain started last night at 6/10 but has increased to 9/10. Unable to ambulate to BR without limping and assistance due to acute pain. Entire left leg more pale, mottled, and lighter in color than right leg. Left leg and foot cooler than right leg and foot. No palpable pedal, posterior tibial, or popliteal pulse in left leg but all pulses present in right leg.

Complete the diagram below by selecting from the choices to specify what **one** potential condition the client may be experiencing, **two** actions the nurse would take to address that condition, and **two** parameters the nurse would monitor to assess the client's progress.

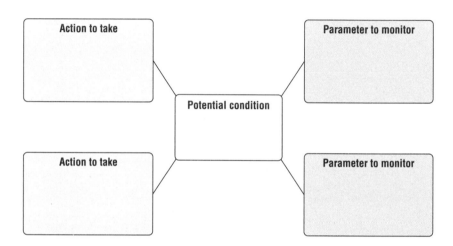

| Actions to Take | Potential Condition | Parameters to Monitor |
|---|---|---|
| Call 911 for transfer to hospital ED | Peripheral artery disease | Vital signs |
| Administer IV unfractionated heparin per protocol | Deep vein thrombosis | Neurovascular status |
| Elevate the client's affect leg on two pillows | Peripheral venous disease | Mobility status |
| Administer analgesic to help manage pain | Acute arterial occlusion | $SpO_2$ |
| Apply warm moist compress to affected leg | //////////////////////////////// | Pain intensity and quality |

**NGN Challenge #2**

The nurse reviews the Nurses Notes for a 59-year-old client admitted to the Emergency Department.

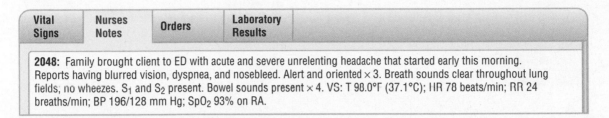

| Vital Signs | Nurses Notes | Orders | Laboratory Results |
|---|---|---|---|

**2048:** Family brought client to ED with acute and severe unrelenting headache that started early this morning. Reports having blurred vision, dyspnea, and nosebleed. Alert and oriented × 3. Breath sounds clear throughout lung fields; no wheezes. $S_1$ and $S_2$ present. Bowel sounds present × 4. VS: T 98.0°F (37.1°C); HR 78 beats/min; RR 24 breaths/min; BP 196/128 mm Hg; $SpO_2$ 93% on RA.

Complete the diagram below by selecting from the choices to specify what **one** potential condition the client may be experiencing, **two** actions the nurse would take to address that condition, and **two** parameters the nurse would monitor to assess the client's progress.

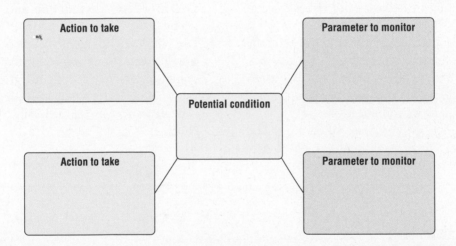

| Actions to Take | Potential Condition | Parameters to Monitor |
|---|---|---|
| Administer IV morphine sulfate for headache | Acute ischemic stroke | Peripheral pulses |
| Monitor HR and BP every 4 hours | Hypertensive crisis | Respiratory rate and effort |
| Keep client in sitting position and administer supplemental oxygen | Pulmonary embolus | aPTT and anti-factor Xa levels |
| Prepare for IV fibrinolytic therapy | Pulmonary hypertension | Blood pressure |
| Give IV antihypertensive drug such as nitroprusside per protocol | /////////////////////////////// | Neurologic status |

# 31 CHAPTER

# *Critical Care of Patients with Shock*

## LEARNING OUTCOMES

1. Plan collaborative care with the interprofessional team to promote perfusion in critically ill patients with shock.
2. Teach adults how to decrease the risk for sepsis and shock.
3. Teach the patient and caregiver(s) about common drugs and other management strategies used for shock.
4. Plan patient- and family-centered nursing interventions to decrease the psychosocial impact caused by shock or its complications.
5. Apply knowledge of anatomy, physiology, and pathophysiology to provide evidence-based care for critically ill patients with shock.
6. Analyze assessment and diagnostic findings to generate solutions and prioritize nursing care for critically ill patients with shock.
7. Organize care coordination and transition management for critically ill patients with shock.
8. Use clinical judgment to plan evidence-based nursing care to promote perfusion and prevent complications in critically ill patients with shock.
9. Incorporate factors that affect health equity into the plan of care for critically ill patients with shock.

## Preliminary Reading

Read and review Chapter 31, pp. 760–780.

## Chapter Review

### Pathophysiology Review

#1. Match the Key Term in Column A with its definition in Column B.

**Column A**

___1. Anaphylaxis
___2. Multiple organ dysfunction syndrome
___3. Sepsis
___4. Septic shock
___5. Sequential organ failure assessment
___6. Shock
___7. Sympathetic tone
___8. Systemic inflammatory response syndrome

**Column B**

A. Widespread abnormal cellular metabolism when oxygen and tissue perfusion cannot maintain cellular function
B. Life-threatening organ dysfunction caused by systemic inflammation and coagulation in response to infection
C. Extreme type of allergic reaction
D. Widespread inflammation that can occur with septic shock
E. Subset of sepsis in which circulatory, cellular, and metabolic alterations are associated with a higher mortality ratc than scpsis alone
F. State of partial vasoconstriction caused by nerves that continuously stimulate vascular smooth muscle
G. Progressive organ dysfunction in two or more body systems requiring medical intervention
H. Assessment tool used to detect organ function and mortality associated with sepsis/septic shock

#2. For each statement, specify if the statement is **true (T)** or **false (F).**

_____1. All body organs are affected by shock and either work harder to adapt and compensate for reduced gas exchange or perfusion or fail to function because of hypoxia.

_____2. Most signs and symptoms of shock are similar regardless of what starts the process or which tissues are affected first.

_____3. Cardiogenic shock occurs when too little circulating blood volume decreases preload and stroke volume, thereby decreasing mean arterial pressure.

_____4. The progressive stage of shock is a life-threatening emergency.

_____5. Increased heart rate is often the first sign of shock.

_____6. Sepsis and septic shock are a major cause of mortality and morbidity and are the most expensive health care problem in the United States.

_____7. Laboratory test results for patients who have sepsis include a rising serum procalcitonin level, an increasing serum lactate level, a normal or low total WBC count, and a decreasing segmented neutrophil level with a rising band neutrophil level.

_____8. The risk of sepsis-related death is highest in young and middle-aged adults.

_____9. Older patients in long-term care settings are at risk for sepsis and septic shock related to urinary tract infections and pneumonia.

_____10. More than one type of shock can be present at the same time.

_____11. When hypoxia or anoxia persists beyond about an hour, patients are at risk for acute kidney injury (AKI).

_____12. Changes in mental status and behavior occur later when a patient is in shock.

_____13. Septic shock can be identified in patients who require vasopressor therapy to maintain a mean arterial pressure (MAP) of at least 65 mm Hg and have a serum lactate level greater than 2 mmol/L (18 mg/dL) despite adequate fluid resuscitation.

_____14. Septic shock is divided into two phases: cold shock and warm shock; the warm shock stage is nearly irreversible.

_____15. Inappropriate clotting with microthrombi forming in some organ capillaries causes hypoxia and reduces organ function occurs in patients who have sepsis.

## Activities

### Activity #1
List three risk factors associated with the development of shock.

1. _____

2. _____

3. _____

### Activity #2
For each statement, specify if the statement is **true (T)** or **false (F).**

_____1. Measuring intake and output is especially important because urine output is reduced during the first stages of shock, even when fluid intake is normal.

_____2. A registered nurse rather than a licensed practical nurse/vocational nurse or assistive personnel should assess the vital signs of a patient who is suspected of having hypovolemic shock.

_____3. Oxygen therapy is used at any stage of shock and is delivered by mask, hood, nasal cannula, endotracheal tube, or tracheostomy tube to maintain an $SpO_2$ between 85% and 90%.

_____4. IV therapy for fluid resuscitation is a primary intervention for hypovolemic shock.

_____5. Identifying sepsis or septic shock in older adults can be challenging as they do not always meet criteria (e.g., fever, tachycardia) because of age-related changes.

_____6. Early detection of sepsis before progression to septic shock is a major nursing responsibility.

_____7. Interventions for sepsis and septic shock focus on identifying the problem as early as possible, correcting the conditions causing it, and preventing complications.

_____8. Best practice for care of clients with sepsis is to measure lactate level; lactate should be remeasured if the initial lactate is elevated (>2 mmol/L).

_____9. Best practice for care of clients with sepsis is to administer broad-spectrum antibiotic therapy within 1 hour of diagnosing the problem.

____10. Patients diagnosed with septic shock typically experience metabolic alkalosis.

## Activity #3

Match the nursing assessment in Column A with the drug in Column B. Any assessment may apply to one or both choices in Column B.

**Column A**

___1. Assess patient for chest pain.
___2. Assess heart rate and rhythm.
___3. Monitor urine output hourly.
___4. Monitor blood glucose levels.
___5. Assess blood pressure every 15 minutes.
___6. Assess IV insertion site for extravasation.

**Column B**

A. Dopamine
B. Dobutamine

## Activity #4

Complete the table by identifying at least one physiologic change associated with hypovolemic shock.

| Body System | Physiologic Change(s) |
|---|---|
| Cardiovascular | |
| Respiratory | |
| Kidney/urinary | |
| Skin | |
| Central nervous system | |

## Learning Assessments

### NCLEX Examination Challenge #1

The nurse is caring for a client who has vital sign changes when compared with this morning. Which assessment finding(s) may indicate early onset of shock? **Select all that apply.**
A. Increased heart rate
B. Increased respiratory rate
C. Increased systolic blood pressure
D. Increased diastolic blood pressure
E. Increased oxygen saturation

### NCLEX Examination Challenge #2

The nurse is caring for a client diagnosed with sepsis and septic shock. Which nursing activity would be the **most appropriate** for the nurse delegate to the licensed practical nurse?
A. Taking frequent vital signs
B. Monitoring central venous pressure
C. Titrating the dopamine drip
D. Monitoring peripheral oxygen saturation

**NGN Challenge #1**

The nurse reviews the Nurses Notes for a 59-year-old client admitted to the ED.

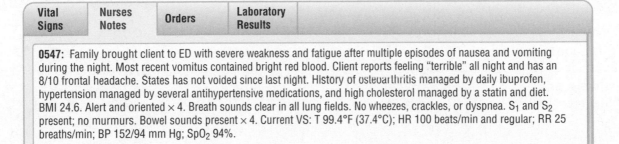

| Vital Signs | Nurses Notes | Orders | Laboratory Results |
|---|---|---|---|

**0547:** Family brought client to ED with severe weakness and fatigue after multiple episodes of nausea and vomiting during the night. Most recent vomitus contained bright red blood. Client reports feeling "terrible" all night and has an 8/10 frontal headache. States has not voided since last night. History of osteoarthritis managed by daily ibuprofen, hypertension managed by several antihypertensive medications, and high cholesterol managed by a statin and diet. BMI 24.6. Alert and oriented × 4. Breath sounds clear in all lung fields. No wheezes, crackles, or dyspnea. $S_1$ and $S_2$ present; no murmurs. Bowel sounds present × 4. Current VS: T 99.4°F (37.4°C); HR 100 beats/min and regular; RR 25 breaths/min; BP 152/94 mm Hg; $SpO_2$ 94%.

Complete the diagram below by selecting from the choices to specify what **one** potential condition the client is at risk for, **two** priority actions the nurse would take to help prevent that condition, and **two** parameters the nurse would monitor to assess the client's progress.

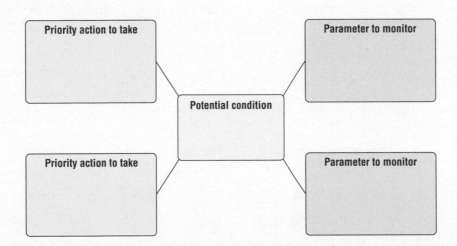

| Priority Actions to Take | Potential Condition | Parameters to Monitor |
|---|---|---|
| Lie the client flat in a supine position | Hypovolemic shock | Vital signs |
| Start two large-bore peripheral IVs | Distributive shock | Neurovascular status |
| Insert a nasogastric tube | Cardiogenic shock | Urinary output |
| Give supplemental oxygen | Septic shock | Lactate level |
| Perform an electrocardiogram | //////////////////////////////// | Capillary refill |

**NGN Challenge #2**

The nurse reviews the assessment findings in the Nursing Flow Sheet for a 77-year-old client admitted to the medical unit last evening for an infected sacral pressure injury with cellulitis.

| Parameter | Current (1720) | 1300 | 0700 |
|---|---|---|---|
| | | | |
| Temperature | 103.6°F (39.8°C) | 103°F (39.4°C) | 102.6°F (39.2°C) |
| Heart rate | 108 beats/min | 106 beats/min | 102 beats/min |
| Respiratory rate | 28 breaths/min | 26 breaths/min | 26 breaths/min |
| Blood pressure | 102/60 mm Hg | 104/52 mm Hg | 106/48 mm Hg |
| $SpO_2$ | 92% | 94% | 94% |
| Capillary refill | 3 sec | 3 sec | 3 sec |
| Urinary output | 350 mL | — | 460 mL |
| Total WBC count | | | 5100/mm$^3$ (5.1 × 10$^9$/L) |
| Serum lactate | 1.8 mmol/L | 1.2 mmol/L | 0.8 mmol/L |

*Table heading: Nursing Flow Sheet*

Complete the following sentence by selecting from the lists of options below.

The nurse analyzes the assessment findings and determines that the client is at high risk for _____1 [Select]_____ as evidenced by a(n) _____2 [Select]_____, _____3 [Select]_____, and _____4 [Select]_____.

| Options for 1 | Options for 2 | Options for 3 | Options for 4 |
|---|---|---|---|
| Cardiogenic shock | Increased WBC count | Increased oxygen saturation | Hypotension |
| Septic shock | Increased respiratory rate | Decreased urinary output | Fever |
| Neurogenic shock | Increased lactate | Increased capillary refill | Decreased WBC count |
| Hypovolemic shock | Decreased oxygen saturation | Tachycardia | Decreased lactate |

# 32
CHAPTER

# *Critical Care of Patients with Acute Coronary Syndromes*

## LEARNING OUTCOMES

1. Plan collaborative care with the interprofessional team to promote perfusion in critically ill patients with acute coronary syndromes.
2. Teach adults how to decrease the risk for acute coronary syndromes.
3. Teach the patient and caregiver(s) about common drugs and other management strategies used for acute coronary syndromes.
4. Plan patient- and family-centered nursing interventions to decrease the psychosocial impact of acute coronary events, especially myocardial infarction (MI).
5. Apply knowledge of anatomy, physiology, and pathophysiology to provide evidence-based nursing care for patients with stable angina, unstable angina, and MI.
6. Analyze assessment and diagnostic findings to generate solutions and prioritize nursing care for patients with acute coronary syndromes.
7. Organize care coordination and transition management for patients with acute coronary syndromes.
8. Use clinical judgment to plan evidence-based nursing care to promote perfusion and prevent complications in critically ill patients with acute coronary syndromes.
9. Incorporate factors that affect health equity into the plan of care for patients with acute coronary syndromes.

## Preliminary Reading

Read and review Chapter 32, pp. 781–809.

## Chapter Review

### Pathophysiology Review

#1. Match the Key Term in Column A with its definition in Column B.

**Column A**

_____1. Acute coronary syndromes
_____2. Angina pectoris
_____3. Atypical angina
_____4. Cardiogenic shock
_____5. Chronic stable angina
_____6. Coronary artery disease
_____7. Ischemia
_____8. Metabolic syndrome
_____9. Myocardial infarction
_____10. Ventricular remodeling

**Column B**

A. Blockage of blood flow through an artery resulting in a lack of oxygen

B. Permanent changes in the size and shape of the left ventricle because of scar tissue after an MI

C. Angina with vague presentation such as indigestion or aching jaw

D. Type of angina characterized by chest discomfort that occurs with moderate to prolonged exertion

E. Injury and necrosis of myocardial tissue caused by abrupt and severe oxygen deprivation

F. Disease affecting the arteries that provide oxygen and nutrients to the myocardium

G. A group of disorders including unstable angina and myocardial infarction

H. Post-MI heart failure in which necrosis of more than 40% of the left ventricle has occurred

I. Chest pain caused by a temporary imbalance between the coronary arteries' ability to supply oxygen and the myocardium's demand for oxygen

J. Collection of related health problems with insulin resistance as the main feature

#2. For each statement, specify if the statement is **true (T)** or **false (F)**.

_____1. When the arteries that supply the myocardium are diseased, the heart cannot pump blood effectively to adequately perfuse vital organs and peripheral tissues.

_____2. Ischemia that occurs with angina is limited in duration and does not cause permanent damage of myocardial tissue.

_____3. When a coronary artery reaches 50% occlusion, blood flow is impaired, creating myocardial ischemia when myocardial demand is increased.

_____4. Stable angina is chest pain or discomfort that occurs at rest or with exertion and causes severe activity limitation.

_____5. Patients presenting with STEMI typically have ST elevation in two contiguous leads on a 12-lead ECG, which indicates myocardial ischemia.

_____6. Patients with anterior wall MIs (AWMIs) have the highest mortality rate because they are most likely to have left ventricular failure and dysrhythmias from damage to the left ventricle.

_____7. Atherosclerosis is the primary factor in the development of coronary artery disease.

_____8. Older adults often present with associated symptoms of myocardial ischemia instead of chest pain or pressure alone.

_____9. Troponins T and I are specific markers for MI and cardiac necrosis.

_____10. The presence of central obesity, high blood pressure, and hyperglycemia when diagnosed with metabolic syndrome presents the highest risk for the development of cardiovascular disease.

## Activities

### Activity #1

List four activities or lifestyle habits the nurse would include in health teaching about how to prevent coronary artery disease.

1. _____

2. _____

3. _____

4. _____

### Activity #2

For each statement, specify if the statement is **true (T)** or **false (F)**.

_____1. For a patient diagnosed with probable MI, the nurse auscultates for an $S_3$ gallop, which often indicates heart failure—a serious and common complication of MI.

_____2. Denial is a common early reaction to chest pain associated with angina or MI.

_____3. An ECG should be obtained within 10 minutes of patient presentation with chest discomfort.

_____4. Before administering nitroglycerin, ensure that the patient has not taken any phosphodiesterase inhibitors for erectile dysfunction, such as sildenafil, within the past 24 to 48 hours.

_____5. If the patient has new-onset angina at home, the nurse teaches them to chew aspirin 650 mg (eight "baby aspirins" that are 81 mg each) immediately and wait for pain to resolve.

_____6. Unless contraindicated, all patients experiencing NSTEMI and STEMI should be discharged on beta-blocker therapy.

_____7. Patients who receive thrombolytics require percutaneous coronary intervention (PCI) for more definitive treatment such as stent placement.

_____8. PCI is performed in the operating suite and combines clot retrieval, coronary angioplasty, and stent placement.

_____9. Patients who undergo PCI are required to take dual antiplatelet therapy (DAPT) consisting of aspirin and a platelet inhibitor.

_____10. For intra arterial blood pressure monitoring, frequent assessment of the arterial site and infusion system is essential.

### Activity #3

Match the drug used for acute coronary syndrome in Column A with a nursing implication of drug administration in Column B. Note that one or more choices in Column B may be used more than once.

**Column A**

_____1. Aspirin
_____2. Isosorbide
_____3. Clopidogrel
_____4. Eptifibatide
_____5. Captopril
_____6. Amlodipine
_____7. Reteplase

**Column B**

A. Monitor for cough and decreased urinary output.
B. Monitor for orthostatic hypotension.
C. Assess neurologic status frequently.
D. Monitor platelet level 4 hours after starting drug and then daily.
E. Teach to report bleeding or excessive bruising.
F. Monitor for peripheral edema.

**Activity #4**

List three signs and symptoms associated with inadequate organ perfusion resulting from decreased cardiac output after a myocardial infarction.

1. _____

2. _____

3. _____

## Learning Assessment

### NCLEX Examination Challenge #1

The nurse is caring for a client who is being discharged to home following an MI and beginning carvedilol CR. What health teaching would the nurse include about this drug? **Select all that apply.**

A. "Do not take your daily dose if your pulse rate is less than 50 beats per minute."
B. "Report any bleeding or unusual bruising to your primary health care provider."
C. "Report frequent dry hacking coughing episodes to your primary health care provider."
D. "Take the drug in the evening with or without food to help prevent side effects."
E. "Report new wheezing, shortness of breath, or edema to your primary health care provider."

### NCLEX Examination Challenge #2

The nurse is caring for a client following a PCI for an occluded coronary artery. For which potential complication(s) of PCI would the nurse monitor? **Select all that apply.**

A. Hypertension
B. Dysrhythmias
C. Hypernatremia
D. Hypokalemia
E. Bleeding from insertion site

## NGN Challenge

### Item #1

The nurse reviews the Nurses Notes for a 74-year-old client admitted to the ED with chest pain.

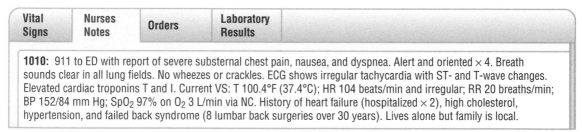

| Vital Signs | Nurses Notes | Orders | Laboratory Results | |
|---|---|---|---|---|

**1010:** 911 to ED with report of severe substernal chest pain, nausea, and dyspnea. Alert and oriented × 4. Breath sounds clear in all lung fields. No wheezes or crackles. ECG shows irregular tachycardia with ST- and T-wave changes. Elevated cardiac troponins T and I. Current VS: T 100.4°F (37.4°C); HR 104 beats/min and irregular; RR 20 breaths/min; BP 152/84 mm Hg; SpO$_2$ 97% on O$_2$ 3 L/min via NC. History of heart failure (hospitalized × 2), high cholesterol, hypertension, and failed back syndrome (8 lumbar back surgeries over 30 years). Lives alone but family is local.

Highlight the relevant client findings that require **immediate** follow-up by the nurse.

### Item #2

The nurse reviews the Nurses Notes for a 74-year-old client admitted to the ED with chest pain.

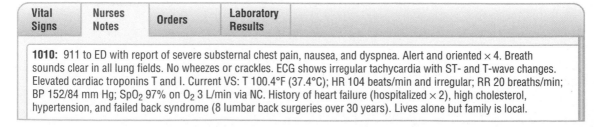

| Vital Signs | Nurses Notes | Orders | Laboratory Results | |
|---|---|---|---|---|

**1010:** 911 to ED with report of severe substernal chest pain, nausea, and dyspnea. Alert and oriented × 4. Breath sounds clear in all lung fields. No wheezes or crackles. ECG shows irregular tachycardia with ST- and T-wave changes. Elevated cardiac troponins T and I. Current VS: T 100.4°F (37.4°C); HR 104 beats/min and irregular; RR 20 breaths/min; BP 152/84 mm Hg; SpO$_2$ 97% on O$_2$ 3 L/min via NC. History of heart failure (hospitalized × 2), high cholesterol, hypertension, and failed back syndrome (8 lumbar back surgeries over 30 years). Lives alone but family is local.

Complete the following sentence by selecting the options in the lists of options below to fill in the blanks. The nurse analyzes the relevant assessment findings to determine that the client most likely has _____1 [Select]_____ as evidenced by _____2 [Select]_____ and _____3 [Select]_____.

| Options for 1 | Options for 2 | Options for 3 |
|---|---|---|
| STEMI | Elevated troponins | Fever |
| NSTEMI | Tachydysrhythmia | Dyspnea |
| Unstable angina | Substernal chest pain | ECG ST- and T-wave changes |

### Item #3

The nurse reviews the Nurses Notes for a 74-year-old client admitted to the ED with chest pain.

| Vital Signs | Nurses Notes | Orders | Laboratory Results |
|---|---|---|---|

**1010:** 911 to ED with report of severe substernal chest pain, nausea, and dyspnea. Alert and oriented × 4. Breath sounds clear in all lung fields. No wheezes or crackles. ECG shows irregular tachycardia with ST- and T-wave changes. Elevated cardiac troponins T and I. Current VS: T 100.4°F (37.4°C); HR 104 beats/min and irregular; RR 20 breaths/min; BP 152/84 mm Hg; $SpO_2$ 97% on $O_2$ 3 L/min via NC. History of heart failure (hospitalized × 2), high cholesterol, hypertension, and failed back syndrome (8 lumbar back surgeries over 30 years). Lives alone but family is local.

Complete the following sentence by selecting the correct word choice in the list below to fill in the blank. The **priority** for the client at this time is to increase _____ to the myocardium to ensure adequate cardiac output.

| Word Choices |
|---|
| Potassium |
| Magnesium |
| Blood flow |
| Iron |

### Item #4

The nurse reviews the Nurses Notes for a 74-year-old client admitted to the ED with chest pain.

| Vital Signs | Nurses Notes | Orders | Laboratory Results |
|---|---|---|---|

**1010:** 911 to ED with report of severe substernal chest pain, nausea, and dyspnea. Alert and oriented × 4. Breath sounds clear in all lung fields. No wheezes or crackles. ECG shows irregular tachycardia with ST- and T-wave changes. Elevated cardiac troponins T and I. Current VS: T 100.4°F (37.4°C); HR 104 beats/min and irregular; RR 20 breaths/min; BP 152/84 mm Hg; $SpO_2$ 97% on $O_2$ 3 L/min via NC. History of heart failure (hospitalized × 2), high cholesterol, hypertension, and failed back syndrome (8 lumbar back surgeries over 30 years). Lives alone but family is local.

Based on the client's probable diagnosis, select five interventions that are appropriate for the client at this time.
A.   Administer nitroglycerin for chest pain.
B.   Start a peripheral IV line.
C.   Have client chew aspirin 325 mg.
D.   Start IV unfractionated heparin drip.
E.   Prepare client for PCI.
F.   Place client on continuous cardiac monitoring.

*Item #5*

The nurse reviews the Nurses Notes for a 74-year-old client admitted to the ED with chest pain.

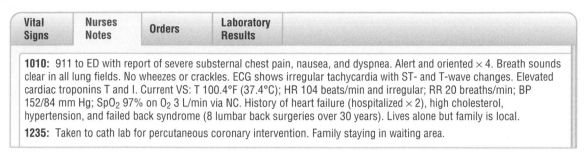

| Vital Signs | Nurses Notes | Orders | Laboratory Results | |
|---|---|---|---|---|

**1010:** 911 to ED with report of severe substernal chest pain, nausea, and dyspnea. Alert and oriented × 4. Breath sounds clear in all lung fields. No wheezes or crackles. ECG shows irregular tachycardia with ST- and T-wave changes. Elevated cardiac troponins T and I. Current VS: T 100.4°F (37.4°C); HR 104 beats/min and irregular; RR 20 breaths/min; BP 152/84 mm Hg; SpO$_2$ 97% on O$_2$ 3 L/min via NC. History of heart failure (hospitalized × 2), high cholesterol, hypertension, and failed back syndrome (8 lumbar back surgeries over 30 years). Lives alone but family is local.

**1235:** Taken to cath lab for percutaneous coronary intervention. Family staying in waiting area.

The nurse plans care for the client's return from percutaneous coronary intervention. Which actions will the nurse include in the postprocedure plan of care? **Select all that apply.**

A.    Monitor for bleeding around the insertion site.
B.    Assess for cardiac dysrhythmias.
C.    Place client in sitting position for 4 hours.
D.    Keep extremity with insertion site straight.
E.    Keep client in bed for several hours per protocol.
F.    Monitor for hypokalemia and hypotension.

*Item #6*

A 74-year-old client visits the cardiologist for follow up 1 week after hospital discharge. The client had a coronary angioplasty with stent placement (PCI) for a NSTEMI. Today the nurse performs an assessment before the client examination by the provider. Indicate which client findings demonstrate that the client's treatment plan was **Effective** (client improved) or **Not Effective** (client did not improve).

| Client Findings on Hospital Admission (Before PCI) | Client Findings Today's Visit | Effective | Not Effective |
|---|---|---|---|
| Severe substernal chest pain | No chest pain since discharge | | |
| Dyspnea | No dyspnea since discharge | | |
| ECG ST- and T-wave changes | ECG: normal sinus rhythm | | |
| HR 104 beats/min and irregular | HR 88 beats/min and regular | | |
| BP 152/84 mm Hg | BP 148/90 mm Hg | | |

# 33
CHAPTER

# *Assessment of the Hematologic System*

## LEARNING OUTCOMES

1. Use knowledge of anatomy and physiology to perform a focused assessment of the hematologic system.
2. Teach evidence-based health promotion activities to help prevent hematologic health problems or trauma.
3. Identify factors that affect health equity for patients with hematologic health problems.
4. Explain how genetic implications and physiologic aging of the hematologic system affect clotting and perfusion.

5. Demonstrate clinical judgment to interpret assessment findings in a patient with a suspected or actual hematologic health problem.
6. Plan evidence-based care and support for patients undergoing diagnostic testing of the hematologic system.

## Preliminary Reading

Read and review Chapter 33, pp. 810–826.

## Chapter Review

### Anatomy & Physiology Review

#1. Label the parts of the erythrocyte (red blood cell) growth pathway using the Anatomy Labels provided after the figure.

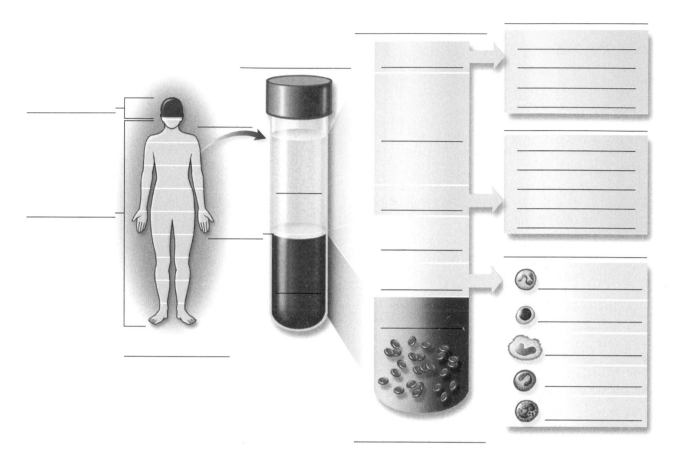

| **Anatomy Labels** |
|---|
| Erythrocyte |
| Polychromatic erythroblast |
| Basophilic erythroblast |
| Proerythroblast |
| Pluripotent stem cell |
| Orthochromatic erythroblast |
| Reticulocyte |
| Proerythroblast |

#2. Provide the normal ranges for the following laboratory tests.

1. Red blood cell count (male) _____ $\times 10^6$/mcL
2. Red blood cell count (female) _____ $\times 10^6$/mcL
3. Hemoglobin (male) _____ g/dL
4. Hemoglobin (female) _____ g/dL
5. Hematocrit (male) _____ %
6. Hematocrit (female) _____ %
7. White blood cell count _____ /mm$^3$
8. Platelet count _____ /mm$^3$
9. D-dimer _____ mcg/mL
10. International normalized ratio (INR) _____
11. Prothrombin time (PT) _____ seconds

## Activities

### Activity #1
List five drugs that are associated with bone marrow suppression.

1. _____

2. _____

3. _____

4. _____

5. _____

### Activity #2
Circle the correct term or phrase that completes each sentence accurately. Only one choice should be selected for each sentence.
1. A prothrombin time of 11 is interpreted to be <u>high/low/normal</u>.
2. A normal percentage of lymphocytes is <u>1–4% or 2–8% or 20–40%.</u>
3. An increased percentage of eosinophils is most likely related to <u>allergies/infection/anemia</u>.
4. Someone who has type O negative blood can receive red blood cells from a donor who has the blood type of <u>O positive/O negative/O positive or O negative</u>.
5. A patient with O+ blood can receive donor blood from a patient with <u>AB blood/A blood/O blood</u>.
6. A patient who is Rh negative is compatible with a donor who is <u>Rh positive/Rh negative/Rh negative or Rh positive.</u>
7. The nurse will monitor a patient with a platelet count of 130,000 for <u>polycythemia vera/malignancy/bone marrow suppression</u>.
8. The nurse will teach a patient with heavy menstrual periods to eat foods higher in <u>Vitamin C/iron/calcium</u>.
9. A patient with a low serum albumin value must be monitored most closely for <u>bruising/fever/edema</u>.
10. The plasma protein type that helps protect the body against infection is <u>albumin/fibrinogen/globulin</u>.

## Activity #3

For each statement, specify if the statement is **true (T)** or **false (F)**.

____1.  Prothrombin and fibrinogen are important to the blood clotting process.

____2.  Red blood cells originate as stem cells.

____3.  White blood cells produce hemoglobin.

____4.  Platelet counts are normally higher in older adults.

____5.  Anticoagulant drugs are used to break down existing clots.

____6.  The normal INR range is 0.8 to 1.2.

____7.  The most common location used for a bone marrow aspiration is the sternum.

____8.  A bone marrow biopsy requires informed consent.

____9.  The Rapid Response Team should be contacted if a crunching sound is heard during a bone marrow aspiration.

___10.  Sterile technique must be observed for a bone marrow aspiration or biopsy.

## Activity #4

List the eight common blood types.

1.  _____

2.  _____

3.  _____

4.  _____

5.  _____

6.  _____

7.  _____

8.  _____

## Learning Assessments

### NCLEX Examination Challenge #1

Which laboratory value for a client receiving an erythrocyte-stimulating agent (ESA) indicates to the nurse that the drug is effective? Refer to the normal values recorded in the Anatomy & Physiology Review Activity #2 above.

A.  INR of 0.9

B.  Platelet count of 160,000/mm³ (160 × 10⁹/L)

C.  WBC count of 8400/mm³ (8.4 × 10⁹/L)

D.  Red blood cell (RBC) count of 4.9 × 10⁶/μL (4.9 × 10¹²/L)

### NCLEX Examination Challenge #2

A client with AB+ blood type is to receive a unit of packed RBCs. When the unit arrives showing that it is from a donor with B negative blood, which action will the nurse take?

A.  Begin the transfusion

B.  Return unit to blood bank

C.  Complete an incident report

D.  Call the health care provider

**NCLEX Examination Challenge #3**

Which type of donor blood does the nurse recognize as compatible with a recipient client whose blood type is O negative? **Select all that apply.**

A. A positive
B. B negative
C. AB positive
D. O negative
E. AB negative

# 34 CHAPTER

# *Concepts of Care for Patients with Hematologic Conditions*

## LEARNING OUTCOMES

1. Plan collaborative care with the interprofessional team to promote perfusion and immunity in patients with hematologic disorders.
2. Teach adults how to decrease the risk for hematologic disorders.
3. Teach the patient and caregiver(s) about common drugs and other management strategies used for hematologic disorders.
4. Plan patient- and family-centered nursing interventions to decrease the psychosocial impact caused by living with a hematologic disorder.
5. Apply knowledge of anatomy, physiology, and pathophysiology to provide evidence-based care

for patients with hematologic disorders affecting perfusion and immunity.
6. Analyze assessment and diagnostic findings to generate solutions and prioritize nursing care for patients with hematologic disorders.
7. Organize care coordination and transition management for patients with hematologic disorders.
8. Use clinical judgment to plan evidence-based nursing care to promote perfusion and immunity and prevent complications in patients with hematologic disorders.
9. Incorporate factors that affect health equity into the plan of care for patients with hematologic disorders.

## Preliminary Reading

Read and review Chapter 34, pages 827–864.

## Chapter Review

### Pathophysiology Review

#1. Match the type of anemia Column A with its description in Column B.

| Column A | | Column B | |
|---|---|---|---|
| ____1. | Aplastic anemia | A. | Caused by antibodies formed against one's own RBC membranes |
| ____2. | Hemolytic anemia | B. | Also known as cobalamin deficiency |
| ____3. | Iron deficiency anemia | C. | Insufficient iron in the body |
| ____4. | Pernicious anemia | D. | Caused by deficiency of intrinsic factor |
| ____5. | Sickle cell anemia | E. | Deficiency of RBCs resulting from bone marrow impairment |
| ____6. | Vitamin $B_{12}$ deficiency anemia | F. | Form of inherited disorder with RBC sickling |

#2. Fill in the chart to indicate precepitating factors associated with each type of transfusion reaction.

| Potential Transfusion Reaction | Precipitating Factor(s) |
|---|---|
| Acute hemolytic transfusion reaction | |
| Acute pain transfusion reaction | |
| Allergic transfusion reaction (mucocutaneous) | |
| Allergic transfusion reaction (anaphylactic transfusion reaction) | |
| Febrile reaction (nonhemolytic) | |
| Transfusion-associated circulatory overload (TACO) | |
| Transfusion-associated graft-versus-host disease | |
| Transfusion-related acute lung injury (TRALI) | |

## Activities

### Activity #1
For each statement, specific if the statement is **true (T)** or **false (F)**.

_____1.   Patients with sickle cell disease develop hemolytic anemia.
_____2.   Iron deficiency anemia is the most common anemia globally.
_____3.   Folic acid deficiency anemia is characterized by paresthesias.
_____4.   Patients with chronic kidney disease can develop anemia of inflammation.
_____5.   Polycythemia vera involves high production of RBCs, leukocytes, and platelets.
_____6.   Leukemia is a type of cancer of the bones.
_____7.   All people visiting a patient with leukemia must wear a mask.
_____8.   Day T-0 is the day that stem cells are infused into the patient.
_____9.   Patients with a platelet value of 120,000/mm$^3$ are at risk for excessive blood clotting.
____10.   Multiple myeloma is cancer of the white blood cells.

### Activity #2
Identify the blood donor groups that are safe for use for each patient/recipient blood group. Choices include:

**O negative, O positive
A negative, A positive
B negative, B positive
AB negative, AB positive**

| Patient (Recipient) Blood Group | Blood Donor Groups |
|---|---|
| O negative | |
| O positive | |
| B negative | |
| B positive | |
| A negative | |
| A positive | |

| Patient (Recipient) Blood Group | Blood Donor Groups |
|---|---|
| AB negative | |
| AB positive | |

## Activity #3

List at least 10 things the nurse will teach a patient about preventing sickle cell crisis.

1. _____

2. _____

3. _____

4. _____

5. _____

6. _____

7. _____

8. _____

9. _____

10. _____

## Activity #4

Provide a description for each phase of stem cell transplantation.

1.   Phase 1 (Conditioning) _____

_____

2.   Phase 2 (Transplant day to engraftment) _____

_____

3.   Phase 3 (Engraftment to day of discharge) _____

_____

4.   Phase 4 (Early convalescence) _____

_____

5.   Phase 5 (Late convalescence) _____

_____

**Activity #5**

Fill in the blanks to complete the sentences about best practice for ensuring patient safety and quality care for older adults receiving a transfusion.

1. Assess the patient's _____, _____, and _____ status prior to transfusion.
2. Use a needle no larger than _____ gauge.
3. Use blood that is less than _____ old.
4. Vital signs must be collected every _____ minutes during the transfusion.
5. Each unit of whole blood, packed RBCs, or plasma is infused between _____ hours.
6. Do not transfuse whole blood, packed RBCs, or plasma for more than _____ hours.
7. When possible, allow _____ hours between infusions of units.
8. Change blood tubing after every _____ units transfused.

## Learning Assessment

### NCLEX Examination Challenge #1

The nurse is caring for a client with sickle cell disease (SCD). Which laboratory value prompts the nurse to notify the health care provider?

A. Hematocrit 41% (range Male: 42%–52% or Female: 37%–47%)
B. Hemoglobin 14.4 g/dL (range Male: 14–18 g/dL or Female: 12–16 g/dL)
C. Platelet count 260,000/mm³ (range 150,000–400,000/mm³)
D. WBC count 20,000/mm³ (range 5000–10,000/mm³)

### NCLEX Examination Challenge #2

An older adult client is receiving a third transfusion of packed RBCs over the past 8 hours. Which **priority** action will the nurse take when the client develops distended neck veins?

A. Slow the infusion rate.
B. Assess circulatory status.
C. Discontinue the transfusion.
D. Document occurrence in the health record.

### NCLEX Examination Challenge #3

Which assessment finding does the nurse expect on assessment of a client newly diagnosed with acute leukemia before initiation of treatment? **Select all that apply.**

A. Fatigue
B. Bone pain
C. Facial flushing
D. Finger clubbing
E. Excessive bruising

## NGN Challenge #1

The nurse is trending laboratory results for a 36-year-old client who reports increasing fatigue despite eating well and walking for 20 minutes three times weekly.

| | Normal Range | April 9, 2023 | October 31, 2022 | May 6, 2022 |
|---|---|---|---|---|
| RBC count | Male: 4.7–6.1<br>Female: 4.2–5.4 | 3.9 | 4.2 | 4.3 |
| Hemoglobin | Male: 14–18 g/dL or 8.7–11.2 mmol/L (SI units)<br>Female: 12–16 g/dL or 7.4–9.9 mmol/L | 12.1 | 12.2 | 13 |
| Hematocrit | Male: 42%–52% or 0.42–0.52 volume fraction (SI units)<br>Female: 37%–47% or 0.37–0.47 volume fraction (SI units) | 35% | 38% | 38% |
| Platelet count | 150,000–400,000/mm$^3$ or 150–400 $\times 10^9$/L (SI units) | 210,000 | 209,000 | 213,000 |
| MCV | 80–95 fL | 78 | 84 | 93 |
| MCH | 27–31 pg | 26 | 28 | 30 |
| Ferritin | Male: 12–300 ng/mL or 12–300 mcg/L (SI units)<br>Female: 10–150 ng/mL or 10–150 mcg/L (SI units) | 8 | 14 | 26 |
| Glycohemoglobin A1C | 4%–5.9% | 5.2% | 5.3% | 5.1% |

Which action will the nurse take at this time? **Select all that apply.**

A. Discuss monoclonal antibody therapy.
B. Recommend limiting red meat in diet.
C. Notify the primary health care provider.
D. Coordinate an appointment with a diabetic educator.
E. Teach that easy bruising may occur because of platelet count.
F. Explain that iron tablets should be taken with Vitamin C.
G. Teach about the use of hydroxyurea to reduce vaso-occlusive occurrences.

**NGN Challenge #2**

The nurse is trending the platelet count for a 53-year-old client who has been undergoing aggressive chemotherapy due to breast cancer.

| | Normal Range | June 11, 2023 | May 6, 2023 | April 1, 2023 |
|---|---|---|---|---|
| Platelet count | 150,000–400,000/mm$^3$ or 150–400 ×10$^9$/L (SI units) | 48,000/mm$^3$ | 75,000/mm$^3$ | 99,000/mm$^3$ |

Select three actions the nurse will take at this time.

A.  Discuss foods high in Vitamin D.
B.  Teach about the risk for bleeding.
C.  Explain the need to assess stool at home.
D.  Demonstrate how to self-inject Vitamin B12.
E.  Teach how to restrict fluid to prevent volume overload.
F.  Recommend increased intake of dark green vegetables.
G.  Discuss a plan for how to recognize an impending sickle cell crisis.
H.  Teach that a Raynaud-like response is possible when counts are this low.

# 35 CHAPTER

# *Assessment of the Nervous System*

## LEARNING OUTCOMES

1. Use knowledge of anatomy and physiology to perform a focused assessment of the nervous system.
2. Teach evidence-based health promotion activities to help prevent neurologic health problems or trauma.
3. Demonstrate clinical judgment to interpret assessment findings in a patient with a neurologic health problem.
4. Identify factors that affect health equity for patients with neurologic health problems.
5. Explain how genetic implications and physiologic aging of the nervous system affect mobility.
6. Interpret assessment findings for patients with a suspected or actual neurologic problem.
7. Plan evidence-based care and support for patients undergoing diagnostic testing of the nervous system.

## Preliminary Reading

Read and review Chapter 35, pp. 865–881.

## Chapter Review

### Anatomy & Physiology Review

#1. Match the major parts of the brain in Column A with their function in Column B.

**Column A**

____1. Occipital lobe
____2. Cerebellum
____3. Frontal lobe
____4. Temporal lobe
____5. Brainstem
____6. Parietal lobe

**Column B**

A. Center for cardiac and respiratory function
B. Sensory and perception center
C. Primary visual center
D. Voluntary movement and balance center
E. Primary motor and speech center
F. Auditory and language center

#2. Using the six parts of the brain listed under Column A in #1, label the location of each part in the figure.

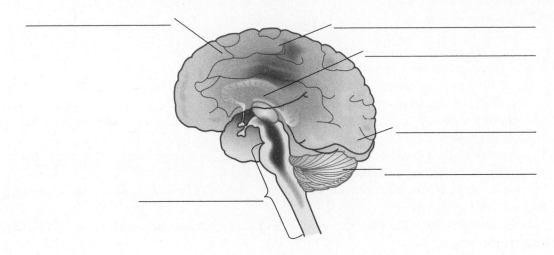

## Activities

### Activity #1
List at least four common physiologic nervous system changes associated with aging.

1. _____

2. _____

3. _____

4. _____

### Activity #2
Complete the sentences with the correct term or phrase.
1. A limitation in mobility or activity that can affect the ability of a patient to perform one or more ADLs is called having a _____.
2. A persistently painful and debilitating condition that involves the trigeminal cranial nerve (CN V) and affects women more than men is known as _____.
3. A commonly used standardized tool to assess a patient's level of consciousness is the _____ _____.
4. Two of the most common reports of individuals with neurologic problems are _____ and _____.
5. The nurse documents an unconscious patient who cannot be aroused despite vigorous or noxious stimulation as _____.
6. Asking the patient to grasp and squeeze the nurse's fingers is one way to assess the patient's _____.
7. If CN III is intact, a patient's pupils should _____ when exposed to light.
8. _____ is an involuntary eye movement that usually causes the eyes to move rapidly from side to side or up and down.

9. A patient's intact cough or gag reflex is a function of CN __ and ___.
10. One of the most common mental health conditions that can result from having an acute or chronic neurologic condition is _____.

## Activity #3
For each statement, specify if the statement is **true (T)** or **false (F).**

_____1. Physical disability occurs more commonly in older adults from Hispanic, American Indian/Alaska Native, and other racial groups when compared to Euro-Caucasian groups.

_____2. Older adults, especially men, have the greatest potential for engaging in risky behaviors that can result in acute neurologic trauma.

_____3. The nurse would teach patients about the need to avoid smoking because nicotine causes decreased blood flow to the brain by vasoconstriction.

_____4. Older adult experience mild to moderate cognitive impairment as a normal or usual changes associated with the aging process.

_____5. The nurse would teach the patient preparing to have cerebral angiography to be NPO for 12 hours before the procedure.

_____6. The nurse would check the patient's serum creatinine level to ensure it is adequate before imaging studies that use contrast medium.

## Activity #4
Match the neurologic diagnostic test is Column A with what it measures in Column B.

| Column A | Column B |
|---|---|
| ___1. CT angiography | A. Identifies nerve and muscle conditions |
| ___2. Electromyography | B. Allows analysis of cerebrospinal fluid |
| ___3. Evoked potentials | C. Measures electrical signals sent to the brain |
| ___4. Electroencephalography | D. Identifies blood vessel narrowing or blockage |
| ___5. Lumbar puncture | E. Records the electrical activity of the brain |

## Learning Assessments

### NCLEX Examination Challenge #1
The nurse is caring for a client who just had a lumbar puncture. What **priority** assessment will the nurse perform?
A. Monitor WBC count for signs of infection.
B. Observe for cerebrospinal fluid leakage at the insertion site.
C. Take vital signs at least every 2 hours.
D. Assess the client's ability to move lower extremities.

### NCLEX Examination Challenge #2
The nurse is caring for a client whose Glasgow Coma Scale score is 15. How will the nurse interpret this assessment findings?
A. The client's is in a stuporous state.
B. The client is in a lethargic state.
C. The client is fully alert and aware.
D. The client's level of consciousness has declined.

### NCLEX Examination Challenge #3
The nurse is caring for a client with brain cancer has new-onset difficulty with speech and right-sided muscle weakness. Which lobe of the brain is most likely affected?
A. Temporal
B. Occipital
C. Parietal
D. Frontal

# 36 CHAPTER

# Concepts of Care for Patients with Conditions of the Central Nervous System: The Brain

## LEARNING OUTCOMES

1. Plan collaborative care with the interprofessional team to promote mobility in patients with Parkinson's disease (PD).
2. Teach adults how to decrease the risk for Alzheimer's disease (AD).
3. Teach the patient and caregiver(s) about common drugs and other management strategies used for migraine headaches and seizures.
4. Plan patient- and family-centered nursing interventions to decrease the psychosocial impact caused by living with AD.
5. Apply knowledge of anatomy, physiology, and pathophysiology to provide evidence-based care for patients with AD affecting cognition.
6. Analyze assessment and diagnostic findings to generate solutions and prioritize nursing care for patients with meningitis.
7. Organize care coordination and transition management for patients with AD.
8. Use clinical judgment to plan evidence-based nursing care to promote mobility and prevent complications in patients with PD.
9. Incorporate factors that affect health equity into the plan of care for patients with AD.

## Preliminary Reading

Read and review Chapter 36, pp. 882–912.

## Chapter Review

### Pathophysiology Review

#1. Match the pathophysiology in Column A with the client condition in Column B.

**Column A**

___1. Neurofibrillary tangles, amyloid-rich neuritic plaques, and vascular degeneration

___2. Widespread degeneration of the substantia nigra decreases dopamine in the brain

___3. Activation of trigeminal nerve pathways that causes pain mediated by calcitonin gene–regulated peptide

___4. Abnormal neuronal activity in the brain, neurotransmitter imbalance, or a combination of both

___5. Pathogens enter the brain or spine, causing central nervous system infection

**Column B**

A. Migraine headache
B. Meningitis
C. Alzheimer's disease
D. Parkinson's disease
E. Epilepsy

#2. Match the type of epileptic seizure in Column A with its description in Column B.

| Column A | Column B |
|---|---|
| ___1. Tonic-clonic | A. Occurs because of activity in the temporal lobe |
| ___2. Atonic (akinetic) | B. Brief jerking of muscles |
| ___3. Myoclonic | C. Sudden loss of muscle tone followed by confusion |
| ___4. Partial | D. Causes muscle rigidity followed by loss of consciousness |
| ___5. Psychomotor | E. Begins in one cerebral hemisphere; can be simple or complex |

## Activities

### Activity #1
For each statement, specify if the statement is **true (T)** or **false (F).**
___1. AD is clinically considered the most common type of dementia.
___2. Dementia is a normal physiologic change of aging.
___3. Veterans who have a traumatic brain injury and/or PTSD are more likely to develop dementia when compared with veterans without these risk factors.
___4. One of the first signs of AD is short-term memory impairment.
___5. Reality orientation is an appropriate intervention for patients who have late-stage dementia.
___6. Cholinesterase inhibitors, such as donepezil, work to improve ADL ability for patients with AD.
___7. The patient with moderate or severe AD requires 24-hour supervision and caregiving.
___8. AD is considered a terminal illness requiring quality end-of-life care.

### Activity #2
List three tips for successful communication with patients who have mild to moderate AD.

1. _____

2. _____

3. _____

### Activity #3
Identify four typical client assessment findings that are associated with PD.

1. _____

2. _____

3. _____

4. _____

## Activity #4

Match the drug in Column A with the client condition for which is it given in Column B. Choices in Column B may be used more than one time.

**Column A**

___1.  Levodopa-carbidopa
___2.  Sumatriptan
___3.  Carbamazepine
___4.  Galcanezumab
___5.  Amantadine
___6.  Selegiline
___7.  Valproic acid

**Column B**

A.   Epilepsy
B.   Parkinson's disease
C.   Migraine headaches

## Activity #5

Many patients with migraine headaches use triptans as abortive drug therapy. As a nurse teaching a patient about these agents, what three health teaching statements would you include?

1. _____

2. _____

3. _____

## Activity #6

Identify three complications for which the nurse monitors when caring for a patient who has bacterial meningitis.

1. _____

2. _____

3. _____

## Learning Assessments

**NCLEX Examination Challenge #1**

The nurse is caring for a client who has a seizure that lasts more than 5 minutes. What actions would the nurse take? **Select all that apply.**

A.   Establish an airway as needed.
B.   Place the client in a sitting position in bed.
C.   Take vital signs every 15 minutes.
D.   Initiate large-bore IV catheter and hang 0.9% sodium chloride.
E.   Administer IV antiepileptic drug per agency or provider protocol.

**NCLEX Examination Challenge #2**

The nurse is caring for a client who has PD who has been taking a levodopa-carbidopa preparation for the past 5 years. For what long-term adverse drug events would the nurse monitor? **Select all that apply.**

A.   Orthostatic hypotension
B.   Acute kidney injury
C.   Psychosis
D.   Dyskinesia
E.   Toxic megacolon

**NCLEX Examination Challenge #3**

The nurse is caring for a client who is in the moderate stage of AD and is admitted to the hospital for possible intestinal obstruction. To assist in planning care, which signs and symptoms related to AD would the nurse anticipate the client to have? **Select all that apply.**

A. Disoriented to time, place, and event
B. Possibly depressed and/or agitated
C. Increasingly dependent in ADLs
D. Has visuospatial deficits and easily gets lost
E. Unable to talk or understand others
F. Incontinent of urine and stool

**NGN Challenge #1**

The nurse reviews the ED admission note for a 74-year-old client.

| Health History | Nurses Notes | Orders | Laboratory Results | |
|---|---|---|---|---|

**1145:** 74-year-old client brought to the ED by the client's partner following a fall at home. Partner states that the client has Parkinson's disease (PD) and uses a walker to ambulate due to gait problems, muscle weakness, and rigidity. Current medications for PD include a levodopa/carbidopa combination and pimavanserin. Client felt dizzy and lightheaded this morning but decided to take a short walk outside near the house. Fell while stepping up to front door. Reported right shoulder pain that radiates down the arm. Client alert and oriented to person only. Rubbing right shoulder and grimacing at times. Lung sounds clear; $S_1$ and $S_2$ present; bowel sounds present × 4. VS: T 98.2°F (36.8°C); HR 94 beats/min; RR 20 breaths/min; BP 98/56 mm Hg; $SpO_2$ 95%.

Complete the diagram by identifying from the choices to specify what condition the client is likely experiencing, **two** potential nursing actions that are appropriate for the condition, and **two** parameters for which the nurse would monitor.

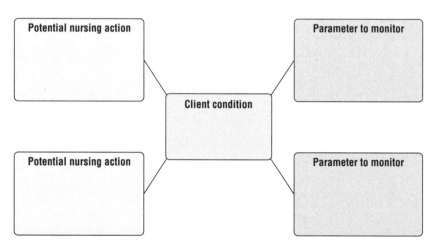

| Potential Nursing Actions | Client Condition | Parameters to Monitor |
|---|---|---|
| Perform frequent orthostatic blood pressure checks | Lewy body dementia | Neurologic status |
| Reorient the client frequently | Delirium | Right arm swelling |
| Hold pimavanserin at this time | Seizure | Positional blood pressures |
| Place the client on fall precautions | Orthostatic hypotension | Client's gait pattern |
| Request a physical therapy consult | ///////////////////////// | Psychotic behaviors |

**NGN Challenge #2**

The nurse assesses and documents findings for a 33-year-old client who visits the urgent care center.

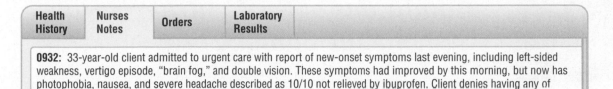

| Health History | Nurses Notes | Orders | Laboratory Results | |
|---|---|---|---|---|

**0932:** 33-year-old client admitted to urgent care with report of new-onset symptoms last evening, including left-sided weakness, vertigo episode, "brain fog," and double vision. These symptoms had improved by this morning, but now has photophobia, nausea, and severe headache described as 10/10 not relieved by ibuprofen. Client denies having any of these symptoms previously. Is concerned about having a stroke because the client's mother died from a severe stroke last year. VS: T 98.2°F (36.8°C); HR 94 beats/min; RR 22 breaths/min; BP 148/68 mm Hg; SpO$_2$ 97%.

Complete the diagram by identifying from the choices to specify what condition the client is likely experiencing, **two** potential nursing actions that are appropriate for the condition, and **two** parameters for which the nurse would monitor before discharge from the urgent care center.

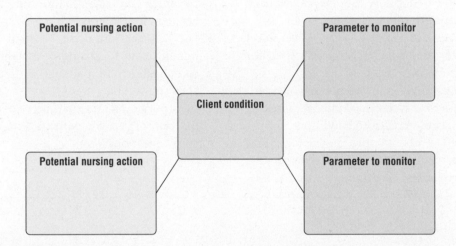

| Potential Nursing Actions | Client Condition | Parameters to Monitor |
|---|---|---|
| Provide supplemental oxygen | Stroke | Blood pressure |
| Have client lie down and close eyes in darkened room | Transient ischemic attack | Oxygen saturation |
| Administer medication for headache | Cerebral aneurysm | Visual acuity |
| Prepare client for head CT scan | Migraine headache | Headache pain intensity level |
| Prepare for transfer to the acute care setting | /////////////////////////////////// | Neurologic status |

# 37 CHAPTER

# *Concepts of Care for Patients with Conditions of the Central Nervous System: The Spinal Cord*

## LEARNING OUTCOMES

1. Plan collaborative care with the interprofessional team to promote mobility, sensory perception, and cognition in patients with multiple sclerosis (MS).
2. Teach adults how to decrease the risk for low back pain and spinal cord injury.
3. Teach the patient and caregiver(s) about common drugs and other management strategies used for MS affecting immunity.
4. Plan patient- and family-centered nursing interventions to decrease the psychosocial impact caused by living with common spinal cord conditions.
5. Apply knowledge of anatomy, physiology, and pathophysiology to provide evidence-based care for patients with spinal cord injury.
6. Analyze assessment and diagnostic findings to generate solutions and prioritize nursing care for patients who have multiple sclerosis.
7. Organize care coordination and transition management for patients living with spinal cord injury.
8. Use clinical judgment to plan evidence-based nursing care to promote sexuality and decrease complications in patients with common spinal cord conditions.
9. Incorporate factors that affect health equity into the plan of care for patients with common spinal cord conditions.

## Preliminary Reading

Read and review Chapter 37, pp. 913–940.

## Chapter Review

### Pathophysiology Review

#1. Match the spinal cord injury in Column A with the type of injury in Column B. Column B options may be used more than once.

**Column A**
____1. Penetrating trauma
____2. Hyperflexion
____3. Ischemia
____4. Hyperextension
____5. Neurogenic shock
____6. Hemorrhage
____7. Vertebral compression

**Column B**
A. Primary spinal cord injury
B. Secondary spinal cord injury

#2. Complete the sentences about multiple sclerosis with the listed choices. Note that not all choices will be used.
1. MS is characterized by periods of _____.
2. Patients with MS have _____ of central nervous system white matter caused by diffuse random or patchy _____.
3. The most common type of MS is _____.
4. Early symptoms of MS include changes in _____, _____, and _____.
5. MS differs from amyotrophic lateral sclerosis (ALS) because ALS leads to death from _____ _____.

| Choices for Sentence Completion |
| --- |
| Mobility |
| Amyloid protein |
| Remissions and exacerbations |
| Nerve injury |
| Primary progressive multiple sclerosis |
| Vision |
| Respiratory muscle paralysis |
| Plaque |
| Sensory perception |
| Relapsing-remitting MS |
| Demyelination |
| Nerve injury |

## Activities

### Activity #1
Match the glossary term in Column A with the definition in Column B.

| Column A | | Column B | |
| --- | --- | --- | --- |
| ____1. | Paraplegia | A. | Changes in peripheral vision, often in patients with MS |
| ____2. | Spinal shock | B. | Spinal nerve root involvement |
| ____3. | Heterotopic ossification | C. | Difficulty swallowing |
| ____4. | Diplopia | D. | Bony overgrowth, often into muscle |
| ____5. | Scotoma | E. | A syndrome that occurs immediately after a spinal cord injury that causes temporary loss of motor, sensory, reflex, and autonomic function |
| ____6. | Neurogenic shock | F. | Paralysis that affects only the lower extremities |
| ____7. | Dysarthria | G. | Difficulty speaking because of facial weakness causing slurred speech |
| ____8. | Tetraplegia (quadriplegia) | H. | Paralysis that affects all four extremities |
| ____9. | Radiculopathy | I. | Occurs from severe spinal cord injury and results in decreased perfusion to major body organs |
| ___10. | Dysphagia | J. | Double vision |

## Activity #2

For each statement, specify if the statement is **true (T)** or **false (F).**

_____1.   Patients with MS are at an increased risk for infection.

_____2.   Patients with MS have muscle flaccidity and atrophy.

_____3.   Airway management is the nursing priority for the patient who has tetraplegia.

_____4.   A Halo fixator is appropriate to manage patients who are paraplegic.

_____5.   Patients with spinal cord injury are at high risk for complications of immobility.

_____6.   Acute lumbosacral back pain usually results from injury or trauma.

_____7.   Complications of minimally invasive surgery for low back pain are rare.

_____8.   If a client experiences cerebrospinal fluid leakage, the nurse should place the client in a flat supine position.

_____9.   One major goal of *Healthy People 2030* is to increase the health and well-being of people living with disabilities, such as spinal cord injury.

___10.   A patient who is paraplegic is usually able to provide self-care without assistance after an appropriate rehabilitation program.

## Activity #3

List three complications of open traditional low back surgery for which the nurse would monitor.

1.   _____

2.   _____

3.   _____

## Activity #4

Match the drug in Column A with the nursing implication in Column B.

**Column A**

___1.   Metaxalone

___2.   Baclofen

___3.   Interferon-beta-1a

___4.   Fingolimod

___5.   Tizanidine

**Column B**

A.   Teach patients to monitor pulse daily because the drug can cause bradycardia.

B.   Be aware that this drug should not be taken by older adults because of anticholinergic effects.

C.   Be aware that this drug can cause liver damage.

D.   Teach patients to rotate injection sites because skin reactions are common.

E.   Monitor for drowsiness and sedation while the patient is taking this drug.

## Activity #5

Identify four health promotion activities that help prevent low back injury.

1.   _____

2.   _____

3.   _____

4.   _____

## Learning Assessments

### NCLEX Examination Challenge #1

The nurse is caring for a client who had an open spinal fusion this morning. The nurse observes that the surgical dressing is damp and has a halo ring around the edge. What is the nurse's **first** action?

A. Notify the surgeon immediately.
B. Place the client in a flat supine position.
C. Contact the Rapid Response Team.
D. Reinforce the dressing with additional gauze.

### NCLEX Examination Challenge #2

The nurse is teaching the client with MS about starting fingolimod. What is the **most important** health teaching the nurse will include about this drug?

A. "Rotate injection sites to prevent site reactions."
B. "Be sure to keep all lab appointments to monitor your liver function."
C. "Avoid large crowds and anyone who has a possible infection."
D. "Take this drug with meals or a food each day."

### NCLEX Examination Challenge #3

The nurse is admitting a client with a complete C5-C6 spinal cord injury to a unit for intensive rehabilitation. What medications would the nurse anticipate the client would be taking? **Select all that apply.**

A. Pantoprazole
B. Morphine sulfate
C. Baclofen
D. Calcium
E. Apixaban
F. Docusate sodium

### NGN Challenge #1

The nurse is caring for a 28-year-old client who was admitted last evening with a T1-T2 spinal cord injury that occurred after a motor vehicle accident. The nurse notes that the client is very drowsy and lethargic. The nurse reviews the vital sign flow sheet data since admission.

*Vital Sign Flow Sheet*

|  | **12 Hours After Admission (0750)** | **6 Hours After Admission (0150)** | **Admission (1950)** |
|---|---|---|---|
| T | 99.8°F (37.7°C) | 99°F (37.2°C) | 98.4°F (36.9°C) |
| HR | 56 beats/min | 98 beats/min | 86 beats/min |
| RR | 24 breaths/min | 20 breaths/min | 18 breaths/min |
| BP | 88/50 mm Hg | 102/58 mm Hg | 114/62 mm Hg |
| SpO$_2$ | 94% | 96% | 97% |
| Urinary output | 120 mL | 200 mL | Urinary catheter inserted |
| Level of consciousness | Drowsy and oriented ×2 | Alert and oriented ×4 | Alert and oriented ×4 |

Complete the following sentence by filling in the blanks using the lists of options below.

The nurse analyzes the data and determines that the client most is most likely experiencing _____1 [Select]_____ as evidenced by _____2 [Select]_____ and _____3 [Select]_____.

| Options for 1 | Options for 2 | Options for 3 |
|---|---|---|
| Autonomic dysreflexia | Fever | Hypotension |
| Neurogenic shock | Tachypnea | Tachycardia |
| Spinal shock | Bradycardia | Disorientation |

**NGN Challenge #2**

The nurse is caring for a 28-year-old client who was admitted last evening with a T1-T2 spinal cord injury that occurred after a motor vehicle accident. The nurse notes that the client is very drowsy and lethargic. The nurse reviews the vital sign flow sheet data since admission.

*Vital Sign Flow Sheet*

| | 12 Hours After Admission (0750) | 6 Hours After Admission (0150) | Admission (1950) |
|---|---|---|---|
| T | 99.8°F (37.7°C) | 99°F (37.2°C) | 98.4°F (36.9°C) |
| HR | 56 beats/min | 98 beats/min | 86 beats/min |
| RR | 24 breaths/min | 20 breaths/min | 18 breaths/min |
| BP | 88/50 mm Hg | 102/58 mm Hg | 114/62 mm Hg |
| SpO$_2$ | 94% | 96% | 97% |
| Urinary output | 120 mL | 200 mL | Urinary catheter inserted |
| Level of consciousness | Drowsy and oriented ×2 | Alert and oriented ×4 | Alert and oriented ×4 |

Based on the assessment findings, the nurse begins planning client care and anticipating orders. Select **five** orders the nurse would anticipate for this client.

A. Initiate supplemental oxygen.
B. Increase the rate of IV fluids.
C. Give dextran.
D. Administer atropine sulfate.
E. Start dopamine infusion.
F. Place the client in a sitting position.

# 38 CHAPTER

# *Critical Care of Patients with Neurologic Emergencies*

## LEARNING OUTCOMES

1. Plan collaborative care with the interprofessional team to promote mobility, sensory perception, perfusion, and cognition in patients with neurologic emergencies.
2. Teach adults how to decrease the risk for traumatic brain injury and stroke.
3. Teach the patient and caregiver(s) about common drugs and other management strategies used for brain tumors affecting mobility and cognition.
4. Plan patient- and family-centered nursing interventions to decrease the psychosocial impact caused by living with traumatic brain injury.
5. Apply knowledge of anatomy, physiology, and pathophysiology to provide evidence-based care for patients with neurologic emergencies.

6. Analyze assessment and diagnostic findings to generate solutions and prioritize nursing care for patients who have neurologic emergencies.
7. Organize care coordination and transition management for patients living with traumatic brain injury.
8. Use clinical judgment to plan evidence-based nursing care to promote perfusion and decrease complications in patients with neurologic emergencies.
9. Incorporate factors that affect health equity into the plan of care for patients with stroke.

## Preliminary Reading

Read and review Chapter 38, pp. 941–974.

## Chapter Review

### Pathophysiology Review

#1. Match the descriptions of strokes in Column A with the stroke type in Column B. Column B options may be used more than once.

**Column A**

___1. Most often occurs from intracerebral or subarachnoid bleeding
___2. Commonly associated with atherosclerotic plaques in intra- or extracranial arteries
___3. Characterized by sudden development of neurologic deficits
___4. Characterized by slow onset of neurologic deficits
___5. Commonly occurs in patients who have atrial fibrillation, heart valve disease, or endocarditis

**Column B**

A. Thrombotic stroke
B. Embolic stroke
C. Hemorrhagic stroke

#2. Match the brain injury in Column A with the type of injury in Column B. Column B options will be used more than once.

**Column A**

___1. Increased intracranial pressure
___2. Intact skull with brain damage
___3. Brain herniation syndromes
___4. Fractured skull
___5. Skull pierced by penetrating object
___6. Hypoxia caused by hypotension
___7. Cardiac dysrhythmias

**Column B**

A. Primary injury
B. Secondary injury

## Activities

### Activity #1

Match the glossary term in Column A with its definition in Column B.

**Column A**

____1. Aphasia
____2. Ataxia
____3. Bruit
____4. Carotid stenosis
____5. Hemianopsia
____6. Papilledema
____7. Ptosis
____8. Spine precautions
____9. Transient ischemic attack
___10. Unilateral neglect

**Column B**

A. Eyelid drooping
B. Edema and hyperemia (increased blood flow) of the optic disk
C. Inability to recognize own physical impairment, especially on one side of the body
D. Lack of muscle control and coordination that affects gait, balance, and walking
E. Hardening and narrowing of the artery, which decreases blood flow
F. Interventions to help protect the spinal cord from primary or secondary injury
G. Problems with speech or language
H. Condition in which the vision of one or both eyes is affected
I. Temporary neurologic dysfunction resulting from brief blood flow interruption to the brain
J. Sound heard over an artery with a stethoscope that indicates narrowed or partially obstructed blood vessel

### Activity #2

Identify at least three symptoms of increasing intracranial pressure for which the nurse monitors in patients who have strokes, traumatic brain injuries, or other brain lesions.

1. _____

2. _____

3. _____

## Activity #3

For each statement, specify if the statement is **true (T)** or **false (F).**

_____1.   Typically, symptoms of a transient ischemic attack (TIA) resolve within 48 hours but may last as long as 72 hours.

_____2.   A stroke is a medical emergency and should be treated immediately to reduce or prevent permanent disability.

_____3.   A major goal of the *Healthy People 2030* initiative is to improve cardiovascular health and reduce deaths from heart disease and stroke.

_____4.   The National Institutes of Health Stroke Scale (NIHSS) is a commonly used valid and reliable assessment tool that nurses complete as soon as possible after the patient arrives in the ED.

_____5.   For selected patients with acute ischemic strokes, early intervention with IV fibrinolytic therapy ("clot-busting drug") is the standard of practice to improve blood flow to viable tissue around the infarction or through the brain.

_____6.   Pinpoint and nonresponsive pupils are indicative of brainstem dysfunction.

_____7.   Generally, head-of-bed elevation in patients with TBI is at 10 to 30 degrees.

_____8.   The nurse's priority in caring for a client who has a TBI is to maintain cerebral perfusion.

_____9.   Nurses need to identify specific determinants of health and educate people of color about the importance of managing diabetes mellitus and hypertension to prevent strokes.

____10.   Drug therapy with mannitol, hypertonic saline, and/or furosemide is used to decrease ICP when a patient has a major brain injury.

## Activity #4

List four essential interventions that nurses and other health staff need to implement to provide patient-centered care for patients who have **physical disability.**

1. _____

2. _____

3. _____

4. _____

## Activity #5

List and describe four of the six core principles of **trauma-informed care** that nurses need to incorporate into their practice.

1. _____

2. _____

3. _____

4. _____

## Activity #6

For each potential complication that could occur in the immediate postoperative period after open craniotomy surgery, identify at least two nursing assessments and/or actions that would be appropriate.

| Potential Complication | Nursing Assessments and/or Actions |
|---|---|
| Cardiac dysrhythmias | 1.<br>2. |
| Syndrome of inappropriate antidiuretic hormone (SIADH) | 1.<br>2. |
| Venous thromboembolism | 1.<br>2. |
| Hypernatremia/diabetes insipidus (DI) | 1.<br>2. |

## Learning Assessments

### NCLEX Examination Challenge #1

The nurse is caring for a client following an open traditional craniotomy to remove a supratentorial brain tumor. In what position would the nurse place the client in bed?

A. In a flat supine position
B. In a Trendelenburg position
C. In a high-Fowler's sitting position
D. In a 30-degree sitting position

### NCLEX Examination Challenge #2

The nurse is teaching a client who had a transient ischemic attack (TIA) about the client's risk for having a stroke. Which risk factors will the nurse include in the health teaching? **Select all that apply.**

A. History of diabetes mellitus
B. BP greater than or equal to 140/90 mm Hg
C. Hemiparesis as a symptom during the client's TIA
D. Alcohol consumption of more than three drinks per week
E. Age greater than 75 years

### NCLEX Examination Challenge #3

The nurse is caring for a client receiving IV alteplase following a new-onset thrombotic stroke. What nursing action is appropriate during the administration of this drug?

A. Perform a neurologic assessment, including vital signs, every 2 hours.
B. Maintain the client's BP to below 130/80 mm Hg.
C. Discontinue drug infusion of the client has a severe headache or bleeding.
D. Administer prescribed IV heparin while the client is receiving alteplase.

### NGN Challenge #1

The nurse reviews the ED admission notes for a 51-year-old client.

| Health History | Nurses Notes | Orders | Laboratory Results | |
|---|---|---|---|---|

**2220:** 51-year-old client brought to the ED by family following a seizure at home. Family states client has a history of lung cancer 2 years ago and hypertension for 10 years. Lung cancer was in remission after treatment with chemotherapy and radiation. Client due for follow-up full-body scan next week. Over the past several months, client had several severe headaches, episodes of recent memory loss, and difficulty finding words during conversation at times. Last week, client reported weakness in the right leg, which created anxiety about driving safety. No history of seizures until seizure occurred after dinner today. Seizure lasted about 50 seconds during which the client moved extremities slightly. Client could not recall event when it ended.

**2230:** Alert and oriented × 2 (person and place). Able to help provide history. Answers questions appropriately; no aphasia or dysarthria. Right leg slightly weaker than left but able to ambulate without ambulatory aid. No headache or other report of pain currently. Lung sounds clear; $S_1$ and $S_2$ present; bowel sounds present × 4. VS: T 98.2°F (36.8°C); HR 82 beats/min; RR 20 breaths/min; BP 158/86 mm Hg; $SpO_2$ 95% on RA.

Complete the diagram by identifying from the choices to specify what condition the client is likely experiencing, **two** potential nursing actions that are appropriate for the condition, and **two** parameters for which the nurse would monitor.

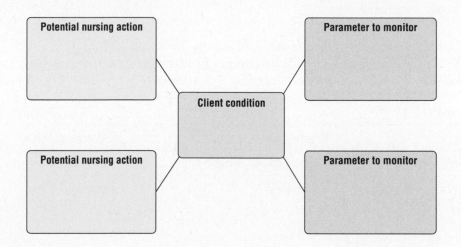

| Potential Nursing Actions | Client Condition | Parameters to Monitor |
|---|---|---|
| Prepare the client for head imaging tests | Stroke | Neurologic status |
| Reorient the client frequently | TIA | Pain assessment |
| Place client on fall precautions | Metastatic brain tumor | GCS score |
| Monitor for signs of increasing intracranial pressure | Epilepsy | Carotid bruits |
| Request a physical therapy consult | /////////////////////////////////// | Occurrence of additional seizure |

**NGN Challenge #2**

A 64-year-old client is admitted to the vascular unit following a carotid artery angioplasty with stenting. The nurse reviews and analyzes the vital sign flow sheet data since admission.

*Vital Sign Flow Sheet*

|  | **3 Hours After Admission (1210)** | **1 Hour After Admission (1010)** | **Admission Postprocedure (0910)** |
|---|---|---|---|
| T | 98.6°F (37°C) | 98.4°F (36.9°C) | 98.4°F (36.9°C) |
| HR | 76 beats/min | 78 beats/min | 80 beats/min |
| RR | 22 breaths/min | 20 breaths/min | 18 breaths/min |
| BP | 146/80 mm Hg | 132/76 mm Hg | 124/74 mm Hg |
| SpO$_2$ | 95% (on RA) | 100% (on O$_2$ 2 L/min) | 100% (on O$_2$ 2 L/min) |
| Urinary output | 270 mL | No additional void | 355 mL |
| Level of consciousness | Drowsy but more difficult to arouse; oriented ×2 (person and place); very restless when awakened | Drowsy but easily awakened; oriented ×4 | Drowsy but easily awakened; oriented ×4 |

Complete the following sentence by filling in the blanks using the lists of options.

The nurse analyzes the assessment data and determines that the client most is most likely experiencing a(n)_____1 [Select]_____ as evidenced by _____2 [Select]_____ and _____3 [Select] _____.

| **Options for 1** | **Options for 2** | **Options for 3** |
|---|---|---|
| Embolic stroke | Bradycardia | Decreased SpO$_2$ |
| Transient ischemic attack | Increased drowsiness | Restlessness |
| Decreased level of consciousness | Tachypnea | Increased BP |

# 39
## CHAPTER

# *Assessment and Concepts of Care for Patients with Eye and Vision Conditions*

## LEARNING OUTCOMES

1. Use knowledge of anatomy and physiology to perform a focused assessment related to visual sensory perception.
2. Teach evidence-based health promotion activities to help prevent visual problems and ear trauma.
3. Explain how genetic implications and physiologic aging affect visual sensory perception.
4. Plan collaborative care with the interprofessional team to promote sensory perception in patients with eye and vision problems.
5. Teach the patient and caregiver(s) about common drugs and other management strategies used for eye and vision problems.
6. Plan patient- and family-centered nursing interventions to decrease the psychosocial impact caused by living with eye and vision problems.
7. Apply knowledge of anatomy, physiology, and pathophysiology to provide evidence-based care for patients with eye and vision problems affecting sensory perception.
8. Analyze assessment and diagnostic findings to generate solutions and prioritize nursing care for patients with eye and vision problems.
9. Organize care coordination and transition management for patients with eye and vision problems.
10. Use clinical judgment to plan evidence-based nursing care to promote sensory perception and prevent complications in patients with eye and vision problems.
11. Incorporate factors that affect health equity into the plan of care for patients with eye and vision problems.

## Preliminary Reading

Read and review Chapter 39, pp. 975–1000.

## Chapter Review

### Pathophysiology Review

#1. Match the Key Term in Column A with its definition in Column B.

| Column A | Column B |
|---|---|
| ___1. Arcus senilis | A. Lens opacity that distorts image projected onto retina |
| ___2. Cataract | B. Corneal inflammation |
| ___3. Glaucoma | C. Nearsightedness |
| ___4. Hyperopia | D. Farsightedness |
| ___5. Keratitis | E. Involuntary, rapid eyeball twitching |
| ___6. Keratoconus | F. Light sensitivity |
| ___7. Myopia | G. Condition related to increased ocular pressure |
| ___8. Nystagmus | H. Opaque, bluish-white ring in cornea's outer edge |
| ___9. Photophobia | I. Corneal degeneration |

#2. For each statement, specify if the statement is **true (T)** or **false (F).**

_____1. Light is changed into nerve impulses in the brain before images are sent to the eye.

_____2. The sclera is the external layer of the eye.

_____3. Tears are produced in the lacrimal gland.

_____4. When the eye overbends light and images converge in front of the retina, myopia occurs.

_____5. Emmetropia occurs when light rays are bent from outside the eye and passed to the retina.

_____6. The ophthalmic artery brings deoxygenated blood to the eye and the orbit.

_____7. The vitreous body collects tears before they are expelled.

_____8. Visual acuity decreases with age because of changes inside the eye.

_____9. Fatty deposits can accumulate in the eye, causing a yellowish tinge.

____10. With age, a patient's far point increases.

## Activities

### Activity #1
Explain changes that occur to these eye structures as a result of the aging process. Use the table on the following page for reference.

1. Appearance: _____

2. Cornea: _____

3. Ocular muscles: _____

4. Lens: _____

5. Iris and pupil: _____

### Activity #2
Fill in the recommended frequency of eye examinations for the patients described.
1. A 34-year-old patient who has not had visual problems in the past _____
2. A 22-year-old patient who has worn contact lenses since the age of 14 years _____
3. A 36-year-old African American patient who had an eye examination 2 years ago _____
4. A 22-year-old White patient who had an eye examination 1 year previously _____
5. A 63-year-old patient who got new glasses after an eye examination 2 years ago _____
6. A 44-year-old patient with type 1 diabetes _____
7. A 69-year-old patient who wears contact lenses and reading glasses _____
8. A 20-year-old patient who had an eye injury at the age of 18 years _____
9. A 27-year-old patient who has never had an eye examination _____
10. A 71-year-old patient who uses reading glasses to knit _____

| Age | Recommended Frequency |
|---|---|
| 20–39 years, in good health with normal vision | Once in the 20s and once in the 30s unless there is an instance of visual impairment, infection, injury, eye pain, or diabetes<br>*Note: For people in this age category who wear contacts, annual examination is recommended |
| 20–39 years, Black | Every 2–4 years |
| 20–39 years, Caucasian | Every 3–5 years |
| 40–64 years, any race | Every 2–4 years |
| 65 years or older, any race | Every 1–2 years |
| People with special risks (e.g., diabetes, eye surgery or trauma, glaucoma) | As recommended by the eye care provider (may be more frequent) |

## Activity #3

Match the diagnostic procedure in Column A with its description or purpose in Column B.

**Column A**

___1.   Corneal staining
___2.   Electroretinography
___3.   Fluorescein angiography
___4.   Gonioscopy
___5.   Ophthalmoscopy
___6.   Optical coherence tomography
___7.   Slit-lamp examination
___8.   Tonometry

**Column B**

A.   Graphs retina's response to light stimulation
B.   Used to assess for corneal trauma or foreign bodies
C.   Application of pressure to the outside of the eye
D.   Helps to determine position of corneal or lens abnormality
E.   Creates a three-dimensional view of the back of the eye
F.   Shows detailed image of eye circulation
G.   Use of ophthalmoscope to view eye structures
H.   Used to discern between open-angle or closed-angle glaucoma

## Activity #4

List activities or actions the nurse will teach patients with increased intraocular pressure to avoid.

1.   _____

2.   _____

3.   _____

4.   _____

5.   _____

6.   _____

7.   _____

8.   _____

9.   _____

**Activity #5**

In a few words, describe each condition and list several signs/symptoms.

1. Cataract

    a. Description _____

    b. Signs/symptoms _____

2. Open-angle glaucoma

    a. Description _____

    b. Signs/symptoms _____

3. Corneal abrasion

    a. Description _____

    b. Signs/symptoms _____

4. Age-related macular degeneration (dry)

    a. Description _____

    b. Signs/symptoms _____

5. Retinal hole

    a. Description _____

    b. Signs/symptoms _____

6. Myopia

    a. Description _____

    b. Signs/symptoms _____

7. Hyperopia

    a. Description _____

    b. Signs/symptoms _____

8. Presbyopia

    a. Description _____

    b. Signs/symptoms _____

9. Astigmatism

    a. Description _____

    b. Signs/symptoms _____

## Learning Assessments

### NCLEX Examination Challenge #1

Which error in refraction does the nurse anticipate when a client reports difficulty seeing objects at a distance?

A. Myopia
B. Hyperopia
C. Emmetropia
D. Astigmatism

### NCLEX Examination Challenge #2

Which sign does the nurse expect when assessing a client for open-angle glaucoma (OAG)?

A. Flashes of light and floaters
B. Gradual loss of visual fields
C. Sudden severe pain around the eyes
D. Brow pain with nausea and vomiting

### NCLEX Examination Challenge #3

Which teaching will the nurse provide to a client who has undergone keratoplasty? **Select all that apply.**

A. Do not bend at the waist.
B. Avoid jogging for several weeks after surgery.
C. Understand that light sensitivity may persist for several days.
D. Report the presence of purulent discharge immediately to the surgeon.
E. Examine the eye daily for the presence of infection or graft rejection.

**NGN Challenge #1**

The nurse reviews the Nurses Notes for a 49-year-old client who has come to the eye care provider reporting difficulty seeing clearly.

| Nurses Notes | Eye Care Provider's Orders | Diagnostic Testing Results | |
|---|---|---|---|
| **1111:** A 49-year-old client here to see provider for visual disturbances. Reports has been having progressive difficulty seeing items at a close distance. When symptoms began several months ago, the problem occurred "sometimes" when reading; client now reports that the problem is consistent. States that vision in one eye is not better or worse than the other. Says, "I think I need new reading glasses." Denies any other changes in vision, eye pain, recent history of eye infection, or trauma. | | | |

Complete the diagram by selecting from the choices to specify what **one** potential condition the client may be experiencing, **two** actions the nurse would take to address that condition, and **two** parameters the nurse would monitor to assess the client's progress.

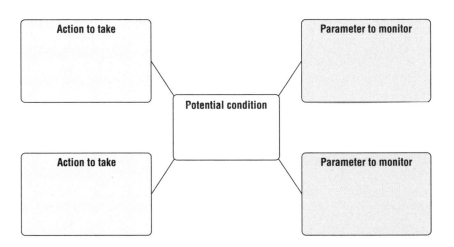

| Actions to Take | Potential Condition | Parameters to Monitor |
|---|---|---|
| Assist with conducting visual acuity testing. | Glaucoma | Intraocular pressure following surgery |
| Prepare for emergency eye surgery. | Presbyopia | Ability to visualize more clearly |
| Obtain fluorescein for corneal staining. | Macular degeneration | Reduction in flashes of light in visual field |
| Assure that gonioscopy has been scheduled. | Retinal detachment | Adherence to filling prescription for corrective lenses |
| Explain age-related changes that occur to the eye. | //////////////////////////////// | Maintenance of using daily eye drops |

## NGN Challenge #2

The nurse reviews the Nurses Notes for a 72-year-old client who has come to the eye care provider reporting difficulty seeing clearly.

| Nurses Notes | Eye Care Provider's Orders | Diagnostic Testing Results | |
|---|---|---|---|

**414:** Client presents to eye care provider reporting progressive difficulty seeing through their left eye. States that since last eye examination (1 year ago), the left eye "doesn't see as good as the right eye." Reports that "blurring" in the left eye occurred initially, and in the last couple of weeks, has noted that it is becoming harder to drive at night, even in areas that are well-lit. Denies any other changes in vision, eye pain, recent history of eye infection, or trauma. Both eyes have clear sclera. No redness, drainage, or signs of infection noted.

Complete the diagram below by selecting from the choices to specify what **one** potential condition the client may be experiencing, **two** actions the nurse would take to address that condition, and **two** parameters the nurse would monitor to assess the client's progress.

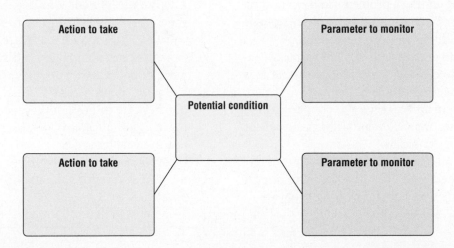

| Actions to Take | Potential Condition | Parameters to Monitor |
|---|---|---|
| Explain that this condition will require antiviral eye drops. | Cataract | Commitment to vascular endothelial growth factor inhibitor therapy |
| Assist with brightness acuity testing. | Myopia | Intraocular pressure |
| Recommend increased intake of lutein. | Astigmatism | Improvement of vision following lens replacement |
| Ask about prolonged use of corticosteroids. | Macular degeneration | Adherence to eye drop therapy following surgery |
| Reassure that this condition occurs periodically and will resolve. | ///////////////////////////////// | Resolution of eye infection |

# 40 CHAPTER

# *Assessment and Concepts of Care for Patients with Ear and Hearing Conditions*

## LEARNING OUTCOMES

1. Use knowledge of anatomy and physiology to perform a focused assessment related to auditory sensory perception.
2. Teach evidence-based health promotion activities to help prevent auditory problems and ear trauma
3. Explain how genetic implications and physiologic aging affect auditory sensory perception.
4. Plan collaborative care with the interprofessional team to promote sensory perception in patients with ear and hearing problems.
5. Teach the patient and caregiver(s) about common drugs and other management strategies used for ear and hearing problems.
6. Plan patient- and family-centered nursing interventions to decrease the psychosocial impact caused by living with ear and hearing problems.

7. Apply knowledge of anatomy, physiology, and pathophysiology to provide evidence-based care for patients with ear and hearing problems affecting sensory perception.
8. Analyze assessment and diagnostic findings to generate solutions and prioritize nursing care for patients with ear and hearing problems.
9. Organize care coordination and transition management for patients with ear and hearing problems.
10. Use clinical judgment to plan evidence-based nursing care to promote sensory perception and prevent complications in patients with ear and hearing problems.
11. Incorporate factors that affect health equity into the plan of care for patients with ear and hearing problems.

## Preliminary Reading

Read and review Chapter 40, pp. 1001–1020.

## Chapter Review
### Pathophysiology Review

#1. Match the Key Term in Column A with its definition in Column B.

**Column A**

_____1. Cerumen
_____2. Frequency
_____3. Grommet
_____4. Intensity
_____5. Myringoplasty
_____6. Myringotomy
_____7. Presbycusis
_____8. Swimmer's ear
_____9. Tinnitus
____10. Vertigo

**Column B**

A. Polyethylene tube placed in tympanic membrane
B. Surgical reconstruction of the eardrum
C. External otitis
D. Quality of sound
E. Continuous ringing or noise perception in the ear
F. Wax that protects and lubricates ear canal
G. Sense of whirling or turning
H. Surgical creation of hole in the eardrum
I. Highness or lowness of tones
J. Sensorineural hearing loss

#2. For each statement, specify if the statement is **true (T)** or **false (F)**.

_____1. Ménière disease is characterized by vertigo, tinnitus, and hearing loss.
_____2. Tinnitus always occurs in both ears.
_____3. The most common cause of an impacted ear canal is cerumen.
_____4. Implanted hearing devices can cause temporary changes in taste sensation.
_____5. People with 20 to 40 dB of hearing loss may have mild difficulty hearing in restaurants.
_____6. Hearing aids should be gently cleaned with alcohol swabs.
_____7. Nurses must teach people to avoid putting anything smaller than their finger in their ears.
_____8. Hearing should improve within a week of stapedectomy.
_____9. Patients with mastoiditis may have a fever and malaise in addition to ear pain.
____10. A vestibular schwannoma is a benign tumor of cranial nerve V.

## Activities
### Activity #1
List changes that occur to these ear structures and findings as a result of the aging process.

1. Pinna: _____

2. Ear canal hair: _____

3. Cerumen: _____

4. Tympanic membrane: _____

5. Hearing acuity: _____

6. Ability to hear high-frequency sounds: _____

**Activity #2**

Identify several nursing adaptations and actions that can be undertaken to address each ear or hearing change that can occur in older adults.

| Ear or Hearing Change | Nursing Adaptations and Actions |
|---|---|
| Pinna | |
| Ear canal hair | |
| Cerumen presence | |
| Tympanic membrane | |
| Hearing acuity | |
| Ability to hear high-frequency sounds | |

**Activity #3**

Place the sounds in order of safe exposure time based on decibel intensity. Sounds should be ranked from safest to least safe.

| Letter for Ranking | Sound |
|---|---|
| A | Motorcycle |
| B | Sirens |
| C | City traffic (from inside a car) |
| D | Nightclub |
| E | Average business office |
| F | Conversational speech |

**Activity #4**

Describe how the nurse will explain the difference between conductive hearing loss and sensorineural hearing loss to a patient. Include pertinent causes and assessment findings that may be present for each disorder.

_____

_____

_____

_____

_____

_____

_____

_____

**Activity #5**
In a few words, explain how the nurse will describe each diagnostic study to a patient.

1. Audiometry

_____

_____

2. Brainstem auditory-evoked response (BAER)

_____

_____

3. Auditory-evoked potential (AEP)

_____

_____

4. Computerized dynamic posturography (CDP)

_____

_____

5. Electronystagmography (ENG)

_____

_____

6. Tympanometry

_____

_____

## Learning Assessments

### NCLEX Examination Challenge #1

Which question will the nurse ask a client to determine if there may be problems with auditory sensory perception? **Select all that apply.**

A. "Have you had any ear trauma or surgery?"
B. "Have you noticed any change in your hearing?
C. "Have you had problems with excessive ear wax?"
D. "Have you had recent pain or itching in your ears?"
E. "Have you been exposed to loud noises in your work?"

### NCLEX Examination Challenge #2

Which action will the nurse take to enhance communication with a client who is hearing-impaired? **Select all that apply.**

A. Sit in adequate light.
B. Use short, simple language.
C. Face the client while speaking.
D. Primarily address the client's caregiver.
E. Talk in a quiet room with minimal distractions.

### NCLEX Examination Challenge #3

The nurse has completed teaching about an acoustic neuroma. Which client response indicates to the nurse that teaching has been understood?

A. "I'm not sure if I want to have chemotherapy and radiation."
B. "This condition is not malignant, so I do not need to worry about it."
C. "The tumor is benign but possible neurological damage sounds scary."
D. "Hearing loss in one ear is not too bad since that is the only thing affected."

**NGN Challenge #1**

The nurse has documented the visit of a 64-year-old client who came in to see the primary health care provider for a routine wellness examination and medication follow-up.

| Nurses Notes | Health Care Provider's Orders | Diagnostic Testing Results | |
|---|---|---|---|

**1503:** Client here with spouse to see provider for routine visit and medication follow-up. Medical history includes hypertension, mild depression, and type 2 diabetes. Medications include amlodipine 5 mg twice daily, lisinopril/hydrochlorothiazide 10 mg/12.5 mg once daily, duloxetine 60 mg daily, and metformin 500 mg twice daily. Reports no health care changes since last appointment 6 months ago. Spouse states, "That isn't true; he can't hear anything anymore." Client says, "Sometimes I have to turn the TV up a little but that's because I'm getting older." Denies any perceived difference in hearing, ear pain or drainage, recent history of ear infection, or trauma. Denies vertigo, nausea, tinnitus. External ears do not show signs of infection or draining. Some cerumen visualized.

Complete the diagram by selecting from the choices to specify what **one** potential condition the client may be experiencing, **two** actions the nurse would take to address that condition, and **two** parameters the nurse would monitor to assess the client's progress.

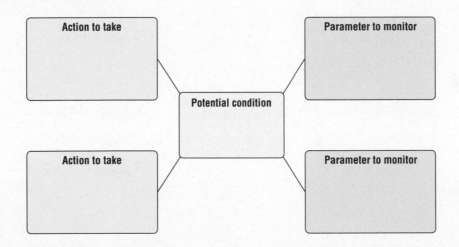

| Actions to Take | Potential Condition | Parameters to Monitor |
|---|---|---|
| Assist with ordering hearing aids. | Tinnitus | Vertigo |
| Refer client to an audiologist. | Ménière disease | Hearing aid fit |
| Prepare for cerumen removal. | Mastoiditis | Presence of cerumen |
| Remind spouse to drive the client home. | Presbycusis | Test results from audiometry testing |
| Explain that computerized dynamic posturography (CDP) test needs to be done. | ///////////////////////////////// | Adherence to use of daily antibiotic ear drops |

**NGN Challenge #2**

The nurse has documented information about a 34-year-old client who is seeing the primary health care provider because of ringing in the ears.

| Nurses Notes | Health Care Provider's Orders | Diagnostic Testing Results |
| --- | --- | --- |

**1618:** Client presents to health care provider reporting over a month of "ringing in the ears." She states it happens without warning, sometimes when she is sitting down and other times when she is standing or walking. It has never occurred when she is driving. There does not seem to be a pattern of the occurrences that she can identify other than the frequency is increasing. When an episode occurs, she says she lies down and closes her eyes and feels like she is spinning. Episodes last between 30 minutes and several hours. Reports nausea during episodes; denies vomiting. States that she feels like she doesn't hear as well since episodes began. Denies any other health changes. Medical history is unremarkable other than two cesarean section deliveries for term infants, 7 and 9 years ago. Alert and oriented × 3. Cranial nerves intact. Lungs clear; heart regular rate and rhythm.

Complete the diagram by selecting from the choices to specify what **one** potential condition the client may be experiencing, **two** actions the nurse would take to address that condition, and **two** parameters the nurse would monitor to assess the client's progress.

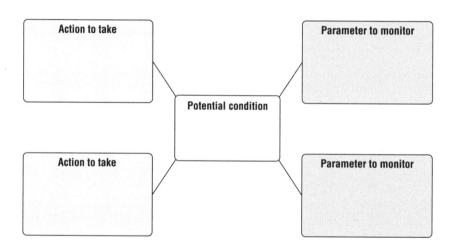

| Actions to Take | Potential Condition | Parameters to Monitor |
| --- | --- | --- |
| Explain that this condition is related to a benign tumor of the vestibulocochlear nerve. | Cerumen accumulation | Appropriate use of antibiotic therapy |
| Teach about intratympanic gentamicin. | Ménière disease | Tumarkin otolithic crisis |
| Plan for labyrinthectomy. | Conductive hearing loss | Recovery following surgical removal of tumor |
| Teach to record a diary of symptoms and episodes. | Nystagmus | Recurrence of inner ear infection |
| Explain how to take diuretic prescription. | ///////////////////////////////// | Adherence to hydrochlorothiazide |

# 41
CHAPTER

# Assessment of the Musculoskeletal System

## LEARNING OUTCOMES

1. Use knowledge of anatomy and physiology to perform a focused assessment of the musculoskeletal system.
2. Teach evidence-based health promotion activities to help prevent musculoskeletal health problems or trauma.
3. Demonstrate clinical judgment to interpret assessment findings in a patient with a musculoskeletal health problems.
4. Identify factors that affect health equity for patients with musculoskeletal health problems.
5. Explain how genetic implications and physiologic aging of the musculoskeletal system affect mobility.
6. Interpret assessment findings for patients with a suspected or actual musculoskeletal problem.
7. Plan evidence-based care and support for patients undergoing diagnostic testing of the musculoskeletal system.

## Preliminary Reading

Read and review Chapter 41, pp. 1021–1030.

## Chapter Review

### Anatomy & Physiology Review

#1. Label the parts of the joint, bone, and supporting structures using the Anatomy Labels provided after the figure.

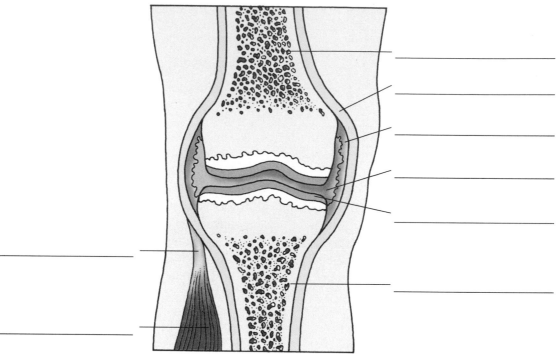

| Anatomy Labels |
|---|
| Articular cartilage |
| Cortical bone |
| Joint |
| Joint capsule |
| Muscle |
| Spongy bone |
| Synovium |
| Tendon |

#2. Complete the sentences by filling in the blanks with terms listed. Not all terms will be used.
1. The bone-forming cells are called the _____.
2. The primary minerals within the bones of the body are _____ and _____.
3. A _____ is a space in which two or more bones come together.
4. _____ joints are freely movable and lubricated with a small amount of fluid.
5. A decrease in the body's Vitamin D level can result in _____ in the adult.
6. Most muscles are surrounded by dense fibrous tissue, or _____, which contains the muscle's blood, lymph, and nerve supply.
7. _____ results when muscles are not regularly exercised.

## Choices for Sentence Completion

| |
|---|
| Calcium |
| Cartilage |
| Fascia |
| Joint |
| Muscle atrophy |
| Muscle spasticity |
| Osteoblasts |
| Osteoclasts |
| Osteomalacia |
| Osteoporosis |
| Phosphorus |
| Synarthrodial |
| Synovial/diarthrodial |
| Vitamin D |

## Activities

### Activity #1
List at least four common physiologic musculoskeletal system changes associated with aging.

1. _____

2. _____

3. _____

4. _____

### Activity #2
Match the Key Term in Column A with the definition in Column B.

**Column A**

____1. Effusion
____2. Kyphosis
____3. Lordosis
____4. Myopathy
____5. Neuropathy
____6. Osteopenia
____7. Physical disability
____8. Scoliosis

**Column B**

A. Problem in nerve tissue often resulting in weakness and decreased sensation
B. Abnormal lateral curvature of the spine
C. Limitation in mobility or activity that can affect one or more ADLs
D. Fluid accumulation, such as in a joint
E. Decreased bone density (bone loss) that occurs as one ages
F. Outward curvature of the thoracic spine causing a "humped back"
G. Problem in muscle tissue often resulting in weakness
H. Inward abnormal curvature of the lumbar spine

## Activity #3
Identify three activities that help promote bone health.

1. _____

2. _____

3. _____

## Activity #4
A client had a repair of an anterior cruciate ligament in the right knee via arthroscopic surgery. Identify three nursing actions that would be included in the client's immediate postoperative care, including discharge teaching.

1. _____

2. _____

3. _____

## Learning Assessments

### NCLEX Examination Challenge #1
The nurse is assessing a client who reports severe pain, warmth, and swelling in the right wrist. What nursing action would be the **priority**?
A. Assess the left wrist.
B. Observe mobility of the right wrist.
C. Palpate the right wrist.
D. Document the client's report.

### NCLEX Examination Challenge #2
The nurse is caring for a young client who has a probable diagnosis of muscular dystrophy. What laboratory findings would the nurse expect for this client? **Select all that apply.**
A. Decreased serum calcium
B. Increased creatine kinase (CK-MM)
C. Increased aldolase
D. Decreased alkaline phosphatase
E. Increased lactate dehydrogenase

### NCLEX Examination Challenge #3
The nurse assesses a client following arthroscopic surgery of the left shoulder. Which client finding would the nurse **immediately** report to the surgeon?
A. Left radial pulse 2+
B. Pain in left shoulder
C. Inability to move left shoulder
D. Numbness and tingling in left hand

# 42

**CHAPTER**

# Concepts of Care for Patients with Musculoskeletal Conditions

## LEARNING OUTCOMES

1. Plan collaborative care with the interprofessional team to promote mobility in patients with osteoporosis.
2. Teach adults how to decrease the risk for osteoporosis.
3. Teach the patient and caregiver(s) about common drugs and other management strategies used for osteoporosis.
4. Plan patient- and family-centered nursing interventions to decrease the psychosocial impact caused by living with bone cancer.
5. Apply knowledge of anatomy, physiology, and pathophysiology to provide evidence-based care

for patients with osteoporosis affecting cellular regulation.
6. Analyze assessment and diagnostic findings to generate solutions and prioritize nursing care for patients with bone infection (osteomyelitis).
7. Organize care coordination and transition management for patients with bone cancer.
8. Use clinical judgment to plan evidence-based nursing care to promote mobility and prevent complications in patients with osteoporosis.
9. Incorporate factors that affect health equity into the plan of care for patients with osteoporosis.

## Preliminary Reading

Read and review Chapter 42, pp. 1031–1048.

## Chapter Review

### Pathophysiology Review

#1. Match the Key Term in Column A with its definition in Column B.

**Column A**

_____1. Bone mineral density
_____2. Dupuytren's contracture
_____3. Fragility fracture
_____4. Ganglion
_____5. Hallux valgus deformity
_____6. Osteomyelitis
_____7. Osteonecrosis
_____8. Osteoporosis
_____9. Paget's disease
____10. Plantar fasciitis

**Column B**

A. Infection in bone caused by pathogens
B. Fracture caused by osteoporosis
C. Chronic, slowly progressive skeletal metabolic bone disorder that causes rapid bone destruction and reformation
D. Condition in which the great toe drifts laterally
E. Amount of mineral in bone
F. Inflammation of the tissue in the foot arch
G. Chronic bone loss that causes decreased bone density, which leads to fractures
H. Flexion contracture of the fourth and fifth fingers
I. Bone tissue death from lack of blood flow
J. Round benign cyst usually on the wrist or foot

#2. For each statement, specify if the statement is **true (T)** or **false (F).**

_____1. If bone infection is misdiagnosed or inadequately treated, chronic osteomyelitis may develop.

_____2. Osteomyelitis may be an acute or chronic client health problem.

_____3. *Osteosarcoma,* or osteogenic sarcoma, is the most common type of benign bone tumor.

_____4. Fragility fractures can occur in clients who have metastatic bone cancer.

_____5. The most common cause of osteomyelitis in older adults occurs in those who have slow-healing foot ulcers.

_____6. Men aged 50 years and older develop osteoporosis as they age because their testosterone levels decrease.

_____7. Calcium loss from bone occurs at a rapid rate when phosphorus intake is high, such as when consuming large amounts of carbonated beverages over time.

_____8. Osteoporosis occurs most often in obese White women.

## Activities

### Activity #1

Identify five risk factors for developing primary osteoporosis.

1. _____

2. _____

3. _____

4. _____

5. _____

### Activity #2

The nurse is preparing to provide health teaching for a client starting on alendronate for osteopenia. List three important teaching points that would be included.

1. _____

2. _____

3. _____

### Activity #3

For each statement, specify if the statement is **true (T)** or **false (F).**

_____1. The *Healthy People 2030* initiative recognizes the need for national attention to the prevention of osteoporosis and fragility fractures.

_____2. Minority groups typically receive less screening and treatment for bone loss, including after experiencing a fracture, when compared with White people.

_____3. The most commonly used screening and diagnostic radiographic test for measuring bone mineral density (BMD) is dual x-ray absorptiometry (DXA).

_____4. Nurses need to teach patients who have osteopenia or osteoporosis to have follow-up DXA scans every 5 years.

_____5. The patient who develops chronic osteomyelitis is placed on antibiotic therapy for more than 3 months.

_____6. Patients who have metastatic bone cancer are usually older adults who have severe, unrelenting pain.

_____7. Dupuytren's contracture is a common disorder of the hand that is most often treated by surgery.

_____8. The priority postoperative nursing action for the client who has a traditional bunionectomy is neurovascular assessment.

## Activity #4

Match the drug in Column A with the health teaching in Column B.

| Column A | | Column B |
|---|---|---|
| ___1. | Calcium | A. Take this drug on an empty stomach and follow by a full glass of water. |
| ___2. | Vitamin D$_3$ | B. Report signs and symptoms of infection. |
| ___3. | Risedronate | C. Take one-third of the daily dose at bedtime. |
| ___4. | Raloxifene | D. Monitor for signs and symptoms of venous thromboembolism. |
| ___5. | Denosumab | E. Check with your health care provider about whether this OTC drug is needed. |

## Learning Assessments

### NCLEX Examination Challenge #1

The nurse is caring for an older female client who has a newly confirmed T-score below −1.5 and a history of two fractures. What interventions would the nurse plan for the client at this time? **Select all that apply.**

A. Inform the client that the primary health care provider will likely prescribe drug therapy to prevent additional bone loss.

B. Teach the client to avoid having more than two alcoholic drinks per day.

C. Teach the client to consume foods high in calcium and/or take a calcium supplement.

D. Remove environmental hazards that could cause falls in the home.

E. Assess additional risk factors that the client may have that contributed to excessive bone loss.

F. Instruct the client to exercise every week, especially by swimming and participating in water aerobics.

### NCLEX Examination Challenge #2

The nurse is caring for a middle-aged adult who has advanced metastatic bone cancer from breast cancer and has intractable pain and weakness. The client's home health nurse would take which of the following **priority** actions?

A. Refer the client and family to the local hospice services for EOL care.

B. Check into how to offer the client medical aid for passive euthanasia.

C. Administer continuous IV opioids per agency protocol.

D. Refer the client to the family's spiritual leader or clergy as requested.

## NGN Challenge #1

The nurse is caring for a 70-year-old client who was admitted last evening with a left draining diabetic foot ulcer that has not healed for more than 6 months. The nurse reviews the vital sign flow sheet data since admission.

### Vital Sign Flow Sheet

| | 12 Hours After Admission (0915) | 6 Hours After Admission (0315) | Admission (2115) |
|---|---|---|---|
| T | 101.8°F (38.8°C) | 100.2°F (37.9°C) | 99.4°F (37.4°C) |
| HR | 86 beats/min | 84 beats/min | 78 beats/min |
| RR | 20 breaths/min | 20 breaths/min | 18 breaths/min |
| BP | 130/86 mm Hg | 122/58 mm Hg | 124/72 mm Hg |
| $SpO_2$ | 94% on RA | 95% on RA | 95% on RA |
| FSBG | 137 mg/dL (7.60 mmol/L) (on insulin sliding scale) | 213 mg/dL (11.82 mmol/L) | 168 mg/dL (9.32 mmol/L) |
| Pain/ neurovascular assessment | 9/10 continuous and throbbing localized (L) ankle pain; worse with movement; nonpalpable (L) pedal pulse; cap refill >3 seconds | 5/10 (after analgesic medication); remains continuous but not as throbbing; nonpalpable (L) pedal pulse; cap refill >3 seconds | 8/10 continuous and worse pain with movement of (L) ankle; 1+ (L) pedal pulse; cap refill >3 seconds |

Complete the following sentence by filling in the blanks using the lists of options listed.

The nurse analyzes the data and determines that the client most is most likely experiencing _____1 [Select]_____ as evidenced by ____2 [Select]_____ and _____3 [Select]_____.

| Options for 1 | Options for 2 | Options for 3 |
|---|---|---|
| Peripheral vascular disease | Hypertension | Fever |
| Osteomyelitis | Draining wound with cellulitis | Tachycardia |
| Hyperosmolar hyperglycemic syndrome | Nonpalpable pedal pulse | Hyperglycemia |

## NGN Challenge #2

The nurse is caring for a 70-year-old client who was admitted last evening with new-onset cellulitis resulting from a left draining diabetic foot ulcer that has not healed for more than 6 months. The nurse reviews the vital sign flow sheet data since admission.

### Vital Sign Flow Sheet

|  | **12 Hours After Admission (0915)** | **6 Hours After Admission (0315)** | **Admission (2115)** |
|---|---|---|---|
| T | 101.8°F (38.8°C) | 100.2°F (37.9°C) | 99.4°F (37.4°C) |
| HR | 86 beats/min | 84 beats/min | 78 beats/min |
| RR | 20 breaths/min | 20 breaths/min | 18 breaths/min |
| BP | 130/70 mm Hg | 122/58 mm Hg | 124/72 mm Hg |
| SpO$_2$ | 94% on RA | 95% on RA | 95% on RA |
| FSBG | 137 mg/dL (7.60 mmol/L) (on insulin sliding scale) | 213 mg/dL (11.82 mmol/L) | 168 mg/dL (9.32 mmol/L) |
| Pain/ neurovascular assessment | 9/10 continuous and throbbing localized (L) ankle pain; worse with movement; nonpalpable (L) pedal pulse; cap refill >3 seconds | 5/10 (after analgesic medication); remains continuous but not as throbbing; nonpalpable (L) pedal pulse; cap refill >3 seconds | 8/10 continuous and worse pain with movement of (L) ankle; 1+ (L) pedal pulse; cap refill >3 seconds |

Based on the client's condition, the nurse begins planning client care. Which of the following nursing actions would be appropriate for this client? **Select all that apply.**

A.   Monitor vital signs every 4 hours.

B.   Give analgesic medication around the clock.

C.   Use sterile technique when changing wound dressing.

D.   Administer IV antibiotic therapy on time for each dose.

E.   Check FSBG levels before every meal and at bedtime.

F.   Initiate supplemental oxygen therapy via nasal cannula.

G.   Elevate ankle on at least two pillows.

# 43 CHAPTER

# *Concepts of Care for Patients with Arthritis and Total Joint Arthroplasty*

## LEARNING OUTCOMES

1. Plan collaborative care with the interprofessional team to promote mobility in patients with arthritis.
2. Teach adults how to decrease the risk for osteoarthritis.
3. Teach the patient and caregiver(s) about common drugs and other management strategies used for rheumatoid arthritis affecting immunity.
4. Plan patient- and family-centered nursing interventions to decrease the psychosocial impact caused by living with arthritis.
5. Apply knowledge of anatomy, physiology, and pathophysiology to provide evidence-based care for patients with rheumatoid arthritis.

6. Analyze assessment and diagnostic findings to generate solutions and prioritize nursing care for patients who have rheumatoid arthritis.
7. Organize care coordination and transition management for patients having total joint arthroplasty.
8. Use clinical judgment to plan evidence-based nursing care to promote mobility and decrease inflammation in patients with rheumatoid arthritis.
9. Incorporate factors that affect health equity into the plan of care for patients with arthritis.

## Preliminary Reading

Read and review Chapter 43, pp. 1049–1078.

## Chapter Review

### Pathophysiology Review

#1. Match the Key Term in Column A with its definition in Column B.

| Column A | Column B |
|---|---|
| ____1. Arthritis | A. Partial joint dislocation |
| ____2. Crepitus | B. Bone spurs caused by irregular bony overgrowth |
| ____3. Exacerbation | C. Joint synovium inflammation |
| ____4. Osteoarthritis | D. Deterioration and loss of joint cartilage |
| ____5. Osteophytes | E. A grating sound caused by loosened joint bone and cartilage |
| ____6. Paresthesia | F. Inflammation of blood vessel walls |
| ____7. Subluxation | G. Diarthrodial joint inflammation |
| ____8. Synovitis | H. Flare-up of disease |
| ____9. Vasculitis | I. Burning and tingling sensations, especially in the extremities |

#2. For each statement, specify if the statement is **true (T)** or **false (F).**

_____1. Osteoarthritis occurs in people who are thin much more commonly than in those who are not thin.

_____2. Osteoarthritis only affects older adults older than aged 65 years.

_____3. In patients who have rheumatoid arthritis, inflammatory responses similar to those occurring in synovial tissue may occur in any organ or body system in which connective tissue is prevalent.

_____4. Gout is the body's inflammatory response to a large amount of uric acid in the blood and other body fluids.

_____5. Patients can experience major organ failure or even death as a result of having rheumatoid arthritis.

## Activities

### Activity #1
Identify three lifestyle habits that can promote joint health and help prevent the development of osteoarthritis.

1. _____

2. _____

3. _____

### Activity #2
List four preoperative instructions the nurse would provide to help prevent infection in the client who has a total hip or knee arthroplasty.

1. _____

2. _____

3. _____

4. _____

### Activity #3
For each statement, specify if the statement is **true (T)** or **false (F).**

_____1. The *Healthy People 2030* initiative recognizes the need for national attention to the reduction and better management of arthritis.

_____2. Although OA is not typically a bilateral, symmetric disease, large bony nodes appear on joints of both hands, especially in women.

_____3. The most common surgical procedure for OA is total joint arthroplasty, also known as total joint replacement (TJR).

_____4. For patients at risk for delirium, Enhanced Recovery After Surgery (ERAS) programs, are common in total joint replacement centers to improve patient outcomes.

_____5. Patient positioning after total hip arthroplasty varies depending on the surgeon who performs the procedure.

_____6. Persistent pain from osteoarthritis is reported to be more severe and disabling among older Blacks when compared with Whites, making them likely to experience decreased mobility, function, and quality of life.

_____7. To help prevent a gouty arthritic attack or flare-up, patients need to avoid red meat, shellfish, and alcohol, especially beer.

_____8.  Chronic arthritis is a major cause of physical disability in adult patients, especially among older adults.

_____9.  Formal preoperative teaching using an interprofessional approach results in optimal postoperative patient outcomes.

_____10.  The most potentially life-threatening postoperative complication of a total hip arthroplasty is wound infection.

## Activity #4

Match the drug in Column A with the health teaching the nurse would provide in Column B.

| Column A | Column B |
|---|---|
| _____1.  Methotrexate | A.  Take this antigout drug with food to prevent GI distress. |
| _____2.  Hydroxychloroquine | B.  Be sure to have follow-up liver tests because this drug can cause hepatic dysfunction. |
| _____3.  Etanercept | C.  Have an eye examination before starting the drug and every 6 months while on it. |
| _____4.  Anakinra | |
| _____5.  Tofacitinib | D.  When taking this oral drug, avoid crowds and people with infection. |
| _____6.  Ibuprofen | E.  Be aware that this drug can cause acute kidney injury over time. |
| _____7.  Colchicine | F.  This drug is administered under medical supervision every 2 weeks. |
| _____8.  Febuxostat | G.  This drug used for chronic gout increases the risk of cardiovascular events. |
| _____9.  Pegloticase | |
| | H.  Report injection site reactions to the primary health care provider. |
| | I.  This drug increases the risk of cardiac events, cancer, and clotting issues. |

## Activity #5

List three ways that patients who have arthritis can protect their joints.

1.  _____

2.  _____

3.  _____

## Activity #6

For each potential complication that could occur after a total knee arthroplasty for an older patient, identify at least two nursing/collaborative actions that would be appropriate.

| Potential Complication | Nursing/Collaborative Actions |
|---|---|
| Venous thromboembolism | 1.<br>2. |
| Skin breakdown | 1.<br>2. |
| Anemia | 1.<br>2. |
| Decreased mobility | 1.<br>2. |

## Activity #7

Arthritis is one of the most common physical disabilities that individuals experience. When caring for a hospitalized patient who has arthritis, identify three nursing interventions that address the patient's disability.

1. _____

2. _____

3. _____

## Learning Assessments

### NCLEX Examination Challenge #1

The nurse assesses an older client who has a long history of osteoarthritis, especially in the hands. Which of the following assessments most likely describes the type of arthritis this client has?
A. Reddened, inflamed finger joints
B. Swollen, spongy metacarpal joints
C. Subcutaneous nodules on metacarpal joints
D. Symmetrical bony nodules on finger joints

### NCLEX Examination Challenge #2

The nurse is planning postoperative care for a client returning from the PACU following a traditional left total hip arthroplasty using an anterior surgical approach. In which position would the nurse place the client?
A. Head of bed at least 60 degrees with legs abducted
B. Head of bed at 15 degrees to 30 degrees with legs in neutral position
C. Head of bed flat with client supine and legs adducted
D. Head of bed in any position as long as legs are abducted

### NCLEX Examination Challenge #3

The nurse is assessing a client who has a severely painful, red, and swollen metatarsal joint of the right great toe for the first time. What drug would the nurse anticipate would need to be administered for this client?
A. Methotrexate
B. Allopurinol
C. Indomethacin
D. Acetaminophen

**NGN Challenge**

*Item #1*

The nurse reviews the 1405 and 1650 rehabilitation unit Nurses Notes entries for a 79-year-old client who had a right posterolateral total hip arthroplasty 5 days ago for osteoarthritis.

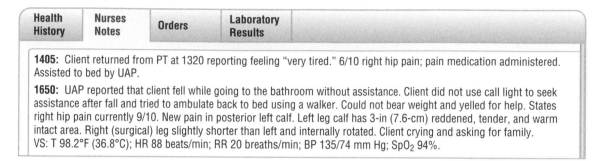

| Health History | Nurses Notes | Orders | Laboratory Results | |
|---|---|---|---|---|

**1405:** Client returned from PT at 1320 reporting feeling "very tired." 6/10 right hip pain; pain medication administered. Assisted to bed by UAP.

**1650:** UAP reported that client fell while going to the bathroom without assistance. Client did not use call light to seek assistance after fall and tried to ambulate back to bed using a walker. Could not bear weight and yelled for help. States right hip pain currently 9/10. New pain in posterior left calf. Left leg calf has 3-in (7.6-cm) reddened, tender, and warm intact area. Right (surgical) leg slightly shorter than left and internally rotated. Client crying and asking for family. VS: T 98.2°F (36.8°C); HR 88 beats/min; RR 20 breaths/min; BP 135/74 mm Hg; SpO$_2$ 94%.

Highlight the client findings in the Nurses Notes that would require **immediate** follow-up by the nurse.

*Item #2*

The nurse reviews the 1405 and 1650 rehabilitation unit Nurses Notes entries for a 79-year-old client who had a right posterolateral total hip arthroplasty 5 days ago for osteoarthritis.

| Health History | Nurses Notes | Orders | Laboratory Results |
|---|---|---|---|

**1405:** Client returned from PT at 1320 reporting feeling "very tired." 6/10 right hip pain; pain medication administered. Assisted to bed by UAP.

**1650:** UAP reported that client fell while going to the bathroom without assistance. Client did not use call light to seek assistance after fall and tried to ambulate back to bed using a walker. Could not bear weight and yelled for help. States right hip pain currently 9/10. New pain in posterior left calf. Left leg calf has 3-in (7.6-cm) reddened, tender, and warm intact area. Right (surgical) leg slightly shorter than left and internally rotated. Alert but oriented ×1 to person. Crying and asking for family. VS: T 98.2°F (36.8°C); HR 88 beats/min; RR 20 breaths/min; BP 135/74 mm Hg; SpO$_2$ 94%.

The nurse analyzes the relevant assessment findings to determine the client's current condition. Complete the sentence to fill in the blanks using the list of word choices listed below.

Based on the assessment findings, the nurse determines that the client most likely has _____ and _____.

| Word Choices |
|---|
| Hypertension |
| Dementia |
| Right hip dislocation |
| Left calf pressure injury |
| Left deep vein thrombosis |

*Item #3*

The nurse reviews the 1405 and 1650 rehabilitation unit Nurses Notes entries for a 79-year-old client who had a right posterolateral total hip arthroplasty 5 days ago for osteoarthritis.

| Health History | Nurses Notes | Orders | Laboratory Results | |
|---|---|---|---|---|

**1405:** Client returned from PT at 1320 reporting feeling "very tired." 6/10 right hip pain; pain medication administered. Assisted to bed by UAP.

**1650:** UAP reported that client fell while going to the bathroom without assistance. Client did not use call light to seek assistance after fall and tried to ambulate back to bed using a walker. Could not bear weight and yelled for help. States right hip pain currently 9/10. New pain in posterior left calf. Left leg calf has 3-in (7.6-cm) reddened, tender, and warm intact area. Right (surgical) leg slightly shorter than left and internally rotated. Alert but oriented ×1 to person. Crying and asking for family. VS: T 98.2°F (36.8°C); HR 88 beats/min; RR 20 breaths/min; BP 135/74 mm Hg; SpO$_2$ 94%.

Complete the sentence to fill in the blanks using the lists of options listed below.

Based on the client's condition, the nurse determines that the ***priority*** for care is most likely managing the client's _____**1 [Select]**_____ because this condition can lead to _____**2 [Select]**_____.

| Options for 1 | Options for 2 |
|---|---|
| Hip dislocation | Pulmonary embolism |
| Hypertension | Hypoperfusion |
| Deep vein thrombosis | Stroke |

*Item #4*

The 79-year-old client was transferred to the local hospital as a direct admission for acute care. The nurse in the acute care unit reviews the most recent notes.

| Health History | Nurses Notes | Orders | Laboratory Results | |
|---|---|---|---|---|

***Rehabilitation Unit***

**1405:** Client returned from PT at 1320 reporting feeling "very tired." 6/10 right hip pain; pain medication administered. Assisted to bed by UAP.

**1650:** UAP reported that client fell while going to the bathroom without assistance. Client did not use call light to seek assistance after fall and tried to ambulate back to bed using a walker. Could not bear weight and yelled for help. States right hip pain currently 9/10. New pain in posterior left calf. Left leg calf has 3-in (7.6-cm) reddened, tender, and warm intact area. Right (surgical) leg slightly shorter than left and internally rotated. Alert but oriented × 1 to person. Crying and asking for family. VS: T 98.2°F (36.8°C); HR 88 beats/min; RR 20 breaths/min; BP 135/74 mm Hg; SpO$_2$ 94%.

***Acute Orthopedic Unit***

**1812:** Admitted to the unit with confirmed right hip prosthesis dislocation and probable left calf deep vein thrombosis; accompanied by family. Current medications include:
- Amlodipine 10 mg orally once a day for hypertension
- Apixaban 5 mg orally once a day to prevent VTE
- Gabapentin 100 mg every 6 hours for surgical painv
- Ibuprofen 400 mg every 4 hours for surgical pain
- MVI 1 tablet orally every morning
- DOSS 200 mg orally every night

Surgeon in to examine client. Client NPO awaiting new orders.

The nurse anticipates the surgeon's orders based on the client's current condition. Which of the following orders would the nurse anticipate to be included? **Select all that apply.**
- Establish peripheral IV access.
- Prepare for administration of moderate sedation.
- Administer supplemental oxygen 2 L/min via nasal cannula.
- Initiate continuous pulse oximetry.
- Maintain continuous cardiac monitoring via telemetry.
- Give IV antibiotic therapy to begin after wound culture obtained.
- Begin drug therapy with a direct oral anticoagulant (DOAC) per protocol.

### Item #5

A 79-year-old client is transported from the acute orthopedic unit to the ED for reduction of right hip prosthesis dislocation under moderate sedation with IV propofol and ketamine. During the procedure, the nurse noted that the client's $SpO_2$ decreased from 94% to 88%, the client's RR decreased to 10 breaths/min, and the end-tidal carbon dioxide level dropped to 26 mm Hg. Select **two** interventions that the nurse would implement based on these client findings.
- Administer supplemental oxygen at 2 L/min via nasal cannula.
- Rub the client's sternum several times until RR increases.
- Speak in a loud voice to remind the client to keep breathing.
- Place the client in a flat supine position.
- Stop the procedure and reschedule for another day.

### Item #6

A 79-year-old client who had a right total hip arthroplasty 2 weeks ago was admitted from the rehabilitation unit to the acute orthopedic unit with a right hip dislocation. The dislocation was reduced under moderate sedation and a splint was applied. The client was also treated for a left deep vein thrombosis (DVT) with IV heparin and transitioned to oral anticoagulation. The nurse preparing to discharge the client later today reviews the client's medical record to determine the effectiveness of collaborative management. Indicate which current assessment findings indicate that the client is **Improving** or **Not Improving/Declining.**

| Previous Client Findings | Current Client Findings (Today) | Improving | Not Improving/ Declining |
|---|---|---|---|
| 9/10 right hip pain | 4/10 right hip pain | | |
| Left swollen calf that is reddened, warm, and tender | Slight redness and tenderness; no swelling | | |
| Alert and oriented ×1 | Alert and oriented ×1 | | |
| Able to ambulate with walker until fall | Not able to ambulate with walker | | |
| BP 135/74 | BP 122/70 | | |
| $SpO_2$ 94% on RA | $SpO_2$ 96% on RA | | |

# Concepts of Care for Patients with Musculoskeletal Trauma

## LEARNING OUTCOMES

1. Plan collaborative care with the interprofessional team to promote mobility, perfusion, and tissue integrity in patients with lower extremity amputations.
2. Teach adults how to decrease the risk for musculoskeletal trauma.
3. Teach the patient and caregiver(s) about common drugs and other management strategies used for amputations affecting sensory perception.
4. Plan patient- and family-centered nursing interventions to decrease the psychosocial impact caused by living with one or more amputations.
5. Apply knowledge of anatomy, physiology, and pathophysiology to provide evidence-based care for patients with fractures.
6. Analyze assessment and diagnostic findings to generate solutions and prioritize nursing care for patients who have amputations.
7. Organize care coordination and transition management for patients having surgery to manage fractures.
8. Use clinical judgment to plan evidence-based nursing care to promote mobility and decrease pain in patients with fractures.
9. Incorporate factors that affect health equity into the plan of care for patients planning amputation.

## Preliminary Reading

Read and review Chapter 44, pp. 1079–1109.

## Chapter Review

### Pathophysiology Review

#1. Match the Key Term in Column A with its definition in Column B.

| Column A | Column B |
|---|---|
| ___1. Acute compartment syndrome | A. Tumor consisting of damaged nerve cells |
| ___2. Amputation | B. Bone break that does not extend through the skin |
| ___3. Closed (simple) fracture | C. Condition caused by continuous use, especially hands and wrist |
| ___4. Fat embolism syndrome | D. Limb-threatening condition that causes decreased circulation |
| ___5. Fracture | E. Globules from yellow bone marrow obstruct blood vessels |
| ___6. Neuroma | F. Persistent unpleasant altered sensation in amputated body part |
| ___7. Phantom limb pain | G. Disruption in the continuity of a bone |
| ___8. Repetitive stress injury | H. Removal of a body part |

#2. For each statement, specify if the statement is **true (T)** or **false (F).**

_____1.  Elective amputations are common among individuals who have diabetes mellitus and peripheral arterial disease.

_____2.  The primary cause of a fracture is trauma from a motor vehicle crash or fall, especially in older adults.

_____3.  The primary type of injury experienced by individuals in military training and service is musculoskeletal trauma.

_____4.  Osteoporosis is the biggest risk factor for hip fractures.

_____5.  An amputation of any part of the lower extremity is generally more incapacitating than one of the arm.

_____6.  Carpal tunnel syndrome (CTS) is the most common type of repetitive stress injury (RSI).

_____7.  CTS is a common condition in which the median nerve in the wrist becomes compressed, causing pain and numbness.

_____8.  Multiple petechiae occur in some patients who have pulmonary embolism from a blood clot.

## Activities

### Activity #1

List five areas the nurse would include in a neurovascular assessment following a tibia–fibula fracture.

1.  _____

2.  _____

3.  _____

4.  _____

5.  _____

### Activity #2

List the six Ps that can occur in a patient who has acute compartment syndrome, a potentially limb-threatening complication associated with musculoskeletal trauma and other conditions.

1.  _____

2.  _____

3.  _____

4.  _____

5.  _____

6.  _____

## Activity #3

For each statement, specify if the statement is **true (T)** or **false (F).**

_____1. The primary management for any fracture is reduction and immobilization.

_____2. Closed bone reduction is the most common nonsurgical method for managing a simple fracture.

_____3. External fixation with closed reduction is used when patients have soft-tissue injury and an open fracture.

_____4. For patients who have an open reduction internal fixation (ORIF) to manage a fracture, assess the pin sites every 8 to 12 hours for drainage, color, odor, and severe redness.

_____5. The nursing priority for the patient who has compression vertebral fractures is pain management.

_____6. Vertebral compression fractures (VCFs) may be treated with vertebroplasty or kyphoplasty in which bone cement is injected into the site.

_____7. Capillary refill is the most reliable assessment to determine adequate perfusion to distal extremities.

_____8. If a patient reports phantom limb pain, the nurse would recognize that the pain is real and should be managed promptly and completely.

_____9. To help prevent musculoskeletal injuries at the workplace, ergonomic office furniture is required by law.

___10. The patient with a torn rotator cuff has shoulder pain and cannot easily abduct the arm at the shoulder.

## Activity #4

Identify three health teaching statements that the nurse would provide to help adults promote health to prevent an elective or traumatic amputation.

1. _____

2. _____

3. _____

## Activity #5

Describe the first-line management for musculoskeletal soft-tissue injuries using RICE:

**R:** _____

**I:** _____

**C:** _____

**E:** _____

## Learning Assessments

### NCLEX Examination Challenge #1

The nurse is caring for a client with an elective right below-the-knee amputation. Which action would be **most** effective in helping to prevent a right hip flexion contracture?

A. Ensure that the client sleeps on a firm mattress.
B. Perform passive range-of-motion exercises to the right hip.
C. Elevate the surgical leg on two firm pillows during the day.
D. Have the client change to a prone position several times a day.

### NCLEX Examination Challenge #2

A client who had a traumatic left lower arm amputation reports severe pain in the left hand. What is the nurse's **best** response?

A. "Your left hand was removed as part of the surgery."
B. "I'll get you some medication that will help reduce your pain."
C. "Can you tell me when the pain is the worst during the day?"
D. "If you take a nap, I think your hand will feel much better."

**NCLEX Examination Challenge #3**

The nurse suspects complex regional pain syndrome for a client who had an ORIF for a right ankle fracture. Which client findings support this condition? **Select all that apply.**

A. Decreased right pedal pulse
B. Right ankle and foot edema
C. Right ankle and foot paresis and tingling
D. Changes in right ankle and foot temperature
E. Intense burning sensation in right ankle and foot

**NGN Challenge**

**Item #1**

The nurse is caring for a 52-year-old client who was admitted yesterday for a closed left tibial fracture.

| Health History | Nurses Notes | Orders | Laboratory Results | |
|---|---|---|---|---|

**0755:** Client reports severe throbbing pain in left lower leg that radiates into the foot. Rates pain at 9/10. Left leg immobilized via splint and bulky gauze wrap after closed fracture reduction. Analgesic administered an hour ago. Left lower leg significantly swollen when compared with right. Right pedal pulse 2+; left pedal pulse 1+. Left leg less pigmented when compared to right. Cap refill >3 seconds in left leg; <3 seconds in right leg. Client alert and oriented × 4. Lung sounds clear in all fields. $S_1$ and $S_2$ present. Bowel sounds present × 4. VS: T 98.2°F (36.8°C); HR 80 beats/min; RR 20 breaths/min; BP 125/66 mm Hg; $SpO_2$ 97% on RA.

Highlight the client findings in the Nurses Notes that would be of immediate concern to the nurse.

**Item #2**

The nurse is caring for a 52-year-old client who was admitted yesterday for a closed left tibial fracture.

| Health History | Nurses Notes | Orders | Laboratory Results | |
|---|---|---|---|---|

**0755:** Client reports severe throbbing pain in left lower leg that radiates into the foot. Rates pain at 7/10. Left leg immobilized via splint and bulky gauze wrap after closed fracture reduction. Analgesic administered an hour ago. Left lower leg significantly swollen when compared with right. Right pedal pulse 2+; left pedal pulse 1+. Left leg less pigmented when compared to right. Cap refill >3 seconds in left leg; <3 seconds in right leg. Client alert and oriented × 4. Lung sounds clear in all fields. $S_1$ and $S_2$ present. Bowel sounds present × 4. VS: T 98.2°F (36.8°C); HR 92 beats/min; RR 20 breaths/min; BP 125/66 mm Hg; $SpO_2$ 97% on RA.

The nurse analyzes the relevant assessment findings to determine the client's current condition. Complete the sentence to fill in the blanks using the lists of options listed below.

Based on the assessment findings, the nurse determines that the client is at high risk for _____1 [Select]_____, which causes _____2 [Select]_____.

| Options for 1 | Options for 2 |
|---|---|
| Cellulitis | Edema |
| Necrotizing fasciitis | Infection |
| Peripheral vascular disease | Clotting |
| Acute compartment syndrome | Hypoperfusion |

*Item #3*

The nurse is caring for a 52-year-old client who was admitted yesterday for a closed left tibial fracture.

| Health History | Nurses Notes | Orders | Laboratory Results | |
|---|---|---|---|---|

**0755:** Client reports severe throbbing pain in left lower leg that radiates into the foot. Rates pain at 7/10. Left leg immobilized via splint and bulky gauze wrap after closed fracture reduction. Analgesic administered an hour ago. Left lower leg significantly swollen when compared to right. Right pedal pulse 2+; left pedal pulse 1+. Left leg less pigmented when compared with right. Cap refill >3 seconds in left leg; <3 seconds in right leg. Client alert and oriented × 4. Lung sounds clear in all fields. $S_1$ and $S_2$ present. Bowel sounds present × 4. VS: T 98.2°F (36.8°C); HR 80 beats/min; RR 20 breaths/min; BP 125/66 mm Hg; $SpO_2$ 97% on RA.

Complete the sentence to fill in the blanks using the list of word choices listed below.

Based on the client's condition, the nurse determines that the *priority* for care is to prevent _____.

| Word Choices |
|---|
| Sepsis |
| Tissue necrosis |
| Hypovolemic shock |
| Complex regional pain syndrome |

*Item #4*

The nurse is caring for a 52-year-old client who was admitted yesterday for a closed left tibial fracture.

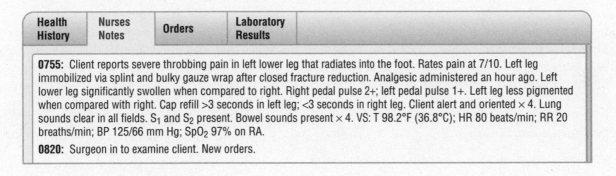

| Health History | Nurses Notes | Orders | Laboratory Results | |
|---|---|---|---|---|

**0755:** Client reports severe throbbing pain in left lower leg that radiates into the foot. Rates pain at 7/10. Left leg immobilized via splint and bulky gauze wrap after closed fracture reduction. Analgesic administered an hour ago. Left lower leg significantly swollen when compared to right. Right pedal pulse 2+; left pedal pulse 1+. Left leg less pigmented when compared with right. Cap refill >3 seconds in left leg; <3 seconds in right leg. Client alert and oriented × 4. Lung sounds clear in all fields. $S_1$ and $S_2$ present. Bowel sounds present × 4. VS: T 98.2°F (36.8°C); HR 80 beats/min; RR 20 breaths/min; BP 125/66 mm Hg; $SpO_2$ 97% on RA.

**0820:** Surgeon in to examine client. New orders.

The nurse begins to develop a plan of care for the client. Select **three** orders by the surgeon that the nurse would anticipate at this time to include in the plan.

A. Administer new analgesic for pain.
B. Perform neurovascular checks every hour.
C. Elevate left leg on two pillows.
D. Remove splint and bulky dressing.
E. Keep heels off the bed at all times.
F. Notify surgeon if pedal pulse is nonpalpable.

*Item #5*

The nurse is caring for a 52-year-old client who was admitted yesterday for a closed left tibial fracture.

| Health History | Nurses Notes | Orders | Laboratory Results | |
|---|---|---|---|---|

**0755:** Client reports severe throbbing pain in left lower leg that radiates into the foot. Rates pain at 7/10. Left leg immobilized via splint and bulky gauze wrap after closed fracture reduction. Analgesic administered an hour ago. Left lower leg significantly swollen when compared to right. Right pedal pulse 2+; left pedal pulse 1+. Left leg less pigmented when compared with right. Cap refill >3 seconds in left leg; <3 seconds in right leg. Client alert and oriented × 3. Lung sounds clear in all fields. $S_1$ and $S_2$ present. Bowel sounds present × 4. VS: T 98.2°F (36.8°C); HR 80 beats/min; RR 20 breaths/min; BP 125/66 mm Hg; $SpO_2$ 97% on RA.

**0820:** Surgeon in to examine client. New orders.

**0925:** Medicated for pain at 0845. Pain reduced to 5/10. Continuing to monitor circulation in left leg every hour. Client made NPO and IV fluids initiated.

**1155:** Client reports intense stabbing pain in left lower leg that radiates into the foot. Rates pain at 10/10 and states new onset of painful tingling and numbness. Left lower leg edema extending into ankle. Right pedal pulse 2+; left pedal pulse nonpalpable. Cap refill >3 seconds in left leg; <3 seconds in right leg. Surgeon notified and client prepared for fasciotomy.

The nurse prepares the client for surgery. Which nursing actions would be included as part of this preparation? **Select all that apply.**

A.  Maintain NPO status for client.
B.  Notify family about impending surgery.
C.  Ask client about understanding of the surgery.
D.  Confirm that client signed informed consent.
E.  Continue to monitor neurovascular status.

*Item #6*

A 52-year-old client had an open fasciotomy for acute compartment syndrome 10 days ago and is being seen in the surgeon's office for follow-up. The nurse in the surgeon's office interviews and screens the client before the client is seen by the surgeon. The nurse compares the current client findings with previous findings when the client was hospitalized. Indicate which current findings indicate that the client is **Improving** or **Not Improving**.

| Previous Client Findings | Current Client Findings (Today) | Improving | Not Improving |
|---|---|---|---|
| Severe pain reported at 10/10 | Pain reported at 2/10 | | |
| Left leg capillary refill >3 seconds | Left leg capillary refill <3 seconds | | |
| Left nonpalpable pedal pulse | Left pedal pulse 1+ | | |
| Left lower leg and ankle edema | Left lower leg and ankle edema | | |

# 45
CHAPTER

# Assessment of the Gastrointestinal System

## LEARNING OUTCOMES

1. Use knowledge of anatomy and physiology to perform a focused assessment of the gastrointestinal system.
2. Teach evidence-based health promotion activities to help prevent gastrointestinal health problems or trauma.
3. Identify factors that affect health equity for patients with gastrointestinal health problems.
4. Explain how genetic implications and physiologic aging of the gastrointestinal affect (concept).
5. Interpret assessment findings for patients with a suspected or actual gastrointestinal problem.
6. Plan evidence-based care and support for patients undergoing diagnostic testing of the gastrointestinal system.

## Preliminary Reading

Read and review Chapter 45, pp. 1110–1127.

## Chapter Review

### Anatomy & Physiology Review

#1. Label the parts of the gastrointestinal system using the Anatomy Labels provided after the figure.

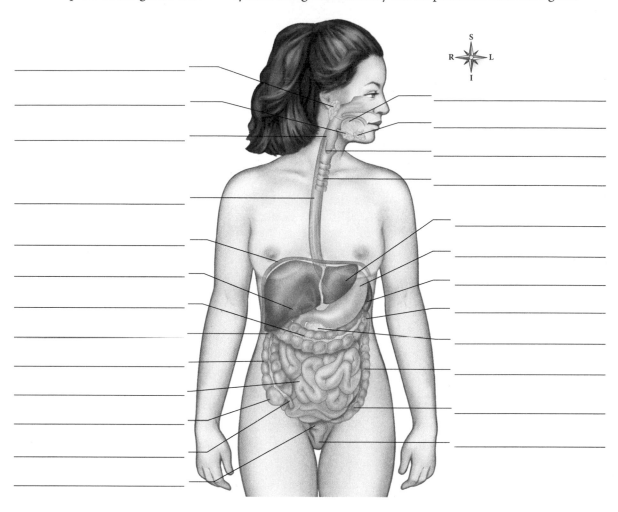

(From Patton KT, & Thibodeau GA. (2022). *Anatomy & physiology* (11th ed.). St. Louis: Elsevier.)

| Anatomy Labels |
| --- |
| Jejunum |
| Salivary glands |
| Colon |
| Esophagus |
| Rectum |
| Duodenum |
| Gallbladder |
| Mouth |
| Parotid gland |

| Anatomy Labels |
| --- |
| Anus |
| Ileum |
| Pancreas |

#2.  Identify key body structures that are located in each abdominal quadrant from the list.

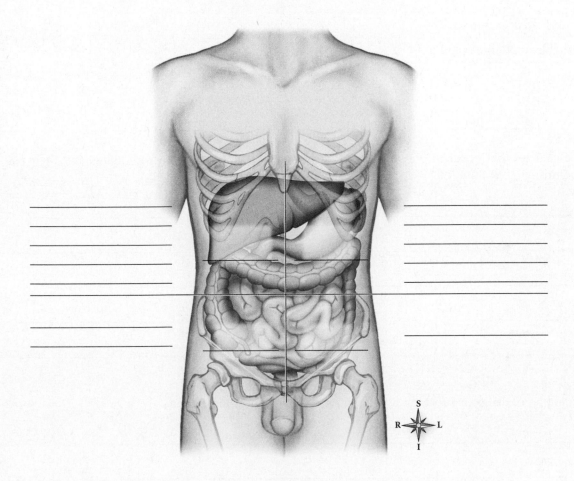

(From Patton KT, & Thibodeau GA. (2022). *Anatomy & physiology* (11th ed.). St. Louis: Elsevier.)

| Key Body Structures |
| --- |
| Majority of the liver |
| Left lobe of the liver |
| Sigmoid colon |
| Appendix |
| Gallbladder |
| Spleen |

| Key Body Structures |
|---|
| Duodenum |
| Stomach |
| Cecum |
| Splenic flexure of the colon |
| Head of pancreas |
| Body and tail of pancreas |
| Hepatic flexure of the colon |

## Activities

### Activity #1

List five changes that occur in the gastrointestinal system that are associated with aging, and their associated implications.

1. _____

2. _____

3. _____

4. _____

5. _____

### Activity #2

Give examples of drugs or substances that irritate the gastrointestinal system.

1. _____

2. _____

3. _____

4. _____

### Activity #3

Complete the sentences with the correct term or phrase.

1. When the nurse hears high-pitched bowel sounds that are above an obstruction, _____ will be documented.
2. When a patient passes gas, the nurse will document that the patient has _____.
3. When the nurse hears an audible swishing sound during abdominal auscultation, the nurse will document that a _____ was heard.
4. When the patient is supposed to refrain from eating or drinking, the nurse will record that the patient's status is _____.
5. When fatty stools are assessed, the nurse will document that the patient has _____.

## Activity #4

For each statement, specify if the statement is **true (T)** or **false (F)**.

_____1. Asking the patient if they have recently traveled outside of the country can provide valuable health history information.

_____2. Lactose intolerance is a rare condition seldom seen in the United States.

_____3. A food desert is a location that has little access to fresh vegetables and fruits.

_____4. The PQRST mnemonic can be used to conduct a pain assessment for a patient with a gastrointestinal disturbance.

_____5. Jaundice is caused by bile pigments.

_____6. Notifying the primary health care provider immediately if a bulging, pulsating mass in the abdominal area is of critical importance.

_____7. The most reliable method for assessing the return of peristalsis after surgery is the first bowel movement.

_____8. Monitor a patient undergoing esophagogastroduodenoscopy for respiratory depression.

_____9. Common assessment findings after a colonoscopy include pallor, dizziness, and tachycardia.

_____10. A tissue biopsy can be performed during a sigmoidoscopy if needed.

## Activity #5

Fill in the blanks with the diagnostic test that fits this description. See choices in the table below.

1. Three-dimensional images of the colon and rectum created by use of an abdominal and pelvic CT scan _____.

2. Endoscopic examination of the rectum and sigmoid colon using a flexible scope _____.

3. Test that measures the presence of blood in the stool from gastrointestinal bleeding _____.

4. Visual examination of the esophagus, stomach, and duodenum by means of a fiberoptic endoscope _____.

5. Direct visualization of the gastrointestinal tract by means of a flexible fiberoptic endoscope _____.

6. Tube insertion that allows viewing and manipulation of internal body areas _____.

7. Procedure in which the bile ducts, pancreatic duct, and gallbladder are visualized through endoscopy _____.

8. Endoscopic examination of the entire large bowel _____.

| Choices |
|---|
| Colonoscopy |
| Endoscopic retrograde cholangiopancreatography |
| Endoscopy |
| Enteroscopy |
| Esophagogastroduodenoscopy |
| Guaiac-based fecal occult blood test |
| Sigmoidoscopy |
| Virtual colonoscopy |

## Learning Assessments

### NCLEX Examination Challenge #1

Which assessment will the nurse perform as the **priority** when a client is given IV midazolam hydrochloride before an esophagogastroduodenoscopy?

A. Determine level of consciousness.
B. Monitor the rate and depth of respirations.
C. Assess the monitor for cardiac dysrhythmias.
D. Auscultate for bowel sounds in all four quadrants.

### NCLEX Examination Challenge #2

Which action will the nurse include when providing care for a client immediately after a colonoscopy? **Select all that apply.**

A. Check vital signs every 15 to 30 minutes.
B. Assess for abdominal pain and guarding.
C. Maintain NPO status until sedation wears off.
D. Keep the top side rails up until the client is alert.
E. Place client in left lateral position to promote passing of flatus.

### NCLEX Examination Challenge #3

The nurse reviews a client's laboratory values and notes a serum potassium level of 3.1 mEq/L. Which factor does the nurse anticipate that has contributed to this value (Reference range 3.5–5.0 mEq/L or 3.5–5.0 mmol/L)?

A. Liver disease
B. Malabsorption
C. Gastric suctioning
D. Acute pancreatitis

# 46
## CHAPTER

# Concepts of Care for Patients with Oral Cavity and Esophageal Conditions

## LEARNING OUTCOMES

1. Plan collaborative care with the interprofessional team to promote tissue integrity and nutrition in patients with oral cavity and esophageal problems.
2. Teach adults how to decrease the risk for oral cavity and esophageal problems.
3. Teach the patient and caregiver(s) about common drugs and other management strategies used for oral cavity and esophageal problems.
4. Plan patient- and family-centered nursing interventions to decrease the psychosocial impact caused by living with oral cavity and esophageal problems.
5. Apply knowledge of anatomy, physiology, and pathophysiology to provide evidence-based care for patients with oral cavity and esophageal problems affecting tissue integrity and nutrition.
6. Analyze assessment and diagnostic findings to generate solutions and prioritize nursing care for patients with oral cavity and esophageal problems.
7. Organize care coordination and transition management for patients with oral cavity and esophageal problems.
8. Use clinical judgment to plan evidence-based nursing care to promote tissue integrity and nutrition and prevent complications in patients with oral cavity and esophageal problems.
9. Incorporate factors that affect health equity into the plan of care for patients with oral cavity and esophageal problems.

## Preliminary Reading

Read and review Chapter 46, pp. 1128–1150.

## Chapter Review

### Pathophysiology Review

#1. Match the Key Term in Column A with its description in Column B.

| Column A | | Column B | |
|---|---|---|---|
| _____1. | Barrett epithelium | A. | Bowel obstruction caused by bowel twisting |
| _____2. | Erythroplakia | B. | Protrusion of stomach through esophageal hiatus of diaphragm into the chest |
| _____3. | Hiatal hernia | C. | Damage to esophageal mucosa in patients with GERD |
| _____4. | Leukoplakia | D. | Velvety red mucosal lesion |
| _____5. | Reflux esophagitis | E. | Salivary gland inflammation |
| _____6. | Regurgitation | F. | Backward flow of stomach contents into esophagus |
| _____7. | Sialadenitis | G. | Very dry mouth from reduction in saliva flow |
| _____8. | Stomatitis | H. | Columnar epithelium in the lower esophagus |
| _____9. | Volvulus | I. | Inflammation of the oral mucosa with ulceration(s) |
| ___10. | Xerostomia | J. | White patchy lesion on a mucous membrane |

#2. List 10 factors that contribute to lower esophageal sphincter pressure.

1. _____

2. _____

3. _____

4. _____

5. _____

6. _____

7. _____

8. _____

9. _____

10. _____

## Activities

### Activity #1

For each statement, specify if the statement is **true (T)** or **false (F)**.

_____1. The risk for oral cavity disorders is increased in people who eat foods high in sugar content.

_____2. Aphthous stomatitis is also known as secondary stomatitis.

_____3. The nurse teaches all patients to brush and floss at least twice daily.

_____4. 2% viscous lidocaine is an example of drug therapy used for oral pain management.

_____5. Oral hairy leukoplakia is often found in patients with Epstein-Barr virus (EBV).

_____6. Basal cell carcinoma of the mouth usually occurs inside the cheek.

____7.  Use disposable foam brushes when caring for a patient with oral cancer.

____8.  Patients with GERD benefit from the development of Barrett epithelium.

____9.  Following a laparoscopic Nissen fundoplication, teach patients to avoid driving for a week.

___10.  Cancer of the esophagus is painful even in its early stages.

## Activity #2

List five actions the nurse will take when caring for a patient with oral cavity problems.

1.  _____

2.  _____

3.  _____

4.  _____

5.  _____

## Activity #3

Provide the actions that are contained within the PASS acronym for dysphagia.

1.  P_____

2.  A_____

3.  S_____

4.  S_____

## Activity #4

Match the type of procedure in Column A with its description in Column B.

**Column A**

___1.  Glossectomy

___2.  Laryngectomy

___3.  Maxillectomy

___4.  Microsurgery

___5.  Pedicle reconstruction

___6.  Tumor resection

**Column B**

A.  Mouth, throat, or mandible reconstruction with patient's own tissue

B.  Removal of entire oral tumor

C.  Removal of part of all of the hard palate

D.  Repair of mouth, throat, or neck after tumor removal

E.  Removal of the larynx and tumor

F.  Removal of the tongue

## Learning Assessments

### NCLEX Examination Challenge #1

Which cause does the nurse recognize as a potential intentional cause for a client's esophageal trauma?

A.  Nasogastric (NG) tube placement

B.  Esophageal ulcers

C.  Struck by a foreign object

D.  Chemical injury

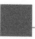 

**NCLEX Examination Challenge #2**

Which action will the nurse teach a client with GERD to minimize symptoms? **Select all that apply.**

A. Restrict caffeinated or carbonated beverages.
B. Eat slowly and chew food thoroughly.
C. Consume 4 to 6 small meals each day.
D. Do not eat for 3 hours before going to bed.
E. Sleep on your side to prevent regurgitation.

**NCLEX Examination Challenge #3**

Which question will the nurse ask as the **priority** to a client suspected of having leukoplakia?

A. "Do you smoke, dip, or chew tobacco products?"
B. "How much alcohol do you drink each day?"
C. "Do you consume many fast food meals?"
D. "How often do you have dental checkups?"

**NGN Challenge**

*Item #1*

The nurse has begun documenting a visit from a 33-year-old client who is establishing care with a new primary health care provider. **Highlight the client findings in the Nurses Notes that require further nursing assessment.**

| Health History | Nurses Notes | Vital Signs | Laboratory Results | |
| --- | --- | --- | --- | --- |

**1202:** Client moved here from another state; wishes to establish care with this primary health care provider. All health records from previous provider are accessible in the electronic health record. Client reports no preexisting medical history other than removal of tonsils as a child. Family history of type 2 diabetes. Lives at home with spouse and 2-year-old child. States, "I feel pretty good overall but lately I've been burping a lot after meals, and I have some burning in my chest." Indicates a preference for fast food because of traveling extensively for work. Drinks 1 to 2 glasses of water daily and about 3 to 4 cans of soda. Denies change in usual dietary habits and bowel or bladder patterns. Denies abdominal pain.

The nurse documents the assessment after obtaining a medical history.

| Health History | Nurses Notes | Vital Signs | Laboratory Results | |
| --- | --- | --- | --- | --- |

**1202:** Client moved here from another state; wishes to establish care with this primary health care provider. All health records from previous provider are accessible in the electronic health record. Client reports no preexisting medical history other than removal of tonsils as a child. Family history of type 2 diabetes. Lives at home with spouse and 2-year-old child. States, "I feel pretty good overall but lately I've been burping a lot after meals, and I have some burning in my chest." Indicates a preference for fast food because of traveling extensively for work. Drinks 1 to 2 glasses of water daily and about 3 to 4 cans of soda. Denies change in usual dietary habits and bowel or bladder patterns. Denies abdominal pain.

Height: 71 in (180 cm); weight: 274 lb (124.3 kg). VS: T 98.6°F (37°C); HR 90 beats/min; RR 18 breaths/min; BP 170/98 mm Hg. SpO$_2$ 99% on RA. Throat clear; mouth without lesions. Heart rate regular; lung sounds clear; bowel sounds present in all quadrants; abdomen nontender on gentle palpation.

*Item #2*

The nurse analyzes the findings to determine the client's condition. Choose the **most likely** options for the information missing from the statement by selecting from the lists of options provided.

The client is at high risk for _____[1] [Select]_____ as evidenced by _____[2] [Select]_____.

| Options for 1 | Options for 2 |
|---|---|
| Esophageal tumor | Heart rate 90 BPM |
| Gas bloat syndrome | Burning in chest |
| Reflux | Blood pressure 170/90 mm Hg |
| Stomatitis | Oral cavity condition |

*Item #3*

The nurse considers the client data to determine the priority for the plan of care. Choose the **most likely** options for the information missing from the statement by selecting from the list of options provided.

The **priority** for the client at this time is to manage _____ to prevent _____.

| Options |
|---|
| Infection Potential |
| Oral Lesions |
| Reflux |
| Barrett Epithelium |
| Esophageal Stricture |

*Item #4*

The nurse is preparing dietary recommendations to teach to the client that may reduce the incidence of reflux. **Select three items the nurse will teach the client to avoid.**

A. Soda
B. Yogurt
C. Applesauce
D. Baked fish
E. Cooked rice
F. Orange juice
G. Fried chicken
H. Mashed potatoes
I. Grilled hamburger

*Item #5*

The client is sent for an upper endoscopy. When the results return, the client is seen 1 week later by the primary health care provider and diagnosed with gastroesophageal reflux disease. A proton pump inhibitor is prescribed. The nurse provides teaching about management of this condition. Which information will the nurse communicate to the client? **Select all that apply.**

A. Try not to bend at the abdomen.
B. Avoid eating 1 hour before bedtime.
C. Keep a food diary to trend symptoms.
D. Avoid foods that contain lots of spices.
E. Weight loss can help minimize symptoms.
F. Prop up on a pillow when lying in bed or on a sofa.
G. Foods with mint as an ingredient should be avoided.
H. Take medication with grapefruit juice to increase absorption.
I. A registered dietitian nutritionist can help with meal planning.
J. Eat 2 to 3 larger meals per day to minimize the work of the GI system.

*Item #6*

Three months later, the client sees their primary health care provider to follow-up. For each client finding, use an X to indicate whether the initial nursing interventions implemented in the emergency department were **Effective** (helped to meet expected outcomes) or **Not Effective** (did not help to meet expected outcomes).

| Previous Client Finding | Current Client Finding | Effective | Not Effective |
|---|---|---|---|
| Burping after meals | Reports incidence of burping has decreased | | |
| Feels burning in chest | Says burning in chest occurs less often than it did previously | | |
| Eats at fast food locations often | Eats at fast food locations often | | |
| Drinks 1 to 2 glasses of water daily | Drinks 3 glasses of water daily | | |
| Consumes 3 to 4 cans of soda daily | Drinks 2 cans of soda daily | | |

# 47 CHAPTER

# *Concepts of Care for Patients with Stomach Conditions*

## LEARNING OUTCOMES

1. Plan collaborative care with the interprofessional team to manage infection in patients with peptic ulcer disease (PUD).
2. Teach adults how to decrease the risk for gastric cancer.
3. Teach the patient and caregiver(s) about common drugs and other management strategies used for PUD.
4. Plan patient- and family-centered nursing interventions to decrease the psychosocial impact caused by living with gastric cancer.
5. Apply knowledge of anatomy, physiology, and pathophysiology to provide evidence-based care for patients with PUD.

6. Analyze assessment and diagnostic findings to generate solutions and prioritize nursing care for patients who have PUD.
7. Organize care coordination and transition management for patients having gastric surgery.
8. Use clinical judgment to plan evidence-based nursing care to promote nutrition and decrease pain and inflammation in patients with gastritis.
9. Incorporate factors that affect health equity into the plan of care for patients with gastric cancer.

## Preliminary Reading

Read and review Chapter 47, pp. 1151–1167.

## Chapter Review

### Pathophysiology Review

#1. Match the Key Term in Column A with its definition in Column B.

| Column A | Column B |
|---|---|
| ___1. Dyspepsia | A. Dark, tarry stool indicating occult blood |
| ___2. Gastritis | B. Acute gastric mucosal lesion that occurs after a medical crisis or trauma |
| ___3. Hematemesis | C. Inflammation of gastric mucosa |
| ___4. Melena | D. Condition that results when GI mucosa is not protected from acid and pepsin |
| ___5. Peptic ulcer disease | E. Epigastric burning sensation or indigestion |
| ___6. Peritonitis | F. Abdominal infection |
| ___7. Stress ulcer | G. Vomiting bright red or coffee-ground blood |

**#2.** For each statement, specify if the statement is **true (T)** or **false (F).**

_____1. Long-term nonsteroidal antiinflammatory drug use creates a high risk for chronic gastritis.

_____2. Most peptic ulcers are caused by *Helicobacter pylori* infection.

_____3. Duodenal ulcers occur more often than other types of GI ulcers.

_____4. Vomiting can cause metabolic acidosis and hyperkalemia.

_____5. Gastric cancer occurs most commonly in people older than 65 years of age.

_____6. Infection with *H. pylori* is the largest risk factor for gastric cancer because it carries the cytotoxin-associated gene A *(CagA)* gene.

_____7. The overall 5-year survival rate of adults with stomach cancer is approximately 30% because most patients have no symptoms until the disease advances.

_____8. Atrophic gastritis is a precancerous patient condition.

## Activities

### Activity #1

List four lifestyle habits that the nurse would include in health teaching to help individuals prevent gastritis.

1. _____

2. _____

3. _____

4. _____

### Activity #2

Match the drug in Column A with its drug classification in Column B. One or more choices in Column B may be used more than once.

**Column A**

___1. Famotidine

___2. Sucralfate

___3. Lansoprazole

___4. Aluminum hydroxide

___5. Tetracycline

___6. Bismuth subsalicylate

**Column B**

A. Antacid

B. Proton pump inhibitor

C. $H_2$-receptor antagonist

D. Antibiotic

E. Mucosal barrier fortifier

### Activity #3

For each statement, specify if the statement is **true (T)** or **false (F).**

_____1. Patients who experience acute gastritis typically have epigastric pain and dyspepsia.

_____2. Esophagogastroduodenoscopy (EGD) with biopsy is the gold standard for diagnosing gastritis.

_____3. Eliminating the causative factor(s) is the primary treatment approach for acute gastritis.

_____4. Upper GI bleeding is a medical emergency that can cause hypovolemic shock if not treated promptly.

_____5. Peptic ulcer perforation is a surgical emergency and can be life threatening.

_____6. For patients who have an upper GI bleed, a nasogastric tube is placed for nutrition and drug therapy.

_____7. Dumping syndrome is a term that refers to a group of vasomotor symptoms that occur after eating in patients who have had upper GI bleeding.

_____8. Nurses need to identify individuals who are at high risk for peptic ulcer disease and gastric cancer and teach them about the need for *H. pylori* screening.

____9.   A common drug regimen to treat *H. pylori* infection is PPI-triple therapy, which includes a PPI plus two antibiotics for 10 to 14 days.

____10.   Patients who have advanced gastric cancer and their families should be referred to a local palliative care program or hospice for symptom management at end-of-life.

## Activity #4
Identify three actions that the patient should implement to prevent dumping syndrome.

1.   _____

2.   _____

3.   _____

## Learning Assessments

### NCLEX Examination Challenge #1
The nurse is caring for a client with a long history of peptic ulcer disease. Which client finding would the nurse report **immediately** to the primary health care provider?
A.   Melena
B.   Epigastric pain
C.   Intolerance to certain foods
D.   Dyspepsia

### NCLEX Examination Challenge #2
The nurse is planning to provide health teaching for a client recently diagnosed with acute gastritis. Which statement by the client indicates a **need for further teaching**?
A.   "I need to avoid caffeine and alcohol, which are stimulants."
B.   "I should eat a better-balanced diet including fruits and vegetables."
C.   "I don't need to stop smoking unless I am diagnosed with cancer."
D.   "I plan to take yoga classes and begin meditating to reduce my stress level."

## NGN Challenge #1

The nurse is caring for a 47-year-old client admitted to the ED.

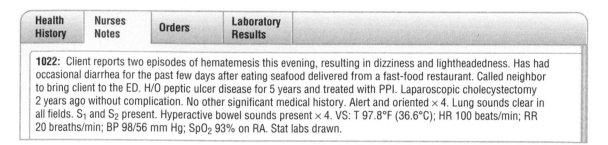

| Health History | Nurses Notes | Orders | Laboratory Results | |
|---|---|---|---|---|

**1022:** Client reports two episodes of hematemesis this evening, resulting in dizziness and lightheadedness. Has had occasional diarrhea for the past few days after eating seafood delivered from a fast-food restaurant. Called neighbor to bring client to the ED. H/O peptic ulcer disease for 5 years and treated with PPI. Laparoscopic cholecystectomy 2 years ago without complication. No other significant medical history. Alert and oriented × 4. Lung sounds clear in all fields. $S_1$ and $S_2$ present. Hyperactive bowel sounds present × 4. VS: T 97.8°F (36.6°C); HR 100 beats/min; RR 20 breaths/min; BP 98/56 mm Hg; $SpO_2$ 93% on RA. Stat labs drawn.

Complete the diagram by selecting from the choices to specify what **one** condition the client is most likely experiencing, **two** actions the nurse would take to address that condition, and **two** parameters the nurse would monitor to assess the client's progress.

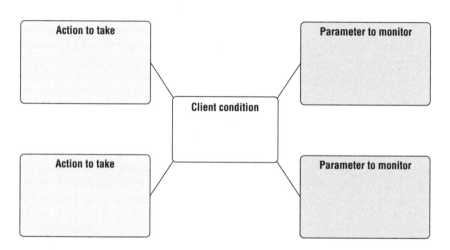

| Actions to Take | Client Condition | Parameters to Monitor |
|---|---|---|
| Maintain intake and output record | Gastroenteritis | Pain intensity and quality |
| Administer supplemental oxygen therapy | Gastric cancer | Vital signs |
| Place client in flat supine position | Upper GI bleeding | Daily body weight |
| Start two large-bore IV lines | Acute gastritis | Urinary output |
| Insert an indwelling urinary catheter | //////////////////////////////// | Hemoglobin and hematocrit |

## NGN Challenge #2

The nurse is caring for a 59-year-old client who was just admitted to the Urgent Care Center.

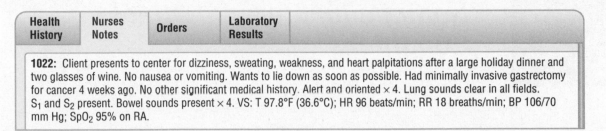

| Health History | Nurses Notes | Orders | Laboratory Results | |
|---|---|---|---|---|

**1022:** Client presents to center for dizziness, sweating, weakness, and heart palpitations after a large holiday dinner and two glasses of wine. No nausea or vomiting. Wants to lie down as soon as possible. Had minimally invasive gastrectomy for cancer 4 weeks ago. No other significant medical history. Alert and oriented × 4. Lung sounds clear in all fields. $S_1$ and $S_2$ present. Bowel sounds present × 4. VS: T 97.8°F (36.6°C); HR 96 beats/min; RR 18 breaths/min; BP 106/70 mm Hg; SpO$_2$ 95% on RA.

Complete the diagram by selecting from the choices to specify what **one** condition the client is most likely experiencing, **two** actions the nurse would take to address that condition, and **two** parameters the nurse would monitor to assess the client's progress.

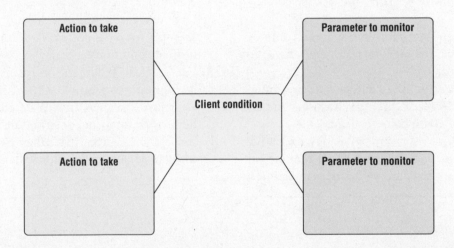

| Actions to Take | Client Condition | Parameters to Monitor |
|---|---|---|
| Place the client in a flat or slightly elevated supine position | Hyponatremia | Similar symptoms in future |
| Infuse a liter of normal saline | Pyloric obstruction | Body weight |
| Administer supplemental oxygen | Pernicious anemia | Reduction or relief of present symptoms |
| Give an IV antiemetic medication | Dumping syndrome | Serum electrolytes |
| Remind the client to avoid alcohol and fluids with meals | //////////////////////////////// | Vital signs |

# 48 CHAPTER

# Concepts of Care for Patients with Noninflammatory Intestinal Conditions

## LEARNING OUTCOMES

1. Plan collaborative care with the interprofessional team to manage elimination in patients with intestinal obstruction.
2. Teach adults how to decrease the risk for colorectal cancer.
3. Teach the patient and caregiver(s) about common drugs and other management strategies used for colorectal cancer.
4. Plan patient- and family-centered nursing interventions to decrease the psychosocial impact caused by living with colorectal cancer.
5. Apply knowledge of anatomy, physiology, and pathophysiology to provide evidence-based care for patients with noninflammatory intestinal conditions.
6. Analyze assessment and diagnostic findings to generate solutions and prioritize nursing care for patients who have noninflammatory intestinal conditions.
7. Organize care coordination and transition management for patients having noninflammatory intestinal conditions.
8. Use clinical judgment to plan evidence-based nursing care to promote elimination and fluid and electrolyte balance and to decrease pain in patients with intestinal obstruction.
9. Incorporate factors that affect health equity into the plan of care for patients with colorectal cancer.

## Preliminary Reading

Read and review Chapter 48, pp. 1168–1190.

## Chapter Review

### Pathophysiology Review

#1. Match the Key Term in Column A with its definition in Column B.

| **Column A** | **Column B** |
|---|---|
| ____1. Borborygmi | A. No passage of stool |
| ____2. Flatulence | B. Weakness in the abdominal muscle wall through which a segment of the bowel protrudes |
| ____3. Hemorrhoids | |
| ____4. Hernia | C. Bowel obstruction or hernia that has compromised blood flow |
| ____5. Intussusception | D. Condition in which the bowel is physically blocked by intestinal problems |
| ____6. Irritable bowel syndrome | |
| ____7. Mechanical obstruction | E. High-pitched bowel sounds above an obstruction |
| ____8. Nonmechanical obstruction | F. Twisting of the intestine |
| ____9. Obstipation | G. Telescoping of a segment of the intestine within itself |
| __10. Intestinal polyps | H. Small growths covered with mucosa and attached to the intestinal wall |
| __11. Strangulated obstruction | |
| __12. Volvulus | I. Excessive gas in the intestines |
| | J. Condition in which peristalsis is decreased or absent in the intestines |
| | K. Swollen or distended veins in the anorectal region |
| | L. Functional GI disorder that causes chronic or recurrent diarrhea |

#2. For each statement, specify if the statement is **true (T)** or **false (F).**

_____1. Bowel obstructions can occur in the small or large bowel and can be either mechanical or nonmechanical (paralytic ileus).

_____2. Obstruction high in the small intestine causes a loss of gastric hydrochloric acid, which can lead to metabolic acidosis.

_____3. A strangulated bowel obstruction causes decreased blood flow to the intestines and can be life-threatening.

_____4. Most colorectal cancers are believed to arise from adenomatous polyps that present as small growths covered with mucosa and are attached to the surface of the intestine.

_____5. The major risk factors for the development of colorectal cancer (CRC) include age younger than 50 years, genetic predisposition, and/or personal or family history of cancer.

_____6. Irritable bowel syndrome is the most common digestive disorder seen in clinical practice.

_____7. Hemorrhoids are unnaturally swollen or distended veins in the anorectal region.

_____8. If a hernia is strangulated, ischemia and obstruction occur in the bowel loop, which can lead to necrosis of the bowel, sepsis, and possibly bowel perforation.

## Activities

### Activity #1

List three actions that the nurse would include in health teaching to help individuals promote bowel health.

1. _____

2. _____

3. _____

**Activity #2**

Match each numbered colostomy location in the figure with its description by letter in the list.

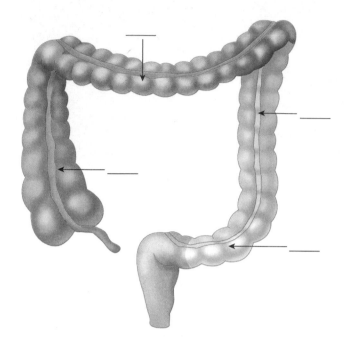

A.  Stool is well-formed and colostomy may not require an appliance at all times.
B.  Stool is liquid and can cause skin irritation because of intestinal enzymes.
C.  Stool is pasty and requires an appliance at all times.
D.  Stool is semiformed and requires an appliance at all times.

**Activity #3**

For each statement, specify if the statement is **true (T)** or **false (F)**.

_____1.   At least every 12 hours, assess the patient with a nasogastric tube (NGT) for proper placement of the tube, tube patency, and output.

_____2.   Weight is the most reliable indicator of fluid balance.

_____3.   Pain is generally less with nonmechanical obstruction than with mechanical obstruction.

_____4.   The *Healthy People 2030* initiative recognizes the need for national attention to the reduction of new cases of cancer and cancer-related illness, disability, and death.

_____5.   Regular screening for colorectal cancer (CRC) is not recommended for individuals who are older than 85 years because of the risks associated with cancer treatment.

_____6.   Although deaths from CRC have decreased over the past 30 years, the 5-year survival rates are lowest for Blacks, especially those younger than 50 years of age, when compared with all other racial groups.

_____7.   As a palliative measure, radiation therapy may be used to control pain, hemorrhage, bowel obstruction, or metastasis to the lung in advanced CRC.

_____8.   Patients who have laparoscopic minimally invasive surgery for CRC usually have a postoperative NGT for decompression.

_____9.   A Salem sump NGT is most effective when connected to low intermittent suction.

___10.   A healthy ostomy stoma should be protruding, moist, and reddish pink.

## Activity #4

Match the drug in Column A with its drug classification in Column B. One or more choices in Column B may be used more than once, but all choices should be used.

**Column A**

___1.  Alosetron
___2.  Alvimopan
___3.  Linaclotide
___4.  Lubiprostone
___5.  Loperamide
___6.  Psyllium hydrophilic mucilloid
___7.  Rifaximin
___8.  Bevacizumab

**Column B**

A.  Antibiotic
B.  Laxative
C.  Bulk-forming drug
D.  Mu opioid receptor antagonist
E.  Antidiarrheal agent
F.  Selective serotonin receptor antagonist
G.  Angiogenesis inhibitor

## Learning Assessments

### NCLEX Examination Challenge #1

The nurse is explaining the procedure for fecal occult blood testing (FOBT). Which statement by the client indicates a **need for further teaching?**

A.  "Do not take drugs like NSAIDs or Vitamin C at least 48 hours before collecting a stool sample."
B.  "Avoid red meat for at least 48 hours before collecting a stool sample."
C.  "Use 2 to 3 different areas in the stool sample for each FOBT."
D.  "Collect a specimen for FOBT for at least 5 consecutive days."

### NCLEX Examination Challenge #2

The nurse is providing discharge teaching for a client who had an abdominoperineal resection for rectal cancer. For which common postoperative complications will the nurse remind the client to anticipate? **Select all that apply.**

A.  Urinary incontinence
B.  Wound infection
C.  Ischemic ostomy stoma
D.  Sexual dysfunction
E.  Obstipation

### NCLEX Examination Challenge #3

The nurse is providing discharge teaching for a client who had a laparoscopic hernioplasty. Which instruction would be the **most important?**

A.  "Apply ice to the surgical area as needed for discomfort."
B.  "Eat high-fiber foods to help prevent constipation."
C.  "Avoid excessive coughing for the next few weeks."
D.  "Rest for a few days after you get home."

NGN Challenge #1

The nurse is caring for a 76-year-old client who had an open exploratory laparotomy and colon resection 2 days ago for colorectal cancer.

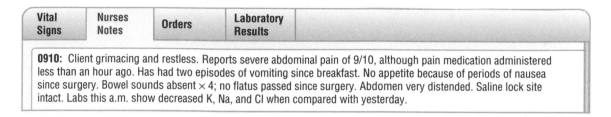

| Vital Signs | Nurses Notes | Orders | Laboratory Results | |
|---|---|---|---|---|

**0910:** Client grimacing and restless. Reports severe abdominal pain of 9/10, although pain medication administered less than an hour ago. Has had two episodes of vomiting since breakfast. No appetite because of periods of nausea since surgery. Bowel sounds absent × 4; no flatus passed since surgery. Abdomen very distended. Saline lock site intact. Labs this a.m. show decreased K, Na, and Cl when compared with yesterday.

| Nurses Notes | Vital Signs | Orders | Laboratory Results | |
|---|---|---|---|---|

**0910:**
T 97.8°F (36.6°C)
HR 108 beats/min
RR 22 breaths/min
BP 116/68 mm Hg
SpO2 95% on RA

Complete the diagram below by selecting from the choices to specify what **one** condition the client is most likely experiencing, **two** actions the nurse would take to address that condition, and **two** parameters the nurse would monitor to assess the client's progress.

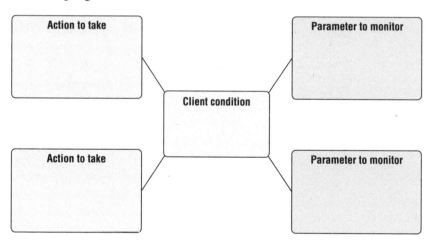

| Actions to Take | Client Condition | Parameters to Monitor |
|---|---|---|
| Place the client in a flat or slightly elevated supine position. | Surgical wound infection | Urinary output |
| Make client NPO and insert NGT to suction. | Mechanical intestinal obstruction | Serum electrolytes |
| Administer supplemental oxygen therapy. | Abdominal hernia | Heart rate and blood pressure |
| Convert saline lock to continuous IV infusion. | Postoperative ileus | Daily weight |
| Restart PCA morphine for pain control. | ///////////////////////////////// | Abdominal distention and pain |

**NGN Challenge #2**

The nurse is caring for a 25-year-old client who presents to the ED.

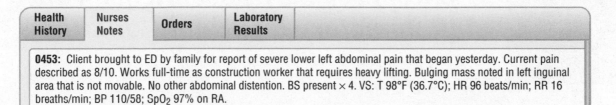

| Health History | Nurses Notes | Orders | Laboratory Results | |
|---|---|---|---|---|

**0453:** Client brought to ED by family for report of severe lower left abdominal pain that began yesterday. Current pain described as 8/10. Works full-time as construction worker that requires heavy lifting. Bulging mass noted in left inguinal area that is not movable. No other abdominal distention. BS present × 4. VS: T 98°F (36.7°C); HR 96 beats/min; RR 16 breaths/min; BP 110/58; SpO$_2$ 97% on RA.

Complete the diagram by selecting from the choices to specify what **one** condition the client is most likely experiencing, **two** actions the nurse would take to address that condition, and **two** parameters the nurse would monitor to assess the client's progress.

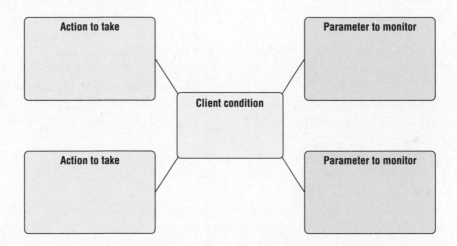

| Actions to Take | Client Condition | Parameters to Monitor |
|---|---|---|
| Prepare the client for surgery as soon as possible. | Irreducible inguinal hernia | Body temperature |
| Make client NPO and insert NGT to suction. | Appendicitis | Surgical site |
| Insert an indwelling urinary catheter. | Umbilical hernia | White blood cell count |
| Initiate peripheral IV access. | Intestinal obstruction | Abdominal assessment |
| Administer antibiotic therapy. | /////////////////////////////// | Oxygen saturation |

# 49
CHAPTER

# Concepts of Care for Patients with Inflammatory Intestinal Conditions

## LEARNING OUTCOMES

1. Plan collaborative care with the interprofessional team to manage inflammation in patients with inflammatory bowel disease (IBD).
2. Teach adults how to decrease the risk for gastroenteritis.
3. Teach the patient and caregiver(s) about common drugs and other management strategies used for chronic IBD.
4. Plan patient- and family-centered nursing interventions to decrease the psychosocial impact caused by living with chronic IBD.
5. Apply knowledge of anatomy, physiology, and pathophysiology to provide evidence-based care for patients with acute and chronic IBD.

6. Analyze assessment and diagnostic findings to generate solutions and prioritize nursing care for patients who have intestinal infection.
7. Organize care coordination and transition management for patients having surgery for IBD.
8. Use clinical judgment to plan evidence-based nursing care to promote elimination and nutrition and decrease pain in patients with chronic IBD.
9. Incorporate factors that affect health equity into the plan of care for patients with chronic IBD.

## Preliminary Reading

Read and review Chapter 49, pp. 1191–1216.

## Chapter Review

### Pathophysiology Review

#1. Match the Key Term in Column A with its definition in Column B.

**Column A**

_____1. Abscess
_____2. Celiac disease
_____3. Crohn's disease
_____4. Diverticulosis
_____5. Effluent
_____6. Fissure
_____7. Fistula
_____8. Gastroenteritis
_____9. Peritonitis
____10. Steatorrhea
____11. Tenesmus
____12. Toxic megacolon

**Column B**

A. Tear, crack, or split in skin and underlying tissue
B. Unpleasant and urgent sensation to defecate
C. Presence of abnormal pouchlike herniations in the intestinal wall
D. Acute inflammation and infection of the lining of the abdominal cavity
E. Acute inflammation and infection with a collection of pus
F. Massive dilation and ileus of the colon causing gangrene and peritonitis
G. Drainage
H. Chronic inflammation of the intestinal wall that can cause atrophy and malabsorption
I. Abnormal opening (tract) between two organs or structures
J. Fatty diarrheal stools
K. Chronic inflammatory disease of the small intestine, most often the terminal ileum
L. Acute inflammation of the stomach and intestines

#2. For each statement, specify if the statement is **true (T)** or **false (F)**.

_____1. Ulcerative colitis and Crohn's disease are the two most common acute inflammatory bowel diseases that affect adults.

_____2. In patients who have undiagnosed or untreated peritonitis, fluid is shifted from the extracellular fluid compartment into the peritoneal cavity, connective tissues, and GI tract.

_____3. Peritonitis is a significant postoperative complication that has a mortality rate of up to 50%.

_____4. Perforation of the appendix results in peritonitis with a temperature of greater than 101°F (38.3°C) and a rise in heart rate.

_____5. Norovirus, which is spread via the respiratory route, is the leading foodborne disease that causes gastroenteritis.

_____6. Older adults with ulcerative colitis are at high risk for impaired fluid and electrolyte balance because of diarrhea, including dehydration and hypokalemia.

_____7. Extraintestinal manifestations of ulcerative colitis include migratory polyarthritis, ankylosing spondylitis, and erythema nodosum.

_____8. Patients with Crohn's disease can become very malnourished and debilitated because of intestinal malabsorption of dietary nutrients.

_____9. Fistula formation is a common complication of ulcerative colitis but is rare in patients who have Crohn's disease.

____10. Examples of complications of ulcerative colitis and Crohn's disease include colorectal cancer, bowel obstruction, hemorrhage, and abscesses.

## Activities

### Activity #1

List three health teaching points the nurse would provide to help prevent the transmission of gastroenteritis.

1. _____

2. _____

3. _____

## Activity #2

For each statement, specify if the statement is **true (T)** or **false (F)**.

_____1. The patient with suspected or confirmed appendicitis should not receive laxatives or enemas, which can cause perforation of the appendix.

_____2. The most classic indication of peritonitis is a rigid, board like abdomen.

_____3. Handwashing and sanitizing surfaces and other environmental items help prevent the spread of gastroenteritis.

_____4. A decreased WBC count, C-reactive protein, or erythrocyte sedimentation rate (ESR) is consistent with bowel inflammation.

_____5. An ileostomy is a procedure in which a loop of the ileum is placed through an opening in the abdominal wall (stoma) for drainage of fecal material into a pouching system worn at all times on the abdomen.

_____6. For patients with a permanent ileostomy, a community ostomy support group can be located by contacting the United Ostomy Associations of America.

_____7. A combination of drug and nutrition therapy with rest is used to decrease the inflammation associated with diverticular disease.

_____8. While diverticulitis is active, provide a high-fiber diet; when the inflammation resolves, provide a low-fiber diet.

_____9. Biologic response modifiers (BRMs) inhibit tumor necrosis factor (TNF)-alpha, which decreases the inflammatory response in patients who have Crohn's disease.

____10. Patients with Crohn's disease are at high risk for fistulas, which can cause major nutritional deficits and fluid and electrolyte imbalances.

## Activity #3

Identify at least three factors that help to explain the poor outcomes of care for non-White individuals who have chronic inflammatory bowel disease.

1. _____

2. _____

3. _____

## Activity #4

Match health teaching in Column A with the drug for which it is appropriate in Column B. One or more drug choices in Column B may be used more than once, but all choices should be used.

**Column A**

____1. "Take folic acid supplements while on this drug."

____2. "Avoid large crowds and anyone with an infection."

____3. "Avoid drinking alcohol while taking this medication."

____4. "Be aware that this drug can cause dizziness."

____5. "Report any neurologic changes immediately to the prescriber."

____6. "Report any injection site reaction, including redness, to the prescriber."

**Column B**

A. Infliximab

B. Metronidazole

C. Natalizumab

D. Paromomycin

E. Sulfasalazine

**Activity #5**
Identify four teaching points that the nurse would include when teaching a patient and family how to care for an ileostomy at home.

1. _____

2. _____

3. _____

4. _____

## Learning Assessments

### NCLEX Examination Challenge #1
The nurse reviews laboratory results for a client diagnosed with Crohn's disease. Which of the following laboratory tests indicating inflammation would the nurse expect to be elevated? **Select all that apply.**
A.   White blood cell count
B.   Blood urea nitrogen
C.   Erythrocyte sedimentation rate
D.   C-reactive protein
E.   Serum creatinine

### NCLEX Examination Challenge #2
The nurse is caring for a client experiencing lower GI bleeding resulting from ulcerative colitis. For which potentially life-threatening complication would the nurse monitor?
A.   Pernicious anemia
B.   Hypovolemic shock
C.   Pulmonary embolus
D.   Toxic megacolon

### NCLEX Examination Challenge #3
The nurse is teaching a client about the special needs for care of an ileostomy. Which statement would the nurse **include** in the health teaching?
A.   "Perform frequent skin care because the effluent contains many enzymes and bile salts, which can quickly irritate and excoriate your skin."
B.   "You won't need to wear a pouch all the time because the stool will be solid or pasty."
C.   "There are no restrictions for your diet except to be sure to consume high-fiber foods to prevent constipation."
D.   "You won't be able to have sexual intercourse while wearing the pouch, but you will be able to find other ways to be intimate."

**NGN Challenge #1**

The nurse is caring for a 36-year-old client who has an exacerbation of Crohn's disease.

| Vital Signs | Nurses Notes | Orders | Laboratory Results |
|---|---|---|---|

**1635:** Client admitted yesterday with Crohn's disease and unintentional weight loss of 10 lb (4.5 kg) during the past 30 days. New open area on skin near umbilicus draining copious effluent; urgent care transferred client to acute medical unit. Pouch in place over draining open area. Reports abdominal pain at 6/10 this afternoon and three diarrheal stools so far today. States has no appetite but pushing to eat "a little something." Dietitian consult today. BMI currently 18.1. IV site intact for continuous fluids.

| Nurses Notes | Flow Sheet | Orders | Laboratory Results |
|---|---|---|---|

| Parameter | 0900 Today | 2000 Yesterday | 0800 Yesterday |
|---|---|---|---|
| T (oral) | 101.4°F (38.6°C) | 101°F (38.3°C) | 100.6°F ( 38.1°C) |
| HR | 100 beats/min | 96 beats/min | 90 beats/min |
| RR | 20 breaths/min | 18 breaths/min | 18 breaths/min |
| BP | 106/62 mm Hg | 108/66 mm Hg | 112/65 mm Hg |
| SpO$_2$ | 95% on RA | 97% on RA | 97% on RA |
| Weight | 125 lb (56.7 kg) | —— | 126 lb (57.2 kg) |
| WBC count* | 19,500 mm$^3$ (19.5 × 10$^9$/L) | —— | 18,350 mm$^3$ (18.35 × 10$^9$/L) |

*Normal WBC: 5000–10,000 mm$^3$ (5–10 × 10$^9$/L).

Complete the sentence with the options listed below.

The nurse analyzes the client data and determines that the client has (a) __1 [Select]___, which could lead to ___2 [Select]___.

| Option 1 | Option 2 |
|---|---|
| Malnutrition | Gangrene |
| Fissure | Sepsis |
| Toxic megacolon | Cachexia |
| Fistula | Acute kidney injury |

**NGN Challenge #2**
The nurse is caring for a 72-year-old client who presents to the ED.

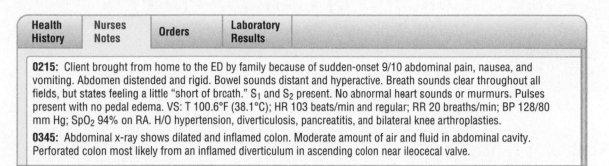

| Health History | Nurses Notes | Orders | Laboratory Results | |
|---|---|---|---|---|

**0215:** Client brought from home to the ED by family because of sudden-onset 9/10 abdominal pain, nausea, and vomiting. Abdomen distended and rigid. Bowel sounds distant and hyperactive. Breath sounds clear throughout all fields, but states feeling a little "short of breath." $S_1$ and $S_2$ present. No abnormal heart sounds or murmurs. Pulses present with no pedal edema. VS: T 100.6°F (38.1°C); HR 103 beats/min and regular; RR 20 breaths/min; BP 128/80 mm Hg; $SpO_2$ 94% on RA. H/O hypertension, diverticulosis, pancreatitis, and bilateral knee arthroplasties.

**0345:** Abdominal x-ray shows dilated and inflamed colon. Moderate amount of air and fluid in abdominal cavity. Perforated colon most likely from an inflamed diverticulum in ascending colon near ileocecal valve.

Complete the diagram by selecting from the choices to specify what **one** condition the client is most likely experiencing, **two** actions the nurse would take to address that condition, and **two** parameters the nurse would monitor to assess the client's progress.

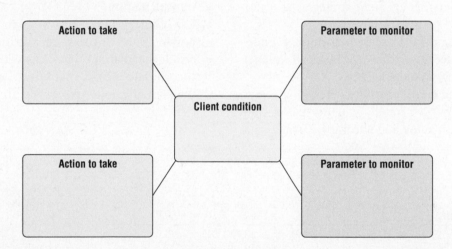

| **Actions to Take** | **Client Condition** | **Parameters to Monitor** |
|---|---|---|
| Administer supplemental oxygen therapy via NC. | Crohn's disease | Serum electrolytes |
| Make client NPO and start peripheral IV access. | Chronic pancreatitis | Red blood cell count |
| Insert an indwelling urinary catheter. | Intestinal obstruction | Gastric pH |
| Prepare the client for surgery immediately. | Peritonitis | Vital signs |
| Administer broad-spectrum antibiotic therapy. | //////////////////////////////// //////////////////////////////// | Urinary output |

# 50
CHAPTER

# *Concepts of Care for Patients with Liver Conditions*

## LEARNING OUTCOMES

1. Plan collaborative care with the interprofessional team to manage inflammation and infection in patients with hepatitis.
2. Teach adults how to decrease the risk for hepatitis.
3. Teach the patient and caregiver(s) about common drugs and other management strategies used for liver disease.
4. Plan patient- and family-centered nursing interventions to decrease the psychosocial impact caused by living with cirrhosis.
5. Apply knowledge of anatomy, physiology, and pathophysiology to provide evidence-based care for patients with acute and chronic hepatitis.

6. Analyze assessment and diagnostic findings to generate solutions and prioritize nursing care for patients who have advanced cirrhosis.
7. Organize care coordination and transition management for patients having surgery for liver transplantation.
8. Use clinical judgment to plan evidence-based nursing care to promote nutrition and manage cellular regulation in patients with cirrhosis.
9. Incorporate factors that affect health equity into the plan of care for patients with liver cancer and cirrhosis.

## Preliminary Reading

Read and review Chapter 50, pp. 1217–1239.

## Chapter Review

### Pathophysiology Review

#1. Match the Key Term in Column A with its definition in Column B.

**Column A**

\_\_\_\_1. Ascites
\_\_\_\_2. Asterixis
\_\_\_\_3. Cirrhosis
\_\_\_\_4. Ecchymosis
\_\_\_\_5. Hepatitis
\_\_\_\_6. Hepatomegaly
\_\_\_\_7. Icterus
\_\_\_\_8. Jaundice
\_\_\_\_9. Petechiae
\_\_\_10. Splenomegaly

**Column B**

A. Yellow coloration of the eye sclerae
B. A disease characterized by widespread fibrotic bands that cause major liver damage
C. Enlarged spleen
D. Yellowish coloration of the skin
E. Collection of free fluid in the peritoneal cavity
F. Inflammation and infection of the liver
G. Round, pinpoint, red-purple hemorrhagic lesions
H. Coarse tremor characterized by rapid hand flapping
I. Liver enlargement
J. Large purple, blue, or yellow bruises

#2. For each statement, specify if the statement is **true (T)** or **false (F)**.

\_\_\_\_1. During early cirrhosis, the liver is usually enlarged and firm.
\_\_\_\_2. Portal hypertension can result in ascites (excessive abdominal [peritoneal] fluid) and prominent abdominal veins.
\_\_\_\_3. Esophageal varices occur when fragile, thin-walled esophageal veins become distended and tortuous from increased portal venous pressure.
\_\_\_\_4. Two of the most common causes of cirrhosis are chronic hepatitis C infection and chronic alcohol use.
\_\_\_\_5. Hepatitis A is the leading cause of cirrhosis and liver cancer in the United States.
\_\_\_\_6. Hepatic encephalopathy may develop slowly in patients with chronic liver disease and go undetected until the later stages.
\_\_\_\_7. Nonalcoholic fatty liver disease is primarily associated with obesity, increased levels of cholesterol and triglycerides, type 2 diabetes mellitus, and metabolic syndrome.
\_\_\_\_8. Chronic hepatitis usually occurs due to hepatitis B virus (HBV) or hepatitis C virus (HCV).
\_\_\_\_9. Scarring from chronic *infection* with either HBV or HCV frequently leads to cirrhosis, which is a risk factor for developing primary liver cancer.
\_\_\_10. Chronic hepatitis A is the most common reason for liver transplants.

## Activities

### Activity #1

List three health teaching points the nurse would provide to help prevent hepatitis A.

1. _____

2. _____

3. _____

## Activity #2

For each statement, specify if the statement is **true (T)** or **false (F).**

_____1.  The patient with early abdominal ascites from cirrhosis is typically placed on a low-sodium diet.

_____2.  Patients with early-stage cirrhosis are typically malnourished and have multiple dietary deficiencies.

_____3.  A paracentesis is an invasive procedure performed to remove abdominal fluid.

_____4.  Nurses should monitor patients for hepatic encephalopathy, which may occur after a transjugular intrahepatic portosystemic shunt (TIPS).

_____5.  The incidence of hepatitis A and hepatitis B is declining as a result of CDC recommendations for vaccination.

_____6.  The *Healthy People 2030* initiative calls for a reduction in deaths from cirrhosis and appropriate management of individuals with hepatitis C.

_____7.  Prothrombin time/international normalized ratio (PT/INR) is prolonged because the liver decreases the production of prothrombin in patients who have cirrhosis.

_____8.  All patients with ascites have the potential to develop spontaneous bacterial peritonitis (SBP) from bacteria in the collected ascitic fluid.

_____9.  Patients with chronic HBV infection often have extrahepatic complications, such as heart disease, polyarthritis, and cognitive impairment.

____10.  For the patient who has undergone liver transplantation, the nurse monitors for clinical signs and symptoms of rejection, such as tachycardia, fever, pain in the right upper quadrant or flank, and jaundice.

## Activity #3

Identify three populations who should receive the hepatitis B vaccine.

1. _____

2. _____

3. _____

## Activity #4

Match the drug in Column A with why it is used for liver conditions in Column B. One or more choices in Column B may be used more than once.

**Column A**

___1.  Propranolol

___2.  Octreotide

___3.  Lactulose

___4.  Cyclosporin A

___5.  Tenofovir

___6.  Furosemide

___7.  Glecaprevir

___8.  Sofosbuvir/velpatasvir

**Column B**

A.  Used to treat hepatitis C infection

B.  Helps to prevent organ transplant rejection

C.  Decreases excess body fluid

D.  Helps prevent bleeding

E.  Used to treat hepatitis B infection

F.  Reduces blood flow by vasoconstriction

G.  Promotes ammonia excretion from the body

## Learning Assessments

### NCLEX Examination Challenge #1

The nurse is caring for a client recently admitted with end-stage liver disease. Which of the following assessment findings would the nurse anticipate for this client? **Select all that apply.**

A. Ascites
B. Jaundice
C. Petechiae
D. Ecchymosis
E. Pruritis
F. Palmar erythema

### NCLEX Examination Challenge #2

The nurse is caring for a client who had a liver transplant 2 days ago. Which client finding would the nurse report to the surgeon **immediately**?

A. Abdominal discomfort since surgery
B. Temperature of 99°F (37.2°C)
C. Nausea and vomiting
D. Elevated liver enzymes

## NGN Challenge

### Item #1

The nurse is caring for a 56-year-old client who was admitted 2 days ago with advanced cirrhosis and esophageal varices.

| Vital Signs | Nurses Notes | Orders | Laboratory Results | |
|---|---|---|---|---|

**1955:** States feeling a "little short of breath" after walking back to bed from the bathroom. Does not usually have this problem except when walking up stairs. States waiting for partner to come to take client home soon to sleep in own bed. Alert and oriented × 1 (to person only); oriented × 4 yesterday. Forgot about being admitted to the hospital. Reoriented to place and time. No adventitious breath sounds. $S_1$ and $S_2$ present; no abnormal heart sounds or murmurs. Severe abdominal distention with distant bowel sounds × 4; abdominal girth increased when compared with yesterday. All peripheral pulses palpable; 1+ bilateral pedal edema. Skin jaundice and icterus present. Reports itchy and dry skin that has worsened with age. VS: T 98°F (36.7°C); HR 89 beats/min; RR 24 breaths/min; BP 140/88 mm Hg; $SpO_2$ 94% on RA.

For each body system listed, click or specify (with an **X**) the client finding that would be of **immediate** concern to the nurse. Each body system **may support more than one finding**.

| Body System | Client Finding |
|---|---|
| Neurologic | o Alert<br>o Oriented ×1 (person)<br>o Forgetfulness |
| Gastrointestinal | o Jaundice<br>o Increased abdominal girth<br>o Distal bowel sounds ×4 |
| Respiratory | o Shortness of breath<br>o RR 24 breaths/min<br>o $SpO_2$ 94% on RA |

*Item #2*

The nurse is caring for a 56-year-old client who was admitted 2 days ago with advanced cirrhosis and esophageal varices.

| Vital Signs | Nurses Notes | Orders | Laboratory Results | |
|---|---|---|---|---|

**1955:** States feeling a "little short of breath" after walking back to bed from the bathroom. Does not usually have this problem except when walking up stairs. States waiting for partner to come to take client home soon to sleep in own bed. Alert and oriented × 1 (to person only); oriented × 4 yesterday. Forgot about being admitted to the hospital. Reoriented to place and time. No adventitious breath sounds. $S_1$ and $S_2$ present; no abnormal heart sounds or murmurs. Severe abdominal distention with distant bowel sounds × 4; abdominal girth increased when compared with yesterday. All peripheral pulses palpable; 1+ bilateral pedal edema. Skin jaundice and icterus present. Reports itchy and dry skin that has worsened with age. VS: T 98°F (36.7°C); HR 89 beats/min; RR 24 breaths/min; BP 140/88 mm Hg; $SpO_2$ 94% on RA.

The nurse analyzes the relevant assessment findings to determine the client's current conditions. Select **four** conditions that the client likely has at this time.

- Upper GI bleeding
- Hepatic encephalopathy
- Respiratory distress
- Heart failure
- Hypertension
- Pruritis

*Item #3*

The nurse is caring for a 56-year-old client who was admitted 2 days ago with advanced cirrhosis and esophageal varices.

| Vital Signs | Nurses Notes | Orders | Laboratory Results | |
|---|---|---|---|---|

**1955:** States feeling a "little short of breath" after walking back to bed from the bathroom. Does not usually have this problem except when walking up stairs. States waiting for partner to come to take client home soon to sleep in own bed. Alert and oriented × 1 (to person only); oriented × 4 yesterday. Forgot about being admitted to the hospital. Reoriented to place and time. No adventitious breath sounds. $S_1$ and $S_2$ present; no abnormal heart sounds or murmurs. Severe abdominal distention with distant bowel sounds × 4; abdominal girth increased when compared with yesterday. All peripheral pulses palpable; 1+ bilateral pedal edema. Skin jaundice and icterus present. Reports itchy and dry skin that has worsened with age. VS: T 98°F (36.7°C); HR 89 beats/min; RR 24 breaths/min; BP 140/88 mm Hg; $SpO_2$ 94% on RA.

Complete the sentence to fill in the blank using the lists of options listed below.

The nurse determines that the *priority* for the care at this time is to manage the client's_____1 [**Select**]_____ as evidenced by ___2 [**Select**]_____ and _____3 [**Select**]_____.

| Options for 1 | Options for 2 | Options for 3 |
|---|---|---|
| Hepatic encephalopathy | Shortness of breath | Pedal edema |
| Respiratory distress | Tachycardia | Jaundice |
| Heart failure | Elevated blood pressure | Increased abdominal girth |
| Hypertension | Disorientation | Increased respiratory rate |

*Item #4*

The nurse is caring for a 56-year-old client who was admitted 2 days ago with advanced cirrhosis and esophageal varices.

| Vital Signs | Nurses Notes | Orders | Laboratory Results | |
|---|---|---|---|---|

**1955:** States feeling a "little short of breath" after walking back to bed from the bathroom. Does not usually have this problem except when walking up stairs. Reports feeling very drowsy this evening. States waiting for partner to come to take client home soon to sleep in own bed. Alert and oriented × 1 (to person only); oriented × 4 yesterday. Forgot about being admitted to the hospital. Reoriented to place and time. No adventitious breath sounds. $S_1$ and $S_2$ present; no abnormal sounds or murmurs. Severe abdominal distention with distant bowel sounds × 4; abdominal girth increased when compared with yesterday. All peripheral pulses palpable; 1+ bilateral pedal edema. Skin jaundice and icterus present. Reports itchy and dry skin that has worsened with age. VS: T 98°F (36.7°C); HR 89 beats/min; RR 24 breaths/min; B/P 140/88 mm Hg; $SpO_2$ 94% on RA.

**2103:** Alert and oriented × 2. States feeling more shortness of breath while trying to rest and having difficulty finding a comfortable position. VS: T 98.8°F (37.1°C); HR 92 beats/min; RR 26 breaths/min; BP 144/90; $SpO_2$ 93% on RA.

For each potential nursing action, indicate if it is **Indicated** (appropriate for the client at this time to meet expected outcomes) or **Not Indicated** (not appropriate for the client to meet expected outcomes).

| Potential Nursing Actions | Indicated | Not Indicated |
|---|---|---|
| Initiate supplemental oxygen therapy. | | |
| Place the client in a sitting or high-Fowler's position. | | |
| Administer analgesic medication. | | |
| Reorient the client frequentl.y | | |
| Monitor respiratory rate and $SpO_2$ frequently. | | |

*Item #5*

The nurse is caring for a 56-year-old client who was admitted 3 days ago with advanced cirrhosis and esophageal varices.

| Vital Signs | Nurses Notes | Orders | Laboratory Results | |
|---|---|---|---|---|

**Yesterday**

**1955:** States feeling a "little short of breath" after walking back to bed from the bathroom. Does not usually have this problem except when walking up stairs. Reports feeling very drowsy this evening. States waiting for partner to come to take client home soon to sleep in own bed. Alert and oriented × 1 (to person only); oriented × 4 yesterday. Forgot about being admitted to the hospital. Reoriented to place and time. No adventitious breath sounds. $S_1$ and $S_2$ present; no abnormal sounds or murmurs. Severe abdominal distention with distant bowel sounds × 4; abdominal girth increased when compared to yesterday. All peripheral pulses palpable; 1+ bilateral pedal edema. Skin jaundice and icterus present. Reports itchy and dry skin that has worsened with age. VS: T 98°F (36.7°C); HR 89 beats/min; RR 24 breaths/min; BP 140/88 mm Hg; $SpO_2$ 94% on RA.

**2103:** Alert and oriented × 2. States feeling more shortness of breath while trying to rest and having difficulty finding a comfortable position. VS: T 98.8°F (37.1°C); HR 92 beats/min; RR 26 breaths/min; BP 144/90; $SpO_2$ 93% on RA.

**2245:** Oxygen therapy at 3 L/min via NC started. $SpO_2$ 96%.

**Today**

**0610:** Drowsy and oriented × 1 (to person only). States breathing seems "a little easier" while in bed since $O_2$ initiated but sweating profusely. Continues to have shortness of breath when walking to bathroom. Instructed to call for assistance before getting OOB. VS: T 100.4°F (38°C); HR 100 beats/min; RR 26 breaths/min; BP 138/86; $SpO_2$ 94% on $O_2$ at 3 L/min.

Which of the following orders would the nurse anticipate from the primary health care provider based on the latest client findings? **Select all that apply.**

- Begin IV antibiotic therapy.
- Prepare client for paracentesis.
- Prepare client for transfer to ICU.
- Insert nasogastric tube for decompression.
- Draw stat ammonia level.
- Type and crossmatch two units packed RBCs.

*Item #6*

A 56-year-old client with advanced cirrhosis and esophageal varices was taken by family to the primary health care provider's office for follow-up a week after hospital discharge. The nurse reviews the initial Nurses' Notes from the hospital to compare with client findings today.

| Vital Signs | Nurses Notes | Orders | Laboratory Results | |
|---|---|---|---|---|

**Yesterday**

**1955:** States feeling a "little short of breath" after walking back to bed from the bathroom. Does not usually have this problem except when walking up stairs. States waiting for partner to come to take client home soon to sleep in own bed. Alert and oriented × 1 (to person only); oriented × 4 yesterday. Forgot about being admitted to the hospital. Reoriented to place and time. No adventitious breath sounds. $S_1$ and $S_2$ present; no abnormal sounds or murmurs. Severe abdominal distention with distant bowel sounds × 4; abdominal girth increased when compared with yesterday. All peripheral pulses palpable, 1+ bilateral pedal edema. Skin jaundice and icterus present. Reports itchy and dry skin that has worsened with age. VS: T 98°F (36.7°C); HR 89 beats/min; RR 24 breaths/min; BP 140/88 mm Hg; $SpO_2$ 94% on RA.

**2103:** Alert and oriented × 2. States feeling more shortness of breath while trying to rest and having difficulty finding a comfortable position. VS: T 98.8°F (37.1°C); HR 92 beats/min; RR 26 breaths/min; BP 144/90; $SpO_2$ 92% on RA.

**2245:** Oxygen therapy at 3 L/min via NC started. $SpO_2$ 96%.

**0610:** Drowsy and oriented × 1 (to person only). States breathing seems "a little easier" while in bed since $O_2$ initiated but sweating profusely. Continues to have shortness of breath when walking to bathroom. Instructed to call for assistance before getting OOB. VS: T 100.4°F (38°C); HR 100 beats/min; RR 26 breaths/min; BP 138/86 mm Hg; $SpO_2$ 93% on $O_2$ at 3 L/min.

Based on current client findings listed, indicate if the client is **Improving** or **Not Improving**.

| Current Client Findings | Improving | Not Improving |
|---|---|---|
| Alert and oriented ×4 | | |
| Uses continuous ambulatory oxygen therapy | | |
| T 98.4°F (36.9°C) | | |
| RR 20 breaths/min | | |
| $SpO_2$ 97% on $O_2$ at 2 L/min | | |

# 51 CHAPTER

# *Concepts of Care for Patients with Conditions of the Biliary System and Pancreas*

## LEARNING OUTCOMES

1. Plan collaborative care with the interprofessional team to manage inflammation and pain in patients with pancreatitis.
2. Teach adults how to decrease the risk for acute pancreatitis.
3. Teach the patient and caregiver(s) about common drugs and other management strategies used for pancreatic cancer.
4. Plan patient- and family-centered nursing interventions to decrease the psychosocial impact caused by living with pancreatic disorders.
5. Apply knowledge of anatomy, physiology, and pathophysiology to provide evidence-based care for patients with cholecystitis.
6. Analyze assessment and diagnostic findings to generate solutions and prioritize nursing care for patients who have pancreatitis.
7. Organize care coordination and transition management for patients having surgery for cholecystitis.
8. Use clinical judgment to plan evidence-based nursing care to promote nutrition and manage inflammation in patients with pancreatitis.
9. Incorporate factors that affect health equity into the plan of care for patients with pancreatic cancer.

## Preliminary Reading

Read and review Chapter 51, pp. 1240–1261.

## Chapter Review

### Pathophysiology Review

#1. Match the Key Term in Column A with its definition in Column B.

| Column A | Column B |
|---|---|
| ___1. Biliary colic | A. Belching |
| ___2. Cholecystitis | B. Surgical removal of the spleen |
| ___3. Cholelithiasis | C. Inflammation of the gallbladder |
| ___4. Chronic pancreatitis | D. Condition in which infected pancreatic fluid is walled off by fibrous tissue |
| ___5. Eructation | E. Severe right upper abdominal pain caused by duct obstruction or gallstones |
| ___6. Pancreatic pseudocyst | F. Complication of cholecystectomy that causes severe pain and vomiting |
| ___7. Postcholecystectomy syndrome | G. Gallstones |
| ___8. Splenectomy | H. Progressive, destructive disease of the pancreas that has remissions and exacerbations |

#2. For each statement, specify if the statement is **true (T)** or **false (F)**.

_____1. Cholecystitis may be acute or chronic.

_____2. Obesity is a major risk factor for cholelithiasis, especially in women.

_____3. In chronic pancreatitis, four major pathophysiologic processes occur: lipolysis, proteolysis, necrosis of blood vessels, and inflammation.

_____4. The hallmark of pancreatic necrosis is fat necrosis of the cells of the pancreas caused by the enzyme lipase.

_____5. Two life-threatening complications of chronic pancreatitis are infection, causing septic shock, and hemorrhage, causing necrotizing hemorrhagic pancreatitis.

_____6. Two of the most common causes of acute pancreatitis are gallstones and alcohol use.

_____7. Chronic calcifying pancreatitis is primarily caused by alcoholism.

_____8. Venous thromboembolism is a common complication of pancreatic cancer.

_____9. Pancreatic cancer often presents in a slow and vague manner.

___10. The head of the pancreas is the most common site for pancreatic cancer.

## Activities

### Activity #1

List three health teaching points the nurse would provide to help prevent biliary and pancreatic conditions.

1. _____

2. _____

3. _____

### Activity #2

Complete each sentence with the appropriate word(s).

1. A complication associated with cholecystitis caused by cholelithiasis is _____ resulting from biliary obstruction.

2. _____ of the right upper quadrant is the best initial diagnostic test for cholecystitis.

3. The primary symptom of clients who have acute pancreatitis is severe _____.

4. A gray-blue discoloration of the abdomen and periumbilical area is associated with acute _____.

5. In patients with acute pancreatitis, _____ levels usually increase within 12 to 24 hours and remain elevated for 2 to 3 days.

6. The nurse carefully monitors the patient who has acute pancreatitis for respiratory distress because of the possible development of _____.

7. _____ is the standard of care to prevent malnutrition, malabsorption, and excessive weight loss in patients who have chronic pancreatitis.

8. Because of the normal endocrine function of the pancreas, patients who have chronic pancreatitis often develop _____.

9. The _____ procedure is an extensive surgical procedure used most often to treat cancer of the head of the pancreas.

10. The development of a _____ is the most common and most serious postoperative complication of surgery for pancreatic cancer.

## Activity #3

Match the client findings that the nurse should assess in Column A with the client condition with which they are associated in Column B. Conditions in Column B will be used more than once.

**Column A**

___1.   Steatorrhea
___2.   Polyuria
___3.   Acute boring abdominal pain
___4.   Polyphagia
___5.   Highly elevated amylase
___6.   Highly elevated lipase
___7.   Polydipsia

**Column B**

A.   Acute pancreatitis
B.   Chronic pancreatitis

## Activity #4

Identify at least three factors that help to explain the poor outcomes of care for non-White individuals who have pancreatic conditions.

1.  _____

2.  _____

3.  _____

## Learning Assessments

### NCLEX Examination Challenge #1

The nurse is caring for a client who is experiencing severe pain as a result of biliary colic. What is the nurse's **priority** for this client's care?

A.   Assess pain intensity level.
B.   Monitor for signs and symptoms of shock.
C.   Place the client flat in a supine position.
D.   Administer a dose of ursodiol.

### NCLEX Examination Challenge #2

The nurse is caring for a client admitted for acute pancreatitis. What is the nurse's **priority** for this client's care?

A.   Providing nutritional support
B.   Monitoring pancreatic enzyme levels
C.   Managing severe pain
D.   Administering oxygen therapy

## NGN Challenge #1

The nurse reviews the Nurses, Notes and selected Laboratory Results for a 45-year-old client admitted for abdominal pain and anorexia.

| Vital Signs | Nurses Notes | Orders | Laboratory Results | |
|---|---|---|---|---|

**0730:** Admitted to the ED with report of severe abdominal pain that has been continuous since yesterday. Pain radiates to right shoulder or back. Very restless with current reported pain of 10/10. Lying in fetal position. History of cholecystitis, cholelithiasis, GERD, and hypertension. Alert and oriented × 4 but moaning at times. No adventitious breath sounds. $S_1$ and $S_2$ present. Hyperactive bowel sounds × 4. VS: T 99.8°F (37.7°C); HR 89 beats/min; RR 24 breaths/min; BP 158/92 mm Hg; $SpO_2$ 95% on RA. Stat labs drawn.

| Nurses Notes | Laboratory Results | Orders | Vital Signs | |
|---|---|---|---|---|

| Laboratory Test | Result | Normal Range |
|---|---|---|
| WBC total | 19,000 mm³ ($19 \times 10^9$/L) | 5,000–10,000 mm³ ($5–10 \times 10^9$/L) |
| Sodium (Na) | 142 mEq/L (142 mmol/L) | 136–142 mEq/L (136–142 mmol/L) |
| Potassium (K) | 4.3 mEq/L (4.3 mmol/L) | 3.5–5.0 mEq/L (3.5–5.0 mmol/L) |
| Chloride (Cl) | 104 mEq/L (104 mmol/L) | 98–106 mEq/L (98–106 mmol/L) |
| Carbon dioxide | 28 mEq/L (28 mmol/L) | 23–30 mEq/L (23–30 mmol/L) |
| BUN | 26 mg/dL (9.28 mmol/L) | 10–20 mg/dL (3.6–7.1 mmol/L) |
| Creatinine | 1.1 mg/dL (75 mmol/L) | 0.5–1.1 mg/dL (22–75 mmol/L) |
| Glucose | 104 mg/dL (5.78 mmol/L) | 74–106 mg/dL (4.1–5.9 mmol/L) |
| ALT | 75 units/L (75 units/L) | 4–36 units/L (4–36 units/L) |
| Amylase | 415 IU/dL (415 units/L) | 60–120 IU/dL (60–120 units/L) |
| Lipase | 182 units/L (182 units/L) | 0–160 units/L (0–160 units/L) |
| ESR | 64 mm/h (64 mm/h) | 0–20 mm/h (0–20 mm/h) |

Complete the diagram by selecting from the choices to specify what **one** condition the client is most likely experiencing, **two** actions the nurse would take to address that condition, and **two** parameters the nurse would monitor to assess the client's progress.

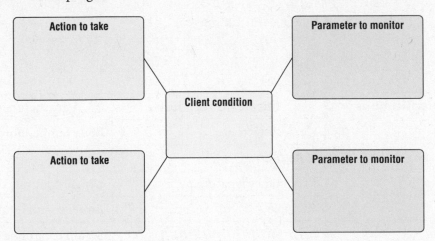

| Actions to Take | Client Condition | Parameters to Monitor |
|---|---|---|
| Administer analgesic medication. | Biliary colic | Serum pancreatic enzyme levels |
| Prepare client for surgery. | Chronic pancreatitis | Cardiac rate and rhythm |

| Actions to Take | Client Condition | Parameters to Monitor |
|---|---|---|
| Initiate supplemental oxygen therapy. | Pancreatic cancer | Pain intensity level |
| Make client NPO and insert NGT. | Acute pancreatitis | Body temperature |
| Administer antibiotic therapy. | ///////////////////////////////// | Serum creatinine and BUN |

### NGN Challenge #2
The nurse is caring for a 63-year-old client in the critical care unit.

| Health History | Nurses Notes | Orders | Laboratory Results |
|---|---|---|---|

**0453:** Returned from PACU after radical surgery to treat pancreatic cancer. Current pain described as 8/10. Very drowsy but can arouse. Abdominal dressing intact. NGT to low continuous suction draining greenish yellow effluent. No adventitious breath sounds. BS absent × 4. VS: T 98°F (36.7°C); HR 81 beats/min; RR 18 breaths/min; BP 106/54; SpO$_2$ 100% on O$_2$ 4 L/min via NC.

Complete the diagram by selecting from the choices to specify what **one** surgery the client most likely had, **two** possible postoperative complications for which the nurse would monitor, and **two** assessments the nurse would perform to monitor for these complications.

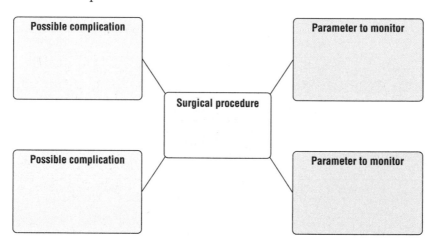

| Possible Complications | Surgical Procedure | Parameters to Monitor |
|---|---|---|
| Diabetes mellitus | Cholecystectomy | Body temperature and pain |
| Acute kidney injury | Colostomy | Blood glucose |
| Diabetes insipidus | Exploratory laparotomy | Urinary output |
| Sepsis | Whipple | Bowel sounds and flatus |
| Bowel obstruction | ///////////////////////////////// | Serum creatinine |

# 52 CHAPTER

# *Concepts of Care for Patients with Malnutrition: Undernutrition and Obesity*

## LEARNING OUTCOMES

1. Plan collaborative care with the interprofessional team to promote nutrition in patients with malnutrition.
2. Teach adults how to decrease the risk for malnutrition.
3. Teach the patient and caregiver(s) about common drugs and other management strategies used for malnutrition.
4. Plan patient- and family-centered nursing interventions to decrease the psychosocial impact caused by living with malnutrition.
5. Apply knowledge of anatomy, physiology, and pathophysiology to provide evidence-based care for patients with malnutrition affecting fluid and electrolyte balance and nutrition.
6. Analyze assessment and diagnostic findings to generate solutions and prioritize nursing care for patients with malnutrition.
7. Organize care coordination and transition management for patients with malnutrition.
8. Use clinical judgment to plan evidence-based nursing care to promote fluid and electrolyte balance and nutrition and prevent complications in patients with malnutrition.
9. Incorporate factors that affect health equity into the plan of care for patients with (disorder).

## Preliminary Reading

Read and review Chapter 52, pp. 1262–1288.

## Chapter Review

### Pathophysiology Review

#1. Match the Key Term in Column A with its description in Column B.

| Column A | | Column B |
|---|---|---|
| ____1. | Anorexia | A. Eating disorder of self-induced starvation |
| ____2. | Anorexia nervosa | B. Inability to tolerate a food (or foods) |
| ____3. | Bariatrics | C. Life-threatening metabolic state when nutrition is restarted |
| ____4. | Binge eating disorder | D. Extreme body wasting and malnutrition |
| ____5. | Body mass index | E. Measure of nutrition not dependent on frame size |
| ____6. | Body surface area | F. Body fat estimation using triceps and subscapular skinfolds |
| ____7. | Bulimia nervosa | G. Loss of appetite for food |
| ____8. | Cachexia | H. Eating disorder involving binging on food and feelings of loss of control |
| ____9. | Food allergy | I. Food reaction that can be life-threatening |
| ___10. | Food intolerance | J. Calorie malnutrition with body fat and protein wastage |
| ___11. | Kwashiorkor | K. Eating disorder of binging and purging |
| ___12. | Marasmus | L. Factor used for appropriate dosage calculation |
| ___13. | Refeeding syndrome | M. Lack of protein quantity and quality despite adequate caloric intake |
| ___14. | Skinfold measurement | N. Medicine branch that manages patients with obesity and related diseases |

#2. List 10 common complications of obesity.

1. _____

2. _____

3. _____

4. _____

5. _____

6. _____

7. _____

8. _____

9. _____

10. _____

#3. List 10 common complications of undernutrition.

1. _____

2. _____

3. _____

4. _____

5. _____

6. _____

7. _____

8. _____

9. _____

10. _____

## Activities

### Activity #1

For each statement, specify if the statement is **true (T)** or **false (F)**.

_____1. Patients with food intolerances are at risk for anaphylactic events.

_____2. The MNA can be used to screen older adults for nutrition concerns.

_____3. Calculation of body mass index requires the nurse to obtain the patient's height and weight.

_____4. Undernutrition occurs when a person is deficient in one nutrient.

_____5. A full nutrition history includes everything a person consumes in 12 hours.

_____6. Total enteral nutrition is delivered through peripheral venous access.

_____7. Long-term feedings are usually delivered via an enterostomal feeding tube.

_____8. Feeding bags and tubes must be changed every 24 to 48 hours.

_____9. Patients should be elevated at least 45 degrees during tube feedings.

___10. Clogged feeding tubes can be cleared by administration of 8 ounces of clear soda.

**Activity #2**

Using the word bank, fill in the type of foods that should be eaten according to the U.S. Department of Agriculture MyPlate.

| Dairy |
|-------|
| Fruits |
| Grains |
| Proteins |
| Vegetables |

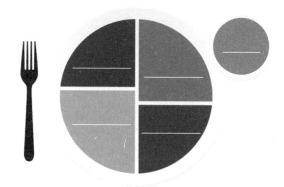

(From U.S. Department of Agriculture. *www.ChooseMyPlate.gov*. https://www.myplate.gov/eat-healthy/what-is-myplate; 2022.)

**Activity #3**

Describe the foods eaten and avoided by each type of vegetarian.

1. Lacto-vegetarian _____

2. Ovo-vegetarian _____

3. Lacto-ovo vegetarian _____

4. Pescatarian _____

5. Vegan _____

## Activity #4

Match the sign or symptom in Column A with the most likely causative nutrient deficiency in Column B.

| Column A | Column B |
|---|---|
| \_\_\_\_1.  Alopecia | A.  Vitamin A |
| \_\_\_\_2.  Conjunctival dryness | B.  Pyridoxine |
| \_\_\_\_3.  Bleeding gums | C.  Vitamin $B_{12}$ |
| \_\_\_\_4.  Bilateral dermatitis | D.  Protein |
| \_\_\_\_5.  Muscle wasting | E.  Vitamin C |
| \_\_\_\_6.  Bone pain | F.  Copper |
| \_\_\_\_7.  Anemia | G.  Zinc |
| \_\_\_\_8.  Cardiac dysrhythmias | H.  Niacin |
| \_\_\_\_9.  Leukopenia | I.  Vitamin D |
| \_\_\_10.  Nausea and vomiting | J.  Magnesium |

## Learning Assessments

### NCLEX Examination Challenge #1

Which action will the nurse take when caring for a client after bariatric surgery to **prevent** complications? **Select all that apply**.

A.   Monitor oxygen saturation.
B.   Apply an abdominal binder.
C.   Place the client in semi-Fowler's position.
D.   Assess skinfolds for redness and excoriation.
E.   Maintain bedrest for the first 24 to 48 hours after surgery.

### NCLEX Examination Challenge #2

Which technique will the nurse teach the family of an 88-year-old female client with severe osteoarthritis, muscle weakness, and dementia to use to improve nutrition? **Select all that apply.**

A.   "Let her feed herself as much as possible even if she uses her fingers."
B.   "Always include some foods that you know she likes for every meal."
C.   "Withhold her pain medications before meals to prevent nausea."
D.   "If she doesn't finish a meal in 20 minutes, take the food away."
E.   "During meals, be sure she has her glasses on and hearing aids in."

### NCLEX Examination Challenge #3

Which assessment will the nurse use as the **most** reliable indicator of a client's fluid status?

A.   Intake and output
B.   Trends in weight
C.   Changes in skin turgor
D.   Presence of dependent edema

**NGN Challenge #1**

A 46-year-old client is being cared for by the nurse on a surgical unit following bariatric surgery yesterday. The nurse reviews and analyzes the flow sheet data since admission to the unit after surgery.

| | 24 Hours After Surgery (1055) | 12 Hours After Surgery (2248) | Admission to Unit Postsurgery (1103) |
|---|---|---|---|
| T | 98.6°F (37.0°C) | 98.4°F (36.9°C) | 98.4°F (36.9°C) |
| HR | 72 beats/min | 74 beats/min | 78 beats/min |
| RR | 18 breaths/min | 16 breaths/min | 18 breaths/min |
| BP | 118/80 mm Hg | 120/76 mm Hg | 106/74 mm Hg |
| SpO$_2$ | 97% (on RA) | 98% (on O$_2$ 2 L/min) | 98% (on O$_2$ 2 L/min) |
| Urinary output | 1482 mL | 1333 mL | 1119 mL |
| Level of consciousness | Easy to arouse; stays awake following assessment; oriented ×4. Walked hallway with support of one assistive personnel. | Easily awakened; oriented ×4. Walked hallway with support of two assistive personnel. | Drowsy but easily awakened; oriented ×4. Resting in bed. |

Based on review of this information, which action will the nurse take at this time? **Select all that apply.**

A. Provide tray with pureed food.
B. Monitor for dumping syndrome.
C. Assess dressing and incision site.
D. Request an order for an antibiotic.
E. Restrict fluid intake to reduce edema.
F. Administer prophylactic anticoagulant.
G. Encourage use of incentive spirometer hourly.
H. Assist client to walk once up and down hallway.

**NGN Challenge #2**

The nurse on a medical unit is preparing to care for an older adult client with nausea and vomiting following radiation treatment. The family reports that the client has lost weight progressively since being diagnosed with cancer and will barely eat anything at this time. She is 5 feet, 3 inches tall (63 cm). An infusion of normal saline is running at 125 cc/hour. She is receiving 8 mg of ondansetron every 8 hours. The nurse reviews data in the electronic health record.

| | Day 3 of Admission | Day 2 of Admission | Day 1 of Admission |
|---|---|---|---|
| T | 98.6°F (37.0°C) | 98.4°F (36.9°C) | 98.4°F (36.9°C) |
| HR | 64 beats/min | 68 beats/min | 62 beats/min |
| RR | 14 breaths/min | 14 breaths/min | 14 breaths/min |
| BP | 90/60 mm Hg | 94/62 mm Hg | 92/66 mm Hg |
| SpO$_2$ | 95% (on RA) | 95% (on O$_2$ 2 L/min) | 96% (on O$_2$ 2 L/min) |
| Weight | 97 pounds (44 kg) | 97.8 pounds (44.4 kg) | 98 pounds (44.5 kg) |

Based this history and assessment, the client is at risk for developing _____ and _____.

| Word Choices |
|---|
| Anorexia Nervosa |
| Dumping Syndrome |
| Kwashiorkor |
| Malnutrition |
| Refeeding Syndrome |
| Undernutrition |

# 53 CHAPTER

# *Assessment of the Endocrine System*

## LEARNING OUTCOMES

1. Use knowledge of anatomy and physiology to perform a focused assessment of the endocrine system.
2. Teach evidence-based health promotion activities to help prevent endocrine health problems or trauma.
3. Identify factors that affect health equity for patients with endocrine health problems.
4. Explain how genetic implications and physiologic aging of the endocrine affect cellular regulation.
5. Interpret assessment findings for patients with a suspected or actual endocrine problem.
6. Plan evidence-based care and support for patients undergoing diagnostic testing of the endocrine system.

## Preliminary Reading

Read and review Chapter 53, pp. 1289–1301.

## Chapter Review

### Anatomy & Physiology Review

#1. Label the parts of the endocrine system using the Anatomy Labels provided after the figures.

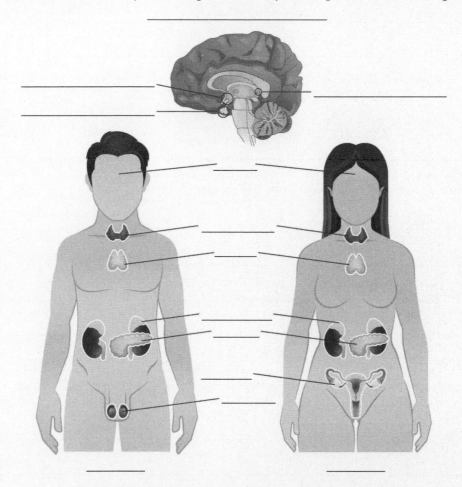

(Used with permission from istockphoto.com, 2020, VectorMine.)

| **Anatomy Labels** |
| --- |
| Adrenal glands |
| Gonads (testes and ovaries) |
| Hypothalamus |
| Pancreas |
| Pineal gland |
| Pituitary gland |
| Thyroid |

#2. Explain how a negative feedback mechanism works.

_____

_____

_____

_____

## Activities

### Activity #1
Explain the key role of each of these components of the endocrine system.

1. Adrenal cortex_____

   _____

2. Adrenal medulla_____

   _____

3. Hypothalamus_____

   _____

4. Pituitary gland_____

   _____

5. Pancreas_____

   _____

6. Parathyroid glands_____

   _____

7. Pineal gland_____

   _____

8. Thyroid gland_____

   _____

## Activity #2

List five changes that occur in the endocrine system that are associated with aging and their associated nursing considerations.

1. _____

2. _____

3. _____

4. _____

5. _____

## Activity #3

Match the component in Column A with its effect in Column B.

**Column A**

____1.  Aldosterone
____2.  Antidiuretic hormone (ADH)
____3.  Epinephrine
____4.  Norepinephrine
____5.  Cortisol
____6.  Insulin
____7.  Thyroxine ($T_4$)
____8.  Triiodothyronine ($T_3$)
____9.  Luteinizing hormone
___10.  Melanocyte-stimulating hormone

**Column B**

A.  Contributes to metabolism with $T_3$
B.  Affects the body's response to stress
C.  Increases glucose uptake by the cells
D.  Acts mainly on beta-adrenergic receptors
E.  Acts mainly on alpha-adrenergic receptors
F.  Contributes to metabolism with $T_4$
G.  Promotes water and electrolyte reabsorption from distal tubules
H.  Maintains extracellular fluid volume and electrolyte composition
I.  Promotes pigmentation
J.  Stimulates testosterone or progesterone secretion

## Activity #4

For each statement, specify if the statement is **true (T)** or **false (F)**.

____1.  The gonads are reproductive endocrine glands that are present at birth.
____2.  Somatostatin inhibits the release of glucagon and insulin from the pancreas.
____3.  PTH activates Vitamin B, which increases the absorption of calcium and phosphorus from the intestines.
____4.  Drug therapy and dietary changes can affect the function of hormones.
____5.  The nurse must assess for thyroid function disruption if a patient has COVID-19.
____6.  Type 2 diabetes occurs when the body destroys the insulin-producing cells in the pancreas.
____7.  Soy products are a good source of dietary iodine.
____8.  A voice change can be indicative of an endocrine problem.
____9.  The patient undergoing a 24-hour urine test should discard their first urine and then begin collecting.
___10.  The glycosylated hemoglobin (A1C) value indicates the average blood glucose level over a period of 1 to 2 weeks.

**Activity #5**

List 10 functions of thyroxine ($T_4$) and triiodothyronine ($T_3$).

1. _____

2. _____

3. _____

4. _____

5. _____

6. _____

7. _____

8. _____

9. _____

10. _____

## Learning Assessments

### NCLEX Examination Challenge #1

Which hormone does the nurse anticipate has decreased in a client with reduced catecholamine levels and decreased cardiac muscle excitability?

A. Insulin
B. Cortisol
C. Oxytocin
D. Glucagon

### NCLEX Examination Challenge #2

Which assessment finding indicates to the nurse the need to assess further for a possible endocrine problem in a 45-year-old client?

A. Received new eyeglasses prescription
B. Father newly diagnosed with prostate cancer
C. Lost 15 pounds in the past 6 weeks without dieting
D. Reports taking oral contraceptives for 2 years without problems

### NCLEX Examination Challenge #3

Which action will the nurse teach to an older female client whose estrogen levels have decreased? **Select all that apply**.

A. Use a skin moisturizer daily.
B. Drink at least 2 L of water daily.
C. Increase your intake of calcium and Vitamin D.
D. Walk a mile a day at least four times per week.
E. Be sure to urinate immediately after sexual intercourse.

# 54 CHAPTER

# *Concepts of Care for Patients with Pituitary and Adrenal Gland Conditions*

## LEARNING OUTCOMES

1. Plan collaborative care with the interprofessional team to promote fluid and electrolyte balance in patients with pituitary and adrenal gland problems.
2. Teach adults how to decrease the risk for pituitary and adrenal gland problems.
3. Teach the patient and caregiver(s) about common drugs and other management strategies used for pituitary and adrenal gland problems.
4. Plan patient- and family-centered nursing interventions to decrease the psychosocial impact caused by living with pituitary and adrenal gland problems.
5. Apply knowledge of anatomy, physiology, and pathophysiology to provide evidence-based care

for patients with pituitary and adrenal gland problems affecting fluid and electrolyte balance.
6. Analyze assessment and diagnostic findings to generate solutions and prioritize nursing care for patients with pituitary and adrenal gland problems.
7. Organize care coordination and transition management for patients with (disorder).
8. Use clinical judgment to plan evidence-based nursing care to promote fluid and electrolyte balance and prevent complications in patients with pituitary and adrenal gland problems.
9. Incorporate factors that affect health equity into the plan of care for patients with pituitary and adrenal gland problems.

## Preliminary Reading

Read and review Chapter 54, pp. 1302–1322.

## Chapter Review

### Pathophysiology Review

#1. Match the Key Term in Column A with its description in Column B.

**Column A**

___1. Acute adrenal insufficiency
___2. Cushing disease
___3. Cushing syndrome
___4. Diabetes insipidus
___5. Hyperaldosteronism
___6. Hypercortisolism
___7. Hyperpituitarism
___8. Syndrome of inappropriate antidiuretic hormone secretion

**Column B**

A. Deficiency of one or more pituitary hormones
B. Secretion of vasopressin even when plasma osmolarity is low or normal
C. A pituitary gland tumor secreting ACTH stimulates overproduction of cortisol
D. Increased secretion of aldosterone with mineralocorticoid excess
E. Life-threatening emergency when body doesn't have enough cortisol and aldosterone
F. Clinical state because of excessive tissue exposure to cortisol and/or glucocorticoids
G. Symptom set caused by excess cortisol sometimes because of ongoing corticosteroid therapy
H. Posterior pituitary gland disorder that causes excessive water loss

#2. List three causes of primary adrenal insufficiency and three causes of secondary adrenal insufficiency.

*Primary*

1. _____

2. _____

3. _____

*Secondary*

1. _____

2. _____

3. _____

#3. Indicate in each box whether the laboratory test will be **high**, **normal to high**, **low**, **normal to low**, or **normal** in the presence of *hypofunction* or *hyperfunction* of the adrenal glands.

| Test | Normal Range | Hypofunction | Hyperfunction |
|---|---|---|---|
| Sodium | 136–145 mEq/L (mmol/L) | | |
| Potassium | 3.5–5.0 mEq/L (mmol/L) | | |
| Glucose (fasting) | 70–110 mg/dL (4–6 mmol/L) | | |
| Calcium | Total: 9–10.5 mg/dL (2.25–2.75 mmol/L) Ionized: 4.5–5.6 mg/dL (1.05–1.30 mmol/L) | | |
| Bicarbonate | 23–30 mEq/L (mmol/L) | | |

| Test | Normal Range | Hypofunction | Hyperfunction |
|---|---|---|---|
| BUN | 10–20 mg/dL (3.6–7.1 mmol/L) | | |
| Cortisol (serum) | 6 a.m. to 8 a.m.: 5–23 mcg/dL (138–635 nmol/L) <br> 4 p.m. to 6 p.m.: 3–13 mcg/dL (83–359 nmol/L) | | |
| Cortisol (salivary) | 7 a.m. to 9 a.m.: 100–750 ng/dL <br> 3 p.m. to 5 p.m.: <401 ng/dL | | |

## Activities

### Activity #1

For each statement, specify if the statement is **true (T)** or **false (F)**.

____1.  Adrenocorticotropic hormone (ACTH) controls release of pituitary hormones.
____2.  Somatostatin is secreted by the hypothalamus.
____3.  In people assigned male at birth, follicle-stimulating hormone stimulates sperm production.
____4.  Release of oocytes is stimulated by luteinizing hormone.
____5.  Oxytocin increases water reabsorption by the kidneys.
____6.  Ejection of breast milk after an infant's birth is stimulated by oxytocin.
____7.  The anterior pituitary secretes antidiuretic hormone.
____8.  The posterior pituitary secretes prolactin.
____9.  Overproduction of growth hormone in adults can lead to acromegaly.
___10.  Prolactin-secreting tumors are the most common type of pituitary adenoma.

### Activity #2

Circle the drugs that can cause syndrome of inappropriate antidiuretic hormone secretion (SIADH).

| | | |
|---|---|---|
| Hydrocodone | Carbamazepine | Fluoxetine |
| Amlodipine | Amitriptyline | Ciprofloxacin |
| Penicillin | Lisinopril | Methoxyflurane |
| Levofloxacin | Halothane | Oxycodone |
| Vincristine | Bupropion | Hydrochlorothiazide |

### Activity #3

List five expected findings in a patient with Cushing syndrome.

1.  _____

2.  _____

3.  _____

4.  _____

5.  _____

**Activity #4**

Fill in each blank to complete the teaching the nurse provides to a patient who has been prescribed cortisol replacement therapy.

- Take your medication with _____ to prevent stomach irritation.
- Weigh yourself _____ and keep a record to show your primary health care provider.
- If you have persistent vomiting or severe diarrhea and cannot take your medication by mouth for _____ to _____ hours, call your primary health care provider.
- Always wear your _____.
- Learn how to self-administer an _____ injection of hydrocortisone in case you cannot take your oral drug.
- Avoid _____ to minimize your chance of getting an infection.

**Learning Assessments**

**NCLEX Examination Challenge #1**

The nurse is caring for a female client receiving hormone replacement therapy with estrogen and progesterone for anterior pituitary hypofunction. Which client statement indicates to the nurse an understanding of drug therapy?
A. "I will switch to vaping instead of smoking cigarettes."
B. "Reducing my use of hot showers and baths may help my dry skin."
C. "If my breast size increases, I will need to have a mammogram done soon."
D. "I will report any leg pain or swelling immediately to my primary health care provider."

**NCLEX Examination Challenge #2**

Which change in a client's condition indicates to the nurse that corticosteroid therapy for acute adrenal insufficiency is effective?
A. Urine output is increased.
B. Client reports not being hungry.
C. Client is alert and oriented.
D. Blood glucose level is 60 mg/dL (3.3 mmol/L).

**NCLEX Examination Challenge #3**

The nurse is caring for a client with syndrome of inappropriate antidiuretic hormone secretion (SIADH) who is on fluid restriction. Which change in laboratory values indicates to the nurse that this intervention is having the desired effect?
A. Decreased hematocrit
B. Increased serum sodium
C. Decreased serum osmolarity
D. Increased urine specific gravity

## NGN Challenge #1

The nurse is reviewing the electronic health record of an 82-year-old client admitted yesterday for a headache rated 8 out of 10 on a 0 to 10 scale and syncope. The client's medical history is positive for generalized anxiety disorder, major depressive disorder, and type 2 diabetes mellitus. She takes sertraline 50 mg daily and metformin 500 mg twice daily. Recently, she began taking oxycodone for chronic back pain that was not resolving with ibuprofen. Surgical history includes bilateral bunionectomy 13 years prior.

| Test | Normal Value | April 23, 2023 2028 | April 23, 2023 0644 | April 22, 2023 1930 |
|---|---|---|---|---|
| Serum sodium | 136–145 mEq/L or 136–145 mmol/L | 118 mEq/L | 124 mEq/L | 132 mEq/L |
| Serum potassium | 3.5–5 mEq/L or 3.5–5 mmol/L | 3.9 | 4.4 | 4.1 |
| Urine pH | 4.6–8 | 7.1 | 6.0 | 6.2 |
| Urine specific gravity | Adult: 1.005–1.03 (usually 1.01–1.025) | 1.040 | 1.029 | 1.020 |
| WBC in urine | 0–4 per low-power field | 2 | 0 | 0 |

Based this history and assessment, the client is at risk for developing _____(1)_____ as evidenced by _____(2)_____.

| Word Choices for 1 |
|---|
| Hyperpituitarism |
| Cushing syndrome |
| Syndrome of inappropriate antidiuretic hormone secretion (SIADH) |
| Acute adrenal insufficiency |

| Word Choices for 2 |
|---|
| History of type 2 diabetes mellitus |
| Potassium value 3.9 mEq/L |
| Urine specific gravity 1.040 |
| 2 WBC in urine |

**NGN Challenge #2**

The nurse coming on shift is reviewing nurses notes from the prior shift for a client on a medical-surgical unit following a motor vehicle crash.

| Vital Signs | Nurses Notes | Health Care Provider's Orders | Laboratory Results | |
|---|---|---|---|---|

**1144:** Admitted to unit following motor vehicle crash. Reports being dizzy and not remembering crash. Can state name, knows she is in the hospital, but cannot remember exact day. Says it is Sunday when it is Monday. Health history positive for COVID-19 9 months prior; she recovered after receiving monoclonal antibody therapy. Other health history unremarkable. Lives at home with her partner who reports that she occasionally drinks a glass of wine but does not use tobacco or illicit drugs. Alert and oriented × 2. PERRLA. HR 62 beats/min, regular without murmur. Lung sounds clear bilaterally. Abdomen nontender. Normal saline infusing at 100 cc/hr. Current VS: T 98.4°F (36.9°C); HR 66 beats/min and regular; RR 16 breaths/min; BP 100/74 mm Hg; SpO$_2$ 97%.

**1310:** Responded to call light pressed by partner who voices concern that client's level of consciousness has changed. Client can give her name after thinking for several seconds. States she is in the hospital after several more seconds. Unable to verbalize day, month, or year. Hands with fine tremors bilaterally. PERRLA. Heart rate 112 beats/min, irregular without murmur. Lung sounds clear bilaterally. Abdomen nontender. Normal saline infusing at 100 cc/hr. Site clean and dry without signs of infection. Current VS: T 98.4°F (36.9°C); HR 112 beats/min and irregular; RR 20 breaths/min; BP 90/68 mm Hg; SpO$_2$ 97%.

Based on review of this information, which action will the nurse take at this time? **Select all that apply.**

A.   Apply heart monitor.

B.   Obtain glucose reading.

C.   Listen closely to heart sounds.

D.   Prepare to administer potassium.

E.   Anticipate administration of IV steroids.

F.   Contact the primary health care provider.

G.   Monitor the client's level of consciousness.

H.   Request laboratory order for serum potassium.

# 55
CHAPTER

# Concepts of Care for Patients with Conditions of the Thyroid and Parathyroid Glands

## LEARNING OUTCOMES

1. Plan collaborative care with the interprofessional team to promote cellular regulation, nutrition, and gas exchange in patients with thyroid and parathyroid problems.
2. Teach adults how to decrease the risk for thyroid and parathyroid problems.
3. Teach the patient and caregiver(s) about common drugs and other management strategies used for thyroid and parathyroid problems.
4. Plan patient- and family-centered nursing interventions to decrease the psychosocial impact caused by living with thyroid and parathyroid problems.
5. Apply knowledge of anatomy, physiology, and pathophysiology to provide evidence-based care for patients with thyroid and parathyroid problems

affecting cellular regulation, nutrition, and gas exchange.
6. Analyze assessment and diagnostic findings to generate solutions and prioritize nursing care for patients with thyroid and parathyroid problems.
7. Organize care coordination and transition management for patients with thyroid and parathyroid problems.
8. Use clinical judgment to plan evidence-based nursing care to promote cellular regulation, nutrition, and gas exchange and to prevent complications in patients with thyroid and parathyroid problems.
9. Incorporate factors that affect health equity into the plan of care for patients with thyroid and parathyroid problems.

## Preliminary Reading

Read and review Chapter 55, pp. 1323–1340.

## Chapter Review

### Pathophysiology Review

#1. Match the Key Term in Column A with its description in Column B.

**Column A**

_____1. Euthyroid
_____2. Exophthalmos
_____3. Goiter
_____4. Hyperparathyroidism
_____5. Hyperthyroidism
_____6. Hypoparathyroidism
_____7. Hypothyroidism
_____8. Myxedema coma
_____9. Tetany
____10. Thyroid storm
____11. Thyroiditis

**Column B**

A. Serious complication of untreated or poorly treated hypothyroidism
B. Decreased parathyroid function
C. Excessive thyroid hormone secretion
D. Hyperexcitability of nerves and muscles
E. Normal or near-normal thyroid function
F. Visibly enlarged thyroid gland
G. Life-threatening condition associated with hyperthyroidism
H. Abnormal protrusion of the eyes
I. Increased parathyroid hormone secretion
J. Reduced or absent thyroid gland hormone secretion
K. Inflammation of the thyroid gland

#2. Indicate in the chart whether the laboratory test is anticipated to be *increased* or *decreased* in hypothyroidism or hyperthyroidism.

| Test | Normal Range (Will Vary by Laboratory) | Hypothyroidism | Hyperthyroidism |
|---|---|---|---|
| Serum $T_3$ | *Age >50 years old:* 40–180 ng/dL (0.6–2.8 nmol/L) | | |
| | *Age 20–50 years old:* 70–205 ng/dL (1.2–3.4 nmol/L) | | |
| Serum $T_4$ (total) | *Males* 4–12 mcg/dL (59–135 nmol/L) | | |
| | *Females* 5–12 mcg/dL (71–142 nmol/L) | | |
| | *Older adults >60 years old* 5–11 mcg/dL (64–142 nmol/L) | | |
| "Direct" free $T_4$ | 0.8–2.8 ng/dL (10–36 pmol/L) | | |

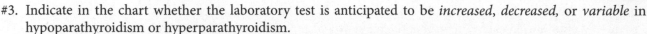

#3. Indicate in the chart whether the laboratory test is anticipated to be *increased*, *decreased*, or *variable* in hypoparathyroidism or hyperparathyroidism.

| Test | Normal Range | Hypoparathyroidism | Hyperparathyroidism |
|---|---|---|---|
| Serum calcium | Total: 9.0–10.5 mg/dL (2.25–2.62 mmol/L)* *Values may be slightly lower in older adults | | |
| Serum magnesium Critical levels <0.5 or >3 mEq/L mg/dL | 1.3–2.1 mEq/L (0.65–1.05 mmol/L) | | |
| Serum parathyroid hormone | 10–65 pg/mL (10–65 ng/L) | | |
| Serum phosphorus Critical level <1 mg/dL | 3–4.5 mg/dL (0.97–1.45 mmol/L) | | |
| Vitamin D | *Male:* 18–64 pg/mL | | |
| | *Females:* 17–78 pg/mL | | |

## Activities

### Activity #1

For each statement, specify if the statement is **true (T)** or **false (F)**.

_____1. Muscle aches, paresthesia, increased sleeping, fatigue, and constipation are associated with hypothyroidism.

_____2. A patient with hypothyroidism will require life-long thyroid hormone replacement therapy.

_____3. Graves' disease is a complication associated with hypothyroidism.

_____4. Radioactive iodine therapy given to patients with hyperthyroidism can induce hypothyroidism.

_____5. Unsealed radioactive isotope therapy requires the patient to avoid close contact with infants, young children, and people who are pregnant.

_____6. The key symptoms of thyroid storm are abdominal pain and diarrhea.

_____7. A complication of calcium treatment is formation of kidney stones.

_____8. Vitamin C is often given together with calcium treatment.

_____9. Numbness or tingling is a symptom of calcium toxicity.

___10. Bisphosphonates can be used for the treatment of hyperparathyroidism.

**Activity #2**
Provide two findings in each system that the nurse would expect to see in a client with hypothyroidism.

1.  Cardiovascular

    a.  _____

    b.  _____

2.  Respiratory

    a.  _____

    b.  _____

3.  Gastrointestinal

    a.  _____

    b.  _____

4.  Metabolic

    a.  _____

    b.  _____

5.  Reproductive

    a.  _____

    b.  _____

6.  Psychosocial

    a.  _____

    b.  _____

7.  Integumentary

    a.  _____

    b.  _____

8.  Neuromuscular

    a.  _____

    b.  _____

**Activity #3**
Provide two findings in each system that the nurse would expect to see in a client with hyperthyroidism.

1. Cardiovascular

   a. _____

   b. _____

2. Gastrointestinal

   a. _____

   b. _____

3. Metabolic

   a. _____

   b. _____

4. Reproductive

   a. _____

   b. _____

5. Psychosocial

   a. _____

   b. _____

6. Integumentary

   a. _____

   b. _____

7. Neuromuscular

   a. _____

   b. _____

## Activity #4

List three causes of hyperparathyroidism and three causes of hypoparathyroidism.

| Hyperparathyroidism | Hypoparathyroidism |
|---|---|
| 1. | 1. |
| 2. | 2. |
| 3. | 3. |

## Learning Assessments

### NCLEX Examination Challenge #1

Which laboratory value does the nurse identify that is likely to be found in a client with untreated hypothyroidism? Refer to the table in NGN Challenge #1 for normal values.

A. Serum $T_3$ of 30 ng/dL
B. Serum calcium of 9.2 mg/dL
C. "Direct" free $T_4$ of 1.4 ng/dL
D. Total serum $T_4$ of 6 mcg/dL

### NCLEX Examination Challenge #2

Which teaching will the nurse provide to a client who has just been prescribed propylthiouracil?

A. Monitor pulse daily for tachycardia.
B. Report urine darkening to the health care provider.
C. Take this drug 1 hour after taking methimazole.
D. This drug must be diluted in a glass of water or beverage.

### NCLEX Examination Challenge #3

Which assessment finding in a client with myxedema coma indicates to the nurse that therapy is effective? **Select all that apply.**

A. $SpO_2$ is 89%.
B. Skin is cool and dry.
C. Pulse is 62 beats/min.
D. Blood pressure is 110/66 mm Hg.
E. Core body temperature is 98.6°F (36.8°C).

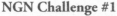

## NGN Challenge #1

The nurse is trending laboratory results for a 29-year-old client with primary hypothyroidism who was started 6 months ago on thyroid replacement therapy.

|  | **Normal Range** | **February 16, 2023** | **August 21, 2022** | **February 10, 2022** |
|---|---|---|---|---|
| Serum $T_3$ | *Age 20–50 years old:* 70–205 ng/dL (1.2–3.4 nmol/L) | 113 ng/dL | 69 ng/dL | 57 ng/dL |
| Serum $T_4$ (total) | *Males* 4–12 mcg/dL (59–135 nmol/L) *Females* 5–12 mcg/dL (71–142 nmol/L) | 11 mcg/dL | 5 mcg/dL | 4 mcg/dL |
| "Direct" free $T_4$ | 0.8–2.8 ng/dL (10–36 pmol/L) | 2.7 ng/dL | 1.1 ng/dL | 0.8 ng/dL |
| TSH | 0.3–5 μU/mL | 3.9 μU/mL | 4.3 μU/mL | 7 μU/mL |

The client states to the nurse, "I feel somewhat better but sometimes I still get somewhat fatigued." Which action will the nurse include in the plan of care? **Select all that apply.**

A.   Teach to moderate calcium in the diet.

B.   Determine if pretibial edema is present or developing.

C.   Contact the primary health care provider for medication adjustment.

D.   Discuss the benefit of consistent mild to moderate exercise.

E.   Recommend temporarily discontinuing medication therapy.

F.   Emphasize the need to continue taking medication as directed.

G.   Conduct assessment of when fatigue occurs and how bothersome it is.

## NGN Challenge #2

The oncoming nurse is preparing to care for a client with hyperparathyroidism who underwent a partial parathyroidectomy 2 days prior. The nurse reviews the most recent notes in the electronic health record from a nurse whose shift just ended.

| Vital Signs | Nurses Notes | Health Care Provider's Orders | Laboratory Results |
|---|---|---|---|

**1855:** Client in bed resting. Alert and oriented. Voice strong without hoarseness. No extremity twitching or movement noted. Client denies pain and sensation tingling anywhere. Percussion over the facial nerve shows very mild contraction of facial muscles. Incision site clean and dry without signs of infection. All other assessment findings within normal parameters. Current VS: T 98.4°F (36.9°C); HR 76 beats/min and regular; RR 20 breaths/min; BP 134/90 mm Hg; SpO$_2$ 96%. Reported these findings to oncoming nurse who is assuming care.

Complete the diagram by selecting from the choices to specify what **one** potential condition the client is at risk for, **two** priority actions the nurse would take to help prevent that condition, and **two** parameters the nurse would monitor to assess the client's progress.

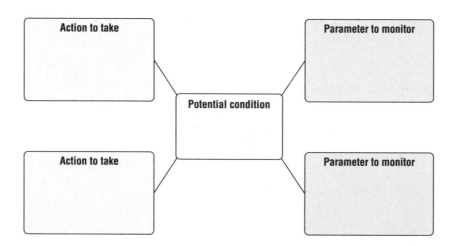

| Priority Actions to Take | Potential Condition | Parameters to Monitor |
|---|---|---|
| Assess for infectious thyroiditis. | Graves' disease | Serum calcium |
| Further assess vocal patterns. | Hypocalcemia | Eyeball protrusion |
| Obtain most recent laboratory results. | Myxedema coma | Presence of tetany |
| Notify the primary health care provider. | Hypercalcemic crisis | Development of Hashimoto thyroiditis |
| Activate the Rapid Response Team. | //////////////////////////// | Effect of propranolol on heart rate |

# 56
CHAPTER

# *Concepts of Care for Patients with Diabetes Mellitus*

## LEARNING OUTCOMES

1. Plan collaborative care with the interprofessional team to promote glucose regulation in patients with diabetes mellitus (DM).
2. Teach individuals at risk for impaired glucose regulation how to prevent or delay development of type 2 DM (T2DM).
3. Teach the patient and caregiver(s) about common drugs and other management strategies used for DM.
4. Plan patient- and family-centered nursing interventions to decrease the psychosocial impact caused by living with DM.
5. Apply knowledge of anatomy, physiology, and pathophysiology to provide evidence-based care for patients with DM affecting glucose regulation.

6. Analyze assessment and diagnostic findings to generate solutions and prioritize nursing care for patients with DM.
7. Organize care coordination and transition management for patients with DM.
8. Use clinical judgment to plan evidence-based nursing care to promote glucose regulation and prevent complications in patients with DM.
9. Incorporate factors that affect health equity into the plan of care for patients with DM.

## Preliminary Reading

Read and review Chapter 56, pp. 1341–1380.

## Chapter Review

### Pathophysiology Review

#1. Match the Key Term related to diabetes pathophysiology in Column A with its definition in Column B.

| Column A | Column B |
|---|---|
| ____1. Diabetic ketoacidosis | A. Conversion of fats to acid products |
| ____2. Diabetic peripheral neuropathy | B. Higher-than-normal (or target) blood glucose |
| ____3. Gastroparesis | C. Growth of new fragile retinal blood vessels that bleed easily and obscure vision |
| ____4. Hyperglycemia | |
| ____5. Hyperglycemic-hyperosmolar state | D. Severe acute complication of diabetes characterized by uncontrolled hyperglycemia, metabolic acidosis, and ketone production |
| ____6. Hypoglycemia | E. Severe acute hyperosmolar state caused by dehydration and hyperglycemia |
| ____7. Ketogenesis | |
| ____8. Ketone bodies | F. Breakdown of body proteins |
| ____9. Proliferative diabetic retinopathy | G. Lower-than-normal (or target) blood glucose |
| ___10. Proteolysis | H. Progressive deterioration of nerve function with the loss of sensory perception |
| | I. Acidic byproduct formed when there is a lack of insulin and fatty acids are used for energy |
| | J. A delay in gastric emptying |

#2. For each statement, specify if the statement is **true (T)** or **false (F)**.

____1. Lack of insulin causes electrolyte imbalance with sodium being most affected.

____2. Lack of insulin causes polyuria, polydipsia, and polyphagia.

____3. Type 1 diabetes mellitus (T1DM) is an autoimmune disorder in which the pancreatic beta cells are destroyed.

____4. Dehydration with diabetes mellitus (DM) leads to hemoconcentration, hypovolemia, poor tissue perfusion, and hypoxia, especially to the brain.

____5. A common acid-base imbalance that occurs in clients who have T1DM is metabolic acidosis.

____6. Macrovascular complications of DM include coronary heart disease, cerebrovascular disease, and peripheral vascular disease.

____7. Microvascular complications of DM lead to nephropathy, neuropathy, and retinopathy.

____8. Chronic hyperglycemia from poor glucose regulation leads to long-term complications.

____9. The most common precipitating factor for diabetic ketoacidosis (DKA) is infection or illness.

___10. If acute confusion or Kussmaul respirations are present, DKA can quickly lead to shock and coma.

___11. Hyperosmolar-hyperglycemic state (HHS) differs from DKA in that ketone levels are absent or low and blood glucose levels are much higher.

___12. Blood glucose levels may exceed 600 mg/dL (33.3 mmol/L), and blood osmolarity may exceed 320 mOsm/L in clients who have HHS.

___13. HHS occurs most often in young and middle-aged adults who have T1DM.

___14. Many females who develop T2DM had gestational diabetes mellitus or glucose intolerance during pregnancy.

___15. Assessing weight and weight change is important because excess weight and obesity are risk factors for T1DM.

## Activities

### Activity #1

Match the term related to diabetes care in Column A with its definition in Column B.

**Column A**

____1. Glycosylated hemoglobin
____2. Oral glucose tolerance test
____3. Blood glucose monitoring
____4. Dawn phenomenon
____5. Continuous blood glucose monitoring
____6. Charcot foot
____7. Glucose regulation
____8. Glycogenolysis
____9. Lipolysis
___10. Kussmaul respirations

**Column B**

A. Process of maintaining blood glucose levels
B. Process of checking a blood glucose level using a glucose meter
C. Diabetes technology system that measures and displays glucose levels continuously
D. Deep and rapid respiratory pattern triggered to reduce blood hydrogen ion concentration by "blowing off" carbon dioxide
E. Standardized test that measures how much glucose attaches to the hemoglobin and is an indicator of glucose control
F. Breakdown of body fats
G. Type of diabetic foot deformity often including hallux valgus
H. Test used to diagnose gestational diabetes mellitus
I. Results from a nighttime release of adrenal hormones that cause blood glucose elevation at 0500 or 0600
J. Breakdown of stored glycogen into glucose

### Activity #2

For each statement, specify if the statement is **true (T)** or **false (F)**.

____1. A glycosylated hemoglobin (A1C) level of ≥6.5% (48 mmol/mol) indicates a diagnosis of diabetes mellitus.

____2. Fasting plasma glucose (fasting blood glucose), along with A1C, can be used to diagnose DM in non-pregnant adults.

____3. Somogyi phenomenon is morning hyperglycemia from the counterregulatory response to nighttime hypoglycemia.

____4. Blood glucose target goals for self-management are set individually for each patient based on the duration of disease, age and life expectancy, other chronic conditions, the severity of cardiovascular disease, and presence of hypoglycemia unawareness.

____5. Patient education for nutrition is based on each patient's nutrition recommendations that consider blood glucose monitoring results, total blood lipid levels, and A1C levels.

____6. Increased physical activity and weight loss reduce the risk for type 1 DM (T1DM) in patients with prediabetes.

____7. When urine ketones are present in a patient who has diabetes mellitus, the patient should not exercise.

____8. The most common surgical intervention for treating T1DM is pancreas transplantation.

____9. Diabetic ketoacidosis is a complication of surgery because diuresis from hyperglycemia can cause dehydration and hypovolemia.

___10. The standards of care for diabetic ulcers are a moist wound environment, débridement of necrotic tissue, and elimination of pressure.

___11. Persistent albuminuria in the range of 30 to 299 mg/24 hours is the earliest stage of nephropathy in T1DM and a marker for the development of nephropathy in T2DM.

___12. Angiotensin-converting enzyme inhibitors reduce the level of albuminuria and the rate of progression of kidney disease.

Activity #3

Match the antidiabetic drug in Column A with its associated health teaching in Column B.

**Column A**

\_\_\_1.  Metformin
\_\_\_2.  Semaglutide
\_\_\_3.  Dapagliflozin
\_\_\_4.  Alogliptin
\_\_\_5.  Glipizide
\_\_\_6.  Pioglitazone
\_\_\_7.  Acarbose
\_\_\_8.  Pramlintide

**Column B**

A.  Teach patients to take this drug only with a meal.
B.  This drug should be injected weekly rather than daily.
C.  Teach patients to take this drug right before or during a meal to prevent hypoglycemia.
D.  Warn patients that this drug commonly causes nausea and vomiting.
E.  Teach patients to avoid alcohol while taking this drug.
F.  Teach patients the symptoms of dehydration, hyponatremia, and urinary tract and yeast infections.
G.  Remind patients that this drug causes weight gain and peripheral edema.
H.  Teach patients to report persistent abdominal pain and nausea associated with pancreatitis.

Activity #4

List four instructions the nurse would provide to a diabetic patient about how to provide meticulous foot care.

1.  _____

2.  _____

3.  _____

4.  _____

Activity #5

Complete the table to identify the onset, peak, and duration of common insulin preparations. Then answer the three questions about insulin therapy.

| Type/Preparation | Onset of Action (minutes) | Peak Action (hours) | Duration of Action (hours) |
|---|---|---|---|
| Insulin lispro | | | |
| Regular insulin | | | |
| NPH insulin | | | |
| Insulin detemir | | | |
| Insulin degludec | | | |

1.  When is the most likely time that the client receiving any type of insulin could experience hypoglycemia? (Onset, peak, or duration of action?)

_____

2.  Which three of the above types of insulin could be used to provide *basal* insulin coverage?

_____

3. What are the components of multiple-component insulin therapy?

_____

_____

_____

## Learning Assessments

### NCLEX Examination Challenge #1

The nurse is caring for a client with a history of uncontrolled diabetes mellitus and finds the client difficult to arouse before dinner. The current finger stick blood glucose (FSBG) is 39 mg/dL (2.16 mmol/L). Which is the **priority** nursing action for the client at this time?

A. Document the client's level of consciousness.
B. Give glucagon per agency protocol.
C. Retake the client's FSBG in 10 minutes.
D. Report the client's condition to the charge nurse.

### NCLEX Examination Challenge #2

A client with a history of type 1 diabetes mellitus presents with a blood glucose of 300 mg/dL (16.7 mmol/L) and is positive for ketone bodies. Which of the following interventions are appropriate for the nurse to implement? **Select all that apply.**

A. Encourage increased oral fluids.
B. Initiate peripheral IV line with fluids.
C. Give short-acting insulin as a bolus.
D. Follow bolus insulin with continuous IV insulin infusion.
E. Draw blood for STAT basic metabolic panel (BMP).
F. Administer glucagon per agency protocol.

### NCLEX Examination Challenge #3

The nurse is teaching a client who was recently diagnosed with COVID-19 infection about managing the client's diabetes mellitus during sick days. Which statement by the client indicates a **need for further teaching?**

A. "I will drink 8 to 12 ounces of sugar-free liquids every 3 to 4 hours while I'm awake."
B. "I will continue to take my insulin unless instructed by my diabetic doctor."
C. "I will let my doctor know if I have a fever of 101.5°F (38.6°C) or higher."
D. "Even if I don't have much appetite, I will try to eat my meals as usual."

## NGN Challenge
### *Item #1*

The nurse is planning care for a newly admitted 78-year-old resident who fell at home without injury on the day before admission to the nursing home a week ago. According to the medical record, the resident has lost 8 lb (3.6 kg) since admission and is being seen by the registered dietitian nutritionist today. Significant medical history includes type 2 diabetes mellitus, controlled at home by metformin, and hypertension, controlled by amlodipine until admission when furosemide was added to the medication regimen. The nurse reviews the latest Nurses Notes and selected laboratory results posted this morning.

| Vital Signs | Nurses Notes | Orders | Laboratory Results | |
|---|---|---|---|---|

**0805:** Drowsy but easily awakened; disoriented and confused this morning. Able to move all extremities but needs assistance getting out of bed because of weakness. Nursing assistant states that client only eats about half of each meal and needs strong encouragement to drink fluids. Refuses supplemental enteral nutrition between meals. Daily urinary output has decreased since admission. Skin and mucous membranes dry with poor skin turgor over sternum. $S_1$ and $S_2$ present; no abnormal or adventitious breath sounds. VS this morning: T 99.6°F (39.3°C); HR 112 beats/min; RR 21 breaths/min; BP 98/76 mm Hg. Medical Director notified of resident condition and lab results.

| Laboratory Test | Results (from Yesterday's Blood Draw) | Normal Reference Range |
|---|---|---|
| Fasting blood glucose (FBG) | 357 mg/dL (19.81 mmol/L) | 74–106 mg/dL (4.1–5.9 mmol/L) |
| Blood urea nitrogen (BUN) | 68 mg/dL (24.28 mmol/L) | 10–20 mg/dL (3.6–7.1 mmol/L) |
| Serum creatinine (Cr) | 1.5 mg/dL (132.63 mmol/L) | 0.6–1.3 mg/dL (53.05–114.95 mmol/L) |
| Blood osmolality | 325 mOsm/kg $H_2O$ (325 mmol/kg) | 285–295 mOsm/kg $H_2O$ (285–295 mmol/kg) |

Highlight the client findings in the Nurses Notes and Laboratory Results that would be of **immediate** concern to the nurse.

*Item #2*

The nurse is planning care for a newly admitted 78-year-old resident who fell at home without injury on the day before admission to the nursing home a week ago. According to the medical record, the client has lost 8 lb (3.6 kg) since admission and is being seen by the registered dietitian nutritionist today. Significant medical history includes type 2 diabetes mellitus, controlled at home by metformin, and hypertension, controlled by amlodipine until admission when furosemide was added to the medication regimen. The nurse reviews the latest Nurses Notes and selected Laboratory Results posted this morning.

| Vital Signs | Nurses Notes | Orders | Laboratory Results | |
|---|---|---|---|---|

**0805:** Drowsy but easily awakened; disoriented and confused this morning. Able to move all extremities but needs assistance getting out of bed because of weakness. Nursing assistant states that client only eats about half of each meal and needs strong encouragement to drink fluids. Refuses supplemental enteral nutrition between meals. Daily urinary output has decreased since admission. Skin and mucous membranes dry with poor skin turgor over sternum. $S_1$ and $S_2$ present; no abnormal or adventitious breath sounds. VS this morning: T 99.6°F (39.3°C); HR 112 beats/min; RR 21 breaths/min; BP 98/76 mm Hg. Medical Director notified of resident condition and lab results.

| Laboratory Test | Results (from Yesterday's Blood Draw) | Normal Reference Range |
|---|---|---|
| Fasting blood glucose (FBG) | 357 mg/dL (19.81 mmol/L) | 74–106 mg/dL (4.1–5.9 mmol/L) |
| Blood urea nitrogen (BUN) | 68 mg/dL (24.28 mmol/L) | 10–20 mg/dL (3.6–7.1 mmol/L) |
| Serum creatinine (Cr) | 1.5 mg/dL (132.63 mmol/L) | 0.6–1.3 mg/dL (53.05–114.95 mmol/L) |
| Blood osmolality | 325 mOsm/kg $H_2O$ (325 mmol/kg) | 285–295 mOsm/kg $H_2O$ |

The nurse analyzes the relevant assessment findings to determine the client's risk for a potentially life-threatening condition. Select the appropriate options from the lists of options to complete the sentence.

The client is at high risk for _____1 [Select]_____ because the client has _____ 2 [Select]_____ and is prescribed _____3 [Select]_____.

| Options for 1 | Options for 2 | Options for 3 |
|---|---|---|
| Diabetic ketoacidosis (DKA) | Hypertension | Metformin |
| Hyperglycemic-hyperosmolar state (HHS) | Chronic kidney disease | Diuretics |
| Metabolic syndrome | Type 2 diabetes mellitus | Amlodipine |

*Item #3*

The nurse is planning care for a newly admitted 78-year-old resident whose medical history includes type 2 diabetes mellitus, for which metformin is prescribed, and hypertension, for which amlodipine and furosemide are prescribed. Based on the review of the Nurses Notes and selected laboratory results, the Medical Director approves a request the resident's transfer via 911 to the local emergency department.

| Vital Signs | Nurses Notes | Orders | Laboratory Results | |
|---|---|---|---|---|

**0805:** Drowsy but easily awakened; disoriented and confused this morning. Able to move all extremities but needs assistance getting out of bed because of weakness. Nursing assistant states that client only eats about half of each meal and needs strong encouragement to drink fluids. Refuses supplemental enteral nutrition between meals. Daily urinary output has decreased since admission. Skin and mucous membranes dry with poor skin turgor over sternum. $S_1$ and $S_2$ present; no abnormal or adventitious breath sounds. VS this morning: T 99.6°F (39.3°C); HR 112 beats/min; RR 21 breaths/min; BP 98/76 mm Hg. Medical Director notified of resident condition and lab results.

| Laboratory Test | Results (from Yesterday's Blood Draw) | Normal Reference Range |
|---|---|---|
| Fasting blood glucose (FBG) | 357 mg/dL (19.81 mmol/L) | 74–106 mg/dL (4.1–5.9 mmol/L) |
| Blood urea nitrogen (BUN) | 68 mg/dL (24.28 mmol/L) | 10–20 mg/dL (3.6–7.1 mmol/L) |
| Serum creatinine (Cr) | 1.5 mg/dL (132.63 mmol/L) | 0.6–1.3 mg/dL (53.05–114.95 mmol/L) |
| Blood osmolality | 325 mOsm/kg $H_2O$ (325 mmol/kg) | 285–295 mOsm/kg $H_2O$ |

On admission to the Emergency Department, the nurse reviews the documentation, assesses the client, and begins to prioritize care. Select **two** priority conditions that need to be addressed immediately.

A.  Dehydration
B.  Hypotension
C.  Hyperglycemia
D.  Tachycardia
E.  Weight loss
F.  Chronic kidney disease

*Item #4*

The nurse is planning care for a 78-year-old client transferred from the local nursing home with a diagnosis of hyperglycemic-hyperosmolar state. For each priority client condition, select potential interventions which are most appropriate to include in this client's plan of care. More than one intervention may be appropriate for each client problem.

| Client Condition | Potential Interventions |
|---|---|
| Dehydration | • Start a peripheral IV with 0.45% NS<br>• Encourage oral fluids as tolerated<br>• Insert an indwelling urinary catheter |
| Hyperglycemia | • Administer IV insulin<br>• Increase metformin dosage<br>• Initiate continuous glucose monitoring |

## Item #5

The nurse is implementing care for a 78-year-old client transferred from the local nursing home with a diagnosis of hyperglycemic-hyperosmolar state. During fluid volume replacement and management of hyperglycemia, which of the following client assessments would the nurse frequently monitor? **Select all that apply.**

A. Serum potassium values
B. Blood glucose values
C. Blood urea nitrogen values
D. Cardiopulmonary congestion
E. Level of consciousness
F. Skin turgor

## Item #6

A 78-year-old client is going to be discharged today back to the local nursing home after a 3-day hospital stay for hyperglycemic-hyperosmolar state (HHS). The nurse performs a client assessment and compares current client findings with admission findings. For each finding, select whether the client's condition has **Improved** or **Not Improved**.

| Admission Client Finding | Current Client Finding | Improved | Not Improved |
|---|---|---|---|
| Drowsy and disoriented | Alert and oriented ×1 | | |
| Weight loss of 8 lb (3.6 kg) | Weight gain of 2.2 lb (1 kg) | | |
| T 99.6°F (39.3°C) | T 98°F (36.7°C) | | |
| HR 112 beats/min | HR 88 beats/min | | |
| BP 98/76 mm Hg | BP 122/72 mm Hg | | |
| FBG 357 mg/dL (19.81 mmol/L) | FBG 146 mg/dL (8.1 mmol/L) | | |
| BUN 68 mg/dL (24.28 mmol/L) | BUN 25 mg/dL (8.93 mmol/L) | | |

# 57 Assessment of the Renal/Urinary System

CHAPTER

## LEARNING OUTCOMES

1. Use knowledge of anatomy and physiology to perform a focused assessment of the renal/urinary system.
2. Teach evidence-based health promotion activities to help prevent urinary/renal health conditions or trauma.
3. Demonstrate clinical judgment to interpret assessment findings in patients with a renal/urinary system health condition.
4. Identify factors that affect health equity for patients with renal/urinary health conditions.
5. Explain how genetic implications and physiologic aging of the renal/urinary system affects elimination, fluid and electrolyte balance, and acid-base balance.
6. Plan evidence-based care and support for patients undergoing diagnostic testing of the renal/urinary system.

## Preliminary Reading

Read and review Chapter 57, pp. 1381–1403.

## Chapter Review

### Anatomy & Physiology Review

#1.  Match the terms in Column A with their definition in Column B.

| Column A | | Column B | |
|---|---|---|---|
| ____1. | Renal cortex | A. | Substance produced by kidneys that assists in blood pressure control |
| ____2. | Glomerulus | B. | Specialized capillary loops in the kidneys |
| ____3. | Glomerular filtration | C. | Voiding or urination |
| ____4. | Tubular reabsorption | D. | Process that keeps urine in normal range of 1 to 3 L/day |
| ____5. | Renin | E. | Outer tissue layer of kidneys |
| ____6. | Erythropoietin | F. | Ability to voluntarily control bladder emptying |
| ____7. | Micturition | G. | First process in urine formation |
| ____8. | Continence | H. | Substance produced by kidneys that triggers red blood cell production in bone marrow |

#2.  Complete the sentences by filling in the blanks with terms listed. Not all terms will be used.
1.  The blood supply to each kidney comes from the _____, which branches off from the abdominal aorta.
2.  The _____ is the functional unit of the kidney and forms urine by filtering waste products and water from the blood.

3. Renin produced by the kidneys converts renin substrate (angiotensinogen) into _____.
4. The point at which the kidney is overwhelmed with glucose and can no longer reabsorb is called the _____ for glucose reabsorption.
5. _____ increases systemic blood pressure with powerful blood vessel–constricting effects and triggers the release of aldosterone from the adrenal glands.
6. _____ is converted to its active form in the kidney.
7. _____is defined as bladder inflammation, most often with infection.
8. The purpose of these nephrons is to _____ urine during times of low fluid intake.

| Choices for Sentence Completion |
|---|
| Aldosterone |
| Angiotensin I |
| Angiotensin II |
| Concentrate |
| Cystitis |
| Dilute |
| Nephron |
| Prostaglandins |
| Renal artery |
| Renal threshold |
| Vitamin D |

## Activities

### Activity #1
List at least three physiologic renal/urinary system changes associated with aging.

1. _____

2. _____

3. _____

### Activity #2
Complete the sentences with the correct term or phrase.
1. Females have a shorter urethra and more commonly develop _____ because bacteria pass more readily into the bladder.
2. An increase in the intensity of color, a change in odor quality, or a decrease in urine clarity may suggest _____.
3. Pain that radiates from the kidneys or ureters into the perineal area, groin, scrotum, or labia is described as _____.
4. _____ is the buildup of nitrogenous waste products in the blood from inadequate elimination as a result of kidney failure.

5. _____ are used to screen for postvoid residual volumes and determine the need for intermittent catheterization based on the amount of urine in the bladder rather than the time between catheterizations.
6. A distended bladder sounds _____ when percussed.
7. No common pathologic condition other than kidney disease increases the serum _____ level.
8. _____ can be calculated from serum creatinine, age, weight, urine creatinine, natal sex, and race.

## Activity #3
For each statement, specify if the statement is **true (T)** or **false (F)**.

_____1. The kidney-ureters-bladder x-study shows gross anatomic features and obvious stones, strictures, calcifications, or obstructions in the urinary tract.
_____2. When contrast is used for renal imaging, the nurse ensures that there is sufficient oral or IV intake to dilute and excrete the contrast medium.
_____3. Contrast medium for any type of imaging test is potentially kidney damaging (nephrotoxic).
_____4. Patients taking metformin are at risk for lactic acidosis when they receive iodinated contrast media.
_____5. A kidney ultrasound is usually performed on a patient with an empty bladder.
_____6. Because of the risk for bleeding after a renal biopsy, coagulation studies such as platelet count, activated partial thromboplastin time (aPTT), prothrombin time (PT), and bleeding time are performed before the procedure.
_____7. Hypertension is the most common complication after a renal biopsy.
_____8. Magnetic resonance angiography is a noninvasive procedure used to detect blockages in large arteries and can determine renal artery stenosis.

## Activity #4
Match the laboratory test is Column A with what it measures or indicates in Column B.

| Column A | Column B |
|---|---|
| ___1. Serum creatinine | A. Measures concentration of urine particles |
| ___2. Blood urea nitrogen | B. Specifically indicates kidney function |
| ___3. Cystatin-C | C. Indicates urinary tract infection |
| ___4. Urine specific gravity | D. Indicates kidney function, dehydration, infection, tissue injury, and/or tissue breakdown |
| ___5. Urine protein | E. If present, indicates glomerular disorders or infection |
| ___6. Urine leukoesterase | F. Measures glomerular filtration rate |

## Learning Assessments

### NCLEX Examination Challenge #1
The nurse is caring for a client following a cystoscopy under deep sedation for removal of a small bladder tumor. What finding would the nurse teach the client to report to the primary health care provider after the procedure?
A. Urethral discomfort
B. Constipation
C. Gross hematuria
D. Increased urinary output

## NCLEX Examination Challenge #2

The nurse is reviewing laboratory results of a urinalysis. Which results would the nurse recognize as **abnormal** in the client's urine? **Select all that apply.**

A. pH of 6
B. Presence of ketones
C. Presence of glucose
D. Presence of bilirubin
E. Protein of 1 mg/dL

## NCLEX Examination Challenge #3

The nurse is reinforcing teaching for the client preparing to have a renal scan. Which statements below are appropriate for the nurse to include? **Select all that apply.**

A. "You will be given an iodine-based contrast medium to help visualize the kidneys."
B. "You don't need to fast or be sedated for this diagnostic test."
C. "You may receive a diuretic like furosemide to better visualize kidney function."
D. "Be sure to drink plenty of fluids after the test to flush out the urinary system."
E. "There is no special follow-up or precautions needed after this test."

# 58

CHAPTER

# Concepts of Care for Patients with Urinary Conditions

## LEARNING OUTCOMES

1. Plan collaborative care with the interprofessional team to promote elimination in patients with urinary conditions.
2. Teach adults how to decrease the risk for urinary conditions.
3. Teach the patient and caregiver(s) about common drugs and other management strategies used for urinary conditions.
4. Plan patient- and family-centered nursing interventions to decrease the psychosocial impact caused by living with urinary conditions.
5. Apply knowledge of anatomy, physiology, and pathophysiology to provide evidence-based care

for patients with urinary conditions affecting elimination.
6. Analyze assessment and diagnostic findings to generate solutions and prioritize nursing care for patients with urinary conditions.
7. Organize care coordination and transition management for patients with urinary conditions.
8. Use clinical judgment to plan evidence-based nursing care to promote elimination and prevent complications in patients with urinary conditions.
9. Incorporate factors that affect health equity into the plan of care for patients with urinary conditions.

## Preliminary Reading

Read and review Chapter 58, pp. 1404–1434.

## Chapter Review

### Pathophysiology Review

#1. Match the Key Term in Column A with its definition in Column B.

| Column A | | Column B | |
|---|---|---|---|
| _____1. | Anuria | A. | Severe flank pain resulting from stones |
| _____2. | Bacteriuria | B. | Enlargement of the ureter |
| _____3. | Cystocele | C. | Presence of bacteria in the urine |
| _____4. | Dysuria | D. | Spread of infection from the urinary tract to the bloodstream |
| _____5. | Hydronephrosis | E. | Pain or burning with urination |
| _____6. | Hydroureter | F. | Scant urine output |
| _____7. | Oliguria | G. | Absence of urine output |
| _____8. | Nephrolithiasis | H. | Involuntary loss of urine |
| _____9. | Renal colic | I. | Herniation of the bladder into the vagina |
| ____10. | Urinary incontinence | J. | Presence of calculi (stones) in the urinary tract |
| ____11. | Urolithiasis | K. | Enlargement of the kidney |
| ____12. | Urosepsis | L. | Formation of stones in the kidney |

#2. For each statement, specify if the statement is **true (T)** or **false (F)**.

_____1. Stress incontinence is the most common type of urinary incontinence and occurs most often in men.

_____2. Overflow incontinence occurs when the detrusor muscle fails to contract and the bladder becomes overdistended.

_____3. Risk for urinary incontinence increases with chronic conditions such as diabetes mellitus, stroke, cognitive impairment, and impaired mobility.

_____4. A recurrent urinary tract infection (UTI) is defined as having two or more infections in 6 months or three or more infections in 1 year.

_____5. When a patient has bacteriuria but no symptoms of infection, it is called colonization or asymptomatic bacteriuria (ABU) and is more common in older adults.

_____6. *Staphylococcus aureus* is the most common organism that causes UTI.

_____7. Family history has a strong association with kidney stone formation and recurrence because of inherited metabolic variations.

_____8. The most common cause of infectious urethritis is sexually transmitted infection.

## Activities

### Activity #1

List three factors that contribute to urinary incontinence in older adults.

1. _____

2. _____

3. _____

### Activity #2

Identify four measures that can minimize the incidence of catheter-associated urinary tract infection (CAUTI).

1. _____

2. _____

3. _____

4. _____

### Activity #3

For each statement, specify if the statement is **true (T)** or **false (F)**.

_____1. Nutrition therapy with weight reduction is helpful for patients who are obese because stress incontinence is made worse by increased abdominal pressure.

_____2. Caffeine and alcohol can cause urinary retention, especially in women.

_____3. The nurse teaches the client with stress or urge incontinence how to perform pelvic floor exercises.

_____4. Habit training (scheduled toileting) is a type of bladder training that is successful in reducing incontinence in cognitively impaired patients.

_____5. For overflow incontinence, the most effective common behavioral interventions are bladder compression and intermittent self-catheterization.

_____6. The stenting method and massage maneuver are examples of bladder compression techniques.

_____7.   Although cystitis is not life-threatening, infection of the urinary tract can lead to life-threatening complications, including pyelonephritis and sepsis.

_____8.   Urinary tract obstruction is an emergency and must be treated immediately to preserve kidney function.

_____9.   Extracorporeal shock wave lithotripsy (SWL) is the use of sound, laser, or dry shock waves to break urinary or kidney stones into small fragments.

_____10.   Most urothelial cancers occur in the bladder.

## Activity #4

Match the drug used for urinary conditions in Column A with relevant health teaching that the nurse would provide for patients in Column B. One or more choices in Column B may be used more than once.

## Column A

___1.   Estrogen vaginal cream
___2.   Oxybutynin
___3.   Midodrine
___4.   Mirabegron
___5.   Duloxetine
___6.   Fluconazole
___7.   Trimethoprim/sulfamethoxazole
___8.   Phenazopyridine

## Column B

A.   Change position slowly due to possible orthostatic hypotension
B.   Take drug with a meal or immediately after a meal
C.   Increase fluid intake while taking this drug
D.   Take entire drug prescription even if symptoms have resolved
E.   Be aware that this drug takes 4 to 6 weeks to work
F.   Monitor blood pressure because this drug can cause hypertension

## Learning Assessments

### NCLEX Examination Challenge #1

A nursing assistant caring for an incontinent older adult asks the nurse about the **best** way to provide care. What is the nurse's best response?

A.   "Put briefs on the client during the day to prevent soiling the bed."
B.   "Reassure the client that it is OK to urinate while in the bed or chair."
C.   "Use the Crede bladder method to help the client empty the bladder."
D.   "Follow the toileting schedule posted in the client's bathroom."

### NCLEX Examination Challenge #2

The nurse is planning teaching a client who is starting trimethoprim/sulfamethoxazole for a urinary tract infection (UTI). Which health teaching would the nurse include? **Select all that apply.**

A.   "Be sure to report a rash to the primary health care provider while taking the drug."
B.   "Monitor your pulse and blood pressure carefully while you're on this drug."
C.   "If you have any known allergies to sulfa drugs, you should not take this drug."
D.   "Drink a full glass of water with every dose of this medication you take."
E.   "This drug will not treat the UTI but will decrease your symptoms."

### NCLEX Examination Challenge #3

The nurse is caring for a client who had a Kock pouch created for treatment of bladder cancer last month. For what complication would the nurse monitor?

A.   Urinary infection
B.   Peritonitis
C.   Urine leakage
D.   Bowel obstruction

## NGN Challenge #1

The nurse assesses a 63-year-old client who has been treated for possible interstitial cystitis under the supervision of the primary health care provider. Today, the client visits a urologist for evaluation.

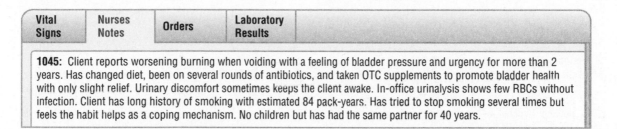

| Vital Signs | Nurses Notes | Orders | Laboratory Results | |
|---|---|---|---|---|

**1045:** Client reports worsening burning when voiding with a feeling of bladder pressure and urgency for more than 2 years. Has changed diet, been on several rounds of antibiotics, and taken OTC supplements to promote bladder health with only slight relief. Urinary discomfort sometimes keeps the client awake. In-office urinalysis shows few RBCs without infection. Client has long history of smoking with estimated 84 pack-years. Has tried to stop smoking several times but feels the habit helps as a coping mechanism. No children but has had the same partner for 40 years.

Complete the diagram by selecting from the choices to specify what **one** condition the client is most likely experiencing, **two** actions the nurse would expect for that condition, and **two** parameters the nurse would monitor to assess the client's progress.

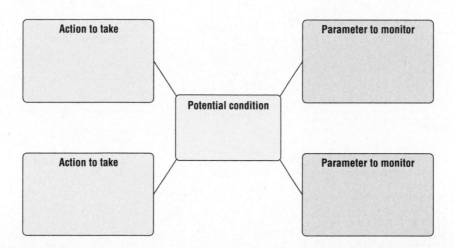

| Actions to Take | Client Condition | Parameters to Monitor |
|---|---|---|
| Reinforce health teaching and schedule a cystoscopy. | Urinary tract infection | Intake and output |
| Teach client about antibiotic administration at home. | Urolithiasis | Bleeding after procedure |
| Reinforce health teaching and schedule lithotripsy. | Bladder cancer | Bladder pain and pressure |
| Refer the client to a formal smoking cessation program. | Cystocele | Vital signs |
| Reinforce health teaching and schedule cystocele repair. | ///////////////////////////////// | Surgical incision integrity |

**NGN Challenge #2**

The nurse is caring for an 85-year-old client residing in a local nursing home who presents to the ED with acute confusion.

| Health History | Nurses Notes | Orders | Laboratory Results | |
|---|---|---|---|---|

**1450:** Client brought to ED by family who report the client having new symptoms of confusion, restlessness, and urinary incontinence. Has not voided since 0800. Is usually able to ambulate with walker, but too weak to use walker this morning. Client currently alert but not oriented or able to communicate appropriately. No facial drooping and able to move all extremities. Dry mucous membranes and lips. Breath sounds clear throughout lung fields; $S_1$ and $S_2$ present. Hyperactive bowel sounds × 4. Current VS: T 100.6°F (38.1°C); HR 102 beats/min; RR 25 breaths/min; BP 106/54; $SpO_2$ 94% on RA.

Complete the diagram by selecting from the choices to specify what **one** condition the client is most likely experiencing, **two** actions the nurse would take to address that condition, and **two** parameters the nurse would monitor to assess the client's progress.

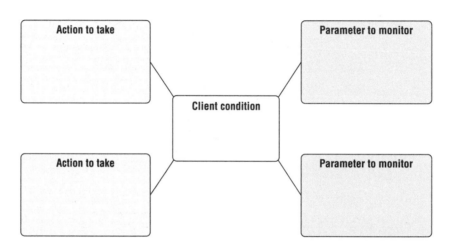

| Actions to Take | Client Condition | Parameters to Monitor |
|---|---|---|
| Administer supplemental oxygen therapy. | Urosepsis | Skin turgor |
| Send sterile urine specimen to laboratory. | Urolithiasis | Heart rate and blood pressure |
| Insert an indwelling urinary catheter. | Pneumonia | Bowel sounds |
| Initiate peripheral IV fluids. | Stroke | Oxygen saturation |
| Administer an antipyretic drug. | ///////////////////////////////// | Body temperature |

# 59 CHAPTER

# *Concepts of Care for Patients with Kidney Conditions*

## LEARNING OUTCOMES

1. Plan collaborative care with the interprofessional team to promote urinary elimination in patients with kidney conditions.
2. Teach adults how to decrease the risk for kidney conditions.
3. Teach the patient and caregiver(s) about common drugs and other management strategies used for kidney conditions.
4. Plan patient- and family-centered nursing interventions to decrease the psychosocial impact caused by living with kidney conditions.
5. Apply knowledge of anatomy, physiology, and pathophysiology to provide evidence-based care for patients with kidney conditions affecting elimination, fluid and electrolyte balance, and acid-base balance.
6. Analyze assessment and diagnostic findings to generate solutions and prioritize nursing care for patients with kidney conditions.
7. Organize care coordination and transition management for patients with kidney disorders.
8. Use clinical judgment to plan evidence-based nursing care to promote urinary elimination and prevent complications in patients with kidney conditions.
9. Incorporate factors that affect health equity into the plan of care for patients with kidney conditions.

## Preliminary Reading

Read and review Chapter 59, pp. 1435–1453.

## Chapter Review

### Pathophysiology Review

#1. Match the Key Term in Column A with its definition in Column B.

**Column A**

____1. Abscess
____2. Acute glomerulonephritis
____3. Nephrosclerosis
____4. Nephrotic syndrome
____5. Polycystic kidney syndrome
____6. Pyelonephritis
____7. Urinary stricture

**Column B**

A. Bacterial infection in the kidney
B. Degenerative kidney disorder resulting from changes in kidney blood vessels
C. Localized collection of pus (infection)
D. Narrowing of the urinary tract
E. Immunologic kidney disorder, which causes massive loss of protein into the urine and decreased plasma albumin level
F. Inflammation of the glomerulus from immune response in kidneys
G. Genetic disorder in which fluid-filled cysts develop in the kidney

#2. For each statement, specify if the statement is **true (T)** or **false (F)**.

_____1. Single episodes of chronic pyelonephritis result from bacterial infection, with or without obstruction or reflux.

_____2. Chronic pyelonephritis usually occurs with structural deformities, urinary stasis, obstruction, or reflux.

_____3. Conditions that lead to urinary stasis include prolonged bedrest and paralysis.

_____4. Acute pyelonephritis involves acute tissue inflammation, local edema, tubular cell necrosis, and possible abscess formation.

_____5. The most common pyelonephritis-causing infecting organism among community-dwelling adults is *Escherichia coli*.

_____6. Young males who are sexually active are the most commonly affected by acute pyelonephritis.

_____7. Acute glomerulonephritis is associated with high blood pressure, progressive kidney damage, and edema.

_____8. The main feature of nephrotic syndrome is increased protein elimination with severe proteinuria (with more than 3.5 g of protein in a 24-hour urine sample).

_____9. Most patients with polycystic kidney disease have low blood pressure caused by kidney ischemia from the enlarging cysts.

____10. Renal artery stenosis from atherosclerosis or blood vessel hyperplasia is the main cause of renovascular disease.

____11. Polycystic kidney disease is a genetic condition, with the most common form being autosomal dominant.

## Activities

### Activity #1
List four common symptoms of acute pyelonephritis.

1. _____

2. _____

3. _____

4. _____

### Activity #2
Complete the statements with the appropriate term(s) from the list provided. Not all terms will be used.

1. In a healthy adult, urine is usually _____.

2. _____ occurs as a complication of an ascending urinary tract infection that spreads from the bladder to the kidneys.

3. A urinalysis for a patient who has acute pyelonephritis shows a positive _____ and _____ dipstick test.

4. The patient who has acute glomerulonephritis typically has _____ and _____ in the urine.

5. A _____ provides a precise diagnosis of glomerulonephritis, assists in determining the prognosis, and helps in outlining treatment.

6. For patients who have nephrosclerosis, management focuses on controlling _____ and reducing albuminuria to preserve kidney function.

7. _____ is the primary method for diagnosing polycystic kidney disease (PKD).

8. Drug therapy with _____ is used to reach a blood pressure below 130/80 mm Hg in all patients with PKD.

9. The cause of hydronephrosis or hydroureter is a(n) _____, which can occur at any location between the collecting duct and the urethral meatus.

10. The most common treatment for renal cell carcinoma is a _____.

| Choices for Sentence Completion |
|---|
| Angiotensin-converting enzyme inhibitors |
| Beta blockers |
| Blood |
| High blood pressure |
| Hydronephrosis |
| Hypotension |
| Kidney biopsy |
| Leukocyte esterase |
| Nephrectomy |
| Nitrite |
| Obstruction |
| Protein |
| Pyelonephritis |
| Sterile |
| Ultrasound |

## Activity #3
For each statement, specify if the statement is **true (T)** or **false (F)**.

_____1. The nurse should assess any older adult who has new-onset confusion for signs and symptoms of urinary or renal infection.

_____2. Glomerulonephritis can lead to acute kidney injury, making it essential to prevent and treat in the older adult who is at greater risk for the condition.

_____3. Penicillin, erythromycin, or azithromycin is prescribed for acute glomerulonephritis (GN) caused by streptococcal infection.

_____4. For patients who have acute GN with fluid overload, hypertension, and edema, diuretics and sodium and water restrictions are prescribed.

_____5. For patients who have chronic GN, the serum creatinine level is elevated, usually greater than 6 mg/dL (500 Mcmol/L).

_____6. In patients who have nephrotic syndrome, ACE inhibitors can decrease protein loss in the urine and cholesterol-lowering drugs can improve blood lipid levels.

_____7.  Patients with PKD often experience hypertension, abdominal and flank pain, ruptured cysts, and infections.

_____8.  Because PKD-related pain is often persistent and associated with multiple factors, an interprofessional pain management approach is helpful.

_____9.  After insertion of a nephrostomy tube, urine drainage may be bloody for the first 3 days after the procedure and should gradually clear.

_____10.  A decrease in blood pressure is an early sign of both hemorrhage and adrenal insufficiency following a nephrectomy.

## Learning Assessments

### NCLEX Examination Challenge #1

The nurse is caring for a client who had a nephrostomy performed this morning during surgery for a ureteral obstruction. Which assessment finding would be the **priority** for the nurse to report to the surgeon immediately?

A.  Incisional pain of 5/10
B.  Dry mucous membranes
C.  No nephrostomy tube drainage
D.  Blood pressure of 108/74

### NCLEX Examination Challenge #2

The nurse is caring for a client who had a left nephrectomy for a cancerous kidney tumor. Which client finding would be of immediate concern to the nurse?

A.  Blood pressure of 90/50
B.  $SpO_2$ of 94% on RA
C.  Shallow but regular respirations
D.  Blood glucose of 110 mg/dL (5.88 mmol/L)

**NGN Challenge #1**

The nurse is caring for a 37-year-old client admitted to the emergency department (ED).

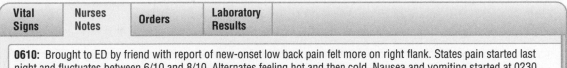

**0610:** Brought to ED by friend with report of new-onset low back pain felt more on right flank. States pain started last night and fluctuates between 6/10 and 8/10. Alternates feeling hot and then cold. Nausea and vomiting started at 0230 and client feels very weak. Alert and oriented × 4. No abnormal heart or lung sounds. Bowel sounds present × 4. VS: T 102.8°F (39.3°C); HR 112 beats/min; RR 20 breaths/min; BP 120/73 mm Hg; SpO₂ 98% on RA. Urinalysis positive for leukocyte esterase and nitrites; white blood cells and bacteria present. Urine sent for culture and sensitivity. KUB shows no abscess, cysts, stones, or anatomic defect. Admitted to the medical unit.

Complete the diagram by selecting from the choices to specify what **one** condition the client is most likely experiencing, **two** actions the nurse would expect for that condition, and **two** parameters the nurse would monitor to assess the client's progress.

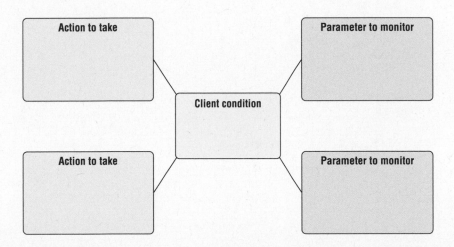

| Actions to Take | Client Condition | Parameters to Monitor |
|---|---|---|
| Prepare client for STAT cystoscopy. | Interstitial cystitis | Urinalysis |
| Begin IV fluids and broad-spectrum antibiotic. | Urolithiasis | Postprocedure bleeding |
| Prepare client for lithotripsy. | Glomerulonephritis | Back/flank pain |
| Administer supplemental oxygen therapy. | Pyelonephritis | Vital signs |
| Administer acetaminophen. | ///////////////////////////////// | SpO₂ levels |

## NGN Challenge #2

The nurse completes the intake for a 46-year-old client visiting the primary health care provider.

| Vital Signs | Nurses Notes | Orders | Laboratory Results | |
|---|---|---|---|---|

**1320:** Came for office visit due to increasing foot and ankle edema and fatigue for the past week. History of systemic lupus erythematosus managed by rheumatologist; has been in remission for 6 months. No other significant medical history. Today client is lethargic but oriented × 4. Able to ambulate independently. $S_1$ and $S_2$ present. Crackles in both lung bases; states that in last few days has shortness of breath when climbing stairs. Bowel sounds present × 4. Notes less urinary output for the past few days but has not had much to eat or drink. VS: T 99°F (37.2°C); HR 88 beats/min; RR 24 breaths/min; 162/98 mm Hg; $SpO_2$ 95% on RA.

Complete the diagram by selecting from the choices to specify what **one** condition the client is most likely experiencing, **two** actions the nurse would take to address that condition, and **two** parameters the nurse would monitor to assess the client's progress.

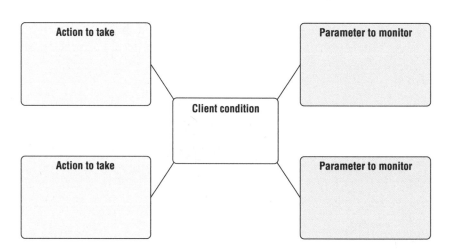

| Actions to Take | Client Condition | Parameters to Monitor |
|---|---|---|
| Administer corticosteroids. | Pyelonephritis | Skin turgor |
| Send sterile urine specimen to laboratory. | Glomerulonephritis | Blood pressure |
| Insert an indwelling urinary catheter. | Renal cell carcinoma | Fluid retention/edema |
| Give diuretics per protocol. | Urolithiasis | Oxygen saturation |
| Administer an antipyretic drug. | //////////////////////////////// | Body temperature |

# 60 CHAPTER

# Concepts of Care for Patients with Acute Kidney Injury and Chronic Kidney Disease

## LEARNING OUTCOMES

1. Plan collaborative care with the interprofessional team to promote urinary elimination in patients with acute kidney injury or chronic kidney disease.
2. Teach adults how to decrease the risk for acute kidney injury and chronic kidney disease.
3. Teach the patient and caregiver(s) about common drugs and other management strategies used for acute kidney injury and chronic kidney disease.
4. Plan patient- and family-centered nursing interventions to decrease the psychosocial impact caused by living with acute kidney injury and chronic kidney disease.
5. Apply knowledge of anatomy, physiology, and pathophysiology to provide evidence-based care for patients with acute kidney injury and chronic

kidney disease affecting urinary elimination, fluid and electrolyte balance, and acid-base balance.
6. Analyze assessment and diagnostic findings to generate solutions and prioritize nursing care for patients with acute kidney injury or chronic kidney disease.
7. Organize care coordination and transition management for patients with acute kidney injury or chronic kidney disease.
8. Use clinical judgment to plan evidence-based nursing care to promote urinary and prevent complications in patients with acute kidney injury and chronic kidney disease.
9. Incorporate factors that affect health equity into the plan of care for patients with acute kidney injury or chronic kidney disease.

## Preliminary Reading

Read and review Chapter 60, pp. 1454–1494.

## Chapter Review

### Pathophysiology Review

#1. Match the Key Term in Column A with its definition in Column B.

| Column A | | Column B |
|---|---|---|
| ___1. | Acute kidney injury | A. | Bone metabolism and structural damage caused by chronic kidney disease |
| ___2. | Azotemia | B. | Rapid reduction in kidney function |
| ___3. | Kussmaul respirations | C. | Urine output less than 400 mL/day |
| ___4. | Oliguria | D. | Systemic clinical and laboratory manifestations of end-stage kidney disease |
| ___5. | Pruritis | E. | Breathing that is fast and deep |
| ___6. | Renal osteodystrophy | F. | Accumulation of nitrogenous wastes in the blood; also called azotemia |
| ___7. | Uremia | G. | Excess of nitrogenous wastes (urea) in the blood H. Itchy skin |
| ___8. | Uremic syndrome | | |

#2. For each statement, specify if the statement is **true (T)** or **false (F).**

_____1. When kidney function declines gradually, it is diagnosed as chronic kidney disease, formerly termed chronic renal failure (CRF).

_____2. Common risk factors for acute kidney injury include shock, cardiac surgery, hypotension, prolonged mechanical ventilation, and sepsis.

_____3. Older adults or adults with diabetes, hypertension, peripheral vascular disease, liver disease, or chronic kidney disease are at higher risk of acute kidney injury if hospitalized.

_____4. Most every patient who develops acute kidney injury has postrenal urinary obstruction.

_____5. Chronic kidney disease is classified into stages based on (glomerular filtration rate [GFR] category.

_____6. CKD is a progressive, irreversible disorder lasting longer than 3 months.

_____7. Stage 3 of CKD is also known as end-stage kidney disease (ESKD).

_____8. CKD affects every physiologic system of the body.

_____9. The two main causes of CKD leading to dialysis or kidney transplantation are hypertension and diabetes mellitus.

_____10. NSAIDs and some antibiotics can cause acute kidney injury.

## Activities

### Activity #1
List three actions that nurses can implement for patients to promote kidney health and prevent kidney injury.

1. _____

2. _____

3. _____

### Activity #2
Complete the table with at least two assessment findings for each body system or process that can be affected by ESKD.

| Body System/Process | Assessment Findings |
| --- | --- |
| Urinary | |
| Neurologic | |
| Integumentary | |
| Cardiovascular | |
| Respiratory | |
| Musculoskeletal | |
| Reproductive | |
| Hematologic | |
| Gastrointestinal | |
| Metabolic | |

**Activity #3**

Complete the statements with the appropriate term(s) from the list provided. Not all terms will be used.

1. Both acute kidney injury and chronic kidney disease may require _____, such as dialysis.
2. Acute kidney injury is defined by the amount of _____ that increases over a short period.
3. A common type of intermittent kidney replacement therapy is _____.
4. Most patients who have chronic kidney disease (CKD) have fluid overload and therefore need _____ and diuretic therapy to manage their fluid balance.
5. For patients who have end-stage kidney disease, the nurse would monitor for signs and symptoms associated with _____, a potentially life-threatening complication of left-sided heart failure.
6. _____ are the most effective drugs to decrease cardiovascular events when patients have CKD and hypertension.
7. _____ in the patient's diet early in the course of CKD may help preserve kidney function.
8. The intake of three electrolytes in the diet needs to be restricted for patients who have CKD: sodium, potassium, and _____.
9. Epoetin alfa is a drug given to help treat the _____ associated with CKD.
10. Phosphate-binding agents help prevent _____ and related injuries in patients who have CKD.

| **Choices for Sentence Completion** |
| --- |
| Anemia |
| Angiotensin-converting enzyme inhibitors |
| Beta blockers |
| Calcium restriction |
| Cor pulmonale |
| Creatinine |
| Fluid restriction |
| Hemodialysis |
| Kidney replacement therapy |
| Phosphorous |
| Protein restriction |
| Pulmonary edema |
| Renal osteodystrophy |

## Activity #4

For each statement, specify if the statement is **true (T)** or **false (F)**.

_____1. An anticoagulant, usually heparin, is delivered into the blood circuit via a pump during hemodialysis.

_____2. The two common choices for long-term vascular access for hemodialysis are an internal arteriovenous (AV) fistula or an AV graft.

_____3. A patient's blood pressure and weight are expected to be reduced as a result of fluid removal during hemodialysis.

_____4. For patients having hemodialysis, a priority for the nurse is to monitor the patient's blood pressure for hypertension, a common complication.

_____5. The nurse ensures that the dialysate is warm to help prevent discomfort during peritoneal dialysis.

_____6. The nurse monitors for indications of peritonitis in patients on peritoneal dialysis (PD), including a cloudy effluent (outflow), fever, and abdominal pain.

_____7. Exit-site infections can occur with any type of PD catheter and can lead to peritonitis and catheter failure.

_____8. Candidates for transplantation have advanced kidney disease, have a reasonable life expectancy, and are medically and surgically fit to undergo the procedure.

_____9. An abrupt decrease in urine output may indicate complications of kidney transplantation, such as rejection, acute kidney injury (AKI), thrombosis, or obstruction.

____10. Bleeding is the most serious complication of transplantation and is the leading cause of graft loss.

## Activity #5

Match each drug used for patients who have chronic kidney disease or kidney transplant in Column A with the indication for its use in Column B. One or more choices in Column B may be used more than once.

**Column A**

____1. Furosemide
____2. Calcium carbonate
____3. Folic acid
____4. Corticosteroids
____5. Calcitriol
____6. Darbepoetin alfa
____7. Cinacalcet
____8. Cyclosporine

**Column B**

A. Suppresses immune response to help prevent kidney transplant rejection
B. Helps manage anemia in patients who have chronic kidney disease
C. Increases urinary output to eliminate excess fluid from the body
D. Binds to phosphate to remove it from the body via the GI system
E. Vitamin D supplement given to help absorb calcium in the intestines
F. Hormone that helps balance calcium and phosphate to prevent renal osteodystrophy

## Learning Assessments

### NCLEX Examination Challenge #1

The nurse is caring for a client with end-stage chronic kidney disease. Which of the following serum laboratory findings would the nurse expect? **Select all that apply.**
A. Elevated creatinine
B. Decreased potassium
C. Decreased calcium
D. Increased phosphorus (phosphate)
E. Decreased hemoglobin

### NCLEX Examination Challenge #2

The nurse is caring for a client with end-stage chronic kidney disease. Which acid-base imbalance would the nurse expect the client to have?
A. Metabolic alkalosis
B. Metabolic acidosis
C. Respiratory alkalosis
D. Respiratory acidosis

## NCLEX Examination Challenge #3

The nurse is caring for a client who has an arteriovenous fistula for hemodialysis. Which nursing precautions are essential when caring for clients with this vascular access? **Select all that apply.**

A. Do not take blood pressure readings using the extremity in which the vascular access is placed.

B. Do not perform venipunctures or start an IV line in the extremity in which the vascular access is placed.

C. Assess the client's distal pulses and circulation in the arm with the access.

D. Palpate for thrills and auscultate for bruits over the vascular access site every 4 hours while the client is awake.

E. Instruct the client not to carry heavy objects or anything that compresses the extremity in which the vascular access is placed.

## NCLEX Examination Challenge #4

The nurse is caring for a client preparing to undergo hemodialysis. Which of the following nursing actions are appropriate for the client's care? **Select all that apply.**

A. Weigh the patient before and after dialysis.

B. Monitor blood pressure, pulse, respirations, and temperature.

C. Assess for indications of hypertension.

D. Assess for headache, nausea, and vomiting.

E. Observe for bleeding at the vascular access site

## NGN Challenge #1

The nurse reviews selected serum Laboratory Results for an 81-year-old client admitted 2 days ago for dehydration and urosepsis.

| Laboratory Test | Today's Results | Yesterday's Results | Admission Results | Normal Reference Range |
|---|---|---|---|---|
| Creatinine | 2.9 mg/dL (256.4 mmol/L) | 2.4 mg/dL (212.2 mmol/L) | 2.0 mg/dL (176.8 mmol/L) | *Male:* 0.6–1.2 mg/dL (53–106 mmol/L) *Female:* 0.5–1.1 mg/dL (44–97 mmol/L) |
| BUN | 47 mg/dL (16.8 mmol/L) | 43 mg/dL (15.4 mmol/L) | 29 mg/dL (10.4 mmol/L) | 10–20 mg/dL (3.6–7.1 mmol/L) |
| Calcium | 8.8 mg/dL (2.2 mmol/L) | 9.1 mg/dL (2.27 mmol/L) | 9.4 mg/dL (2.35 mmol/L) | Total calcium: 9–10.5 mg/dL or 2.25–2.62 mmol/L |
| Phosphorus (inorganic) | 4.7 mg/dL (1.52 mmol/L) | 4.5 mg/dL (1.45 mmol/L) | 4.3 mg/dL (1.34 mmol/L) | 3–4.5 mg/dL or 0.97–1.45 mmol/L |
| Potassium | 5.3 mEq/L (5.3 mmol/L) | 5.2 mEq/L (5.2 mmol/L) | 4.8 mEq/L (4.8 mmol/L) | 3.5–5 mEq/L or (3.5–5 mmol/L) |

Select the **two** laboratory findings that are of **immediate** concern to the nurse.

A. Creatinine (Cr)

B. Blood urea nitrogen (BUN)

C. Calcium (Ca)

D. Phosphorus

E. Potassium (K)

**NGN Challenge #2**

The nurse is caring for an 81-year-old client admitted 2 days ago for dehydration and urosepsis.

| Health History | Nurses Notes | Orders | Laboratory Results |
|---|---|---|---|

**1115:** Alert but not oriented or able to communicate appropriately. Has not voided since 0430 when incontinent of small amount of urine in bed. Able to move all extremities. Dry mucous membranes and lips. Few crackles heard in left lung base; $S_1$ and $S_2$ present. Bowel sounds present × 4. 2+ ankle edema in both feet. Current VS: T 99.2°F (37.3°C); HR 96 beats/min; RR 20 breaths/min; BP 142/94; SpO₂ 94% on O₂ 2 L/min via NC.

| Laboratory Test | Today's Results | Yesterday's Results | Admission Results | Normal Reference Range |
|---|---|---|---|---|
| Creatinine | 2.9 mg/dL (256.4 mmol/L) | 2.4 mg/dL (212.2 mmol/L) | 2.0 mg/dL (176.8 mmol/L) | *Male:* 0.6–1.2 mg/dL (53–106 mmol/L) *Female:* 0.5–1.1 mg/dL (44–97 mmol/L) |
| BUN | 47 mg/dL (16.8 mmol/L) | 43 mg/dL (15.4 mmol/L) | 29 mg/dL (10.4 mmol/L) | 10–20 mg/dL (3.6–7.1 mmol/L) |
| Calcium | 8.8 mg/dL (2.2 mmol/L) | 9.1 mg/dL (2.27 mmol/L) | 9.4 mg/dL (2.35 mmol/L) | Total calcium: 9–10.5 mg/dL or 2.25–2.62 mmol/L |
| Phosphorus (inorganic) | 4.7 mg/dL (1.52 mmol/L) | 4.5 mg/dL (1.45 mmol/L) | 4.3 mg/dL (1.34 mmol/L) | 3–4.5 mg/dL or 0.97–1.45 mmol/L |
| Potassium | 5.3 mEq/L (5.3 mmol/L) | 5.2 mEq/L (5.2 mmol/L) | 4.8 mEq/L (4.8 mmol/L) | 3.5–5 mEq/L or (3.5–5 mmol/L) |

Complete the diagram by selecting from the choices to specify what **one** condition the client is most likely experiencing, **two** actions the nurse would take to address that condition, and **two** parameters the nurse would monitor to assess the client's progress.

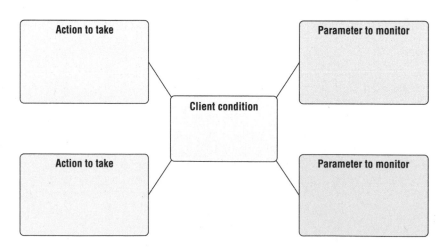

| Actions to Take | Client Condition | Parameters to Monitor |
| --- | --- | --- |
| Decrease IV fluid rate. | Chronic kidney disease | Skin turgor |
| Insert an indwelling urinary catheter. | Pyelonephritis | Vital signs |
| Administer a calcium supplement. | Acute kidney injury | Bowel sounds |
| Initiate continuous cardiac monitoring. | Urolithiasis | Peripheral oxygen saturation |
| Increase oxygen rate to 3 L/min. | ///////////////////////////////// | Urinary output |

# Assessment of the Reproductive System

## LEARNING OUTCOMES

1. Use knowledge of anatomy and physiology to perform a focused assessment of the reproductive system.
2. Teach evidence-based health promotion activities to help prevent reproductive health problems or trauma.
3. Identify factors that affect health equity for patients with reproductive health problems.
4. Explain how genetic implications and physiologic aging of the reproductive system affect sexuality.
5. Interpret assessment findings for patients with a suspected or actual reproductive problem.
6. Plan evidence-based care and support for patients undergoing diagnostic testing of the reproductive system.

## Preliminary Reading

Read and review Chapter 61, pp. 1495–1511.

## Chapter Review

### Anatomy & Physiology Review

#1.  Label the parts of the female genitalia using the Anatomy Labels provided after the figure.

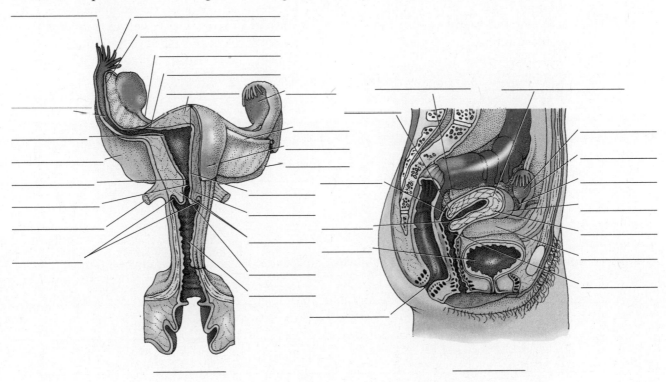

| Anatomy Labels |
|---|
| Anterior fornix |
| Cervix |
| Fallopian tube |
| Ovary |
| Peritoneum |
| Posterior fornix |
| Rectouterine pouch |
| Rectum |
| Round ligament |
| Urinary bladder |
| Uterine body |
| Uterine fundus |
| Utero-ovarian ligament |
| Vesicouterine pouch |

#2 Match the diagnostic test in Column A with its function in Column B.

**Column A**

____1. Colposcopy
____2. Conization
____3. Digital 3D mammography
____4. Dilation and curettage
____5. Hysterosalpingogram
____6. Hysteroscopy
____7. Laparoscopy
____8. Papanicolaou test

**Column B**

A. Removal of tissue in the uterus
B. Locates exact site of lesions for biopsy
C. Fiberoptic camera that visualizes the uterus
D. Removal of a cone-shaped tissue sample
E. Provides direct visualization of the pelvic cavity through an endoscope
F. Cytologic study to detect precancerous and cancerous cells
G. Allows visualization of the breast in slices
H. Provides visualization of cervix, uterus, and fallopian tubes via contrast medium

## Activities

### Activity #1

List five common reproductive changes associated with aging, and associated nursing interventions.

1. _____

2. _____

3. _____

4. _____

5. _____

### Activity #2

Complete the sentences with the correct term that ends in "-itis."
1. _____ can be caused by a history of mumps in men.
2. _____ is often caused by chlamydia and can result in female infertility.
3. Certain factors such as _____ can cause transient rises in PSA.
4. Acute testicular inflammation that arises from trauma or infection is called _____.
5. Pelvic inflammatory disease followed by _____ can cause pelvic scarring, and strictures or adhesions in the fallopian tubes.

### Activity #3

For each statement, specify if the statement is **true (T)** or **false (F)**.
____1. Another name for the female external genitalia is the vagina.
____2. Endometrial biopsies are usually done at the beginning of a menstrual cycle.
____3. Biopsies can differentiate fibrocystic lesions, fibroadenomas, and intraductal papillomas.
____4. Informed consent is necessary when a patient is going to undergo dilation and curettage.
____5. Increased levels of follicle-stimulating hormone can be indicative of polycystic ovaries.
____6. Consumption of sugar-sweetened beverages and highly processed food is linked to colorectal cancer.
____7. Shrinkage of the labia majora is a concerning assessment finding in an older adult woman.
____8. The vas deferens is the first portion of a ductal system that transports sperm.
____9. The risk for sexually transmitted infections decreases as people age.
____10. Certain drugs and supplements can cause changes in libido.

## Activity #4

List pertinent teaching the nurse will provide to a patient who has just undergone cervical biopsy.

_____

_____

_____

_____

_____

_____

_____

## Activity #5

Complete the sentences by filling in the blanks.

1. _____ is the surgical removal of the foreskin.
2. The normal pH in the vagina is 3.8 to 5.0, which is _____ (acidic or alkaline).
3. The ovum is fertilized in the _____ up to 72 hours after release.
4. Benign prostatic hyperplasia (BPH) is enlargement of the _____.
5. Mutation of the _____ or _____ gene increases the overall risk for breast or ovarian cancer.
6. Women between the ages of 25 and 65, or who have had an abnormal Pap test, should be tested for _____.
7. Fluid withdrawn from a breast cyst that is _____ in color may be indicative of cancer.
8. Before a prostate biopsy, the patient who is anxious may be medicated with an _____ drug.
9. A patient who is having a prostate biopsy will usually be prescribed some type of _____ drug prophylactically to reduce the risk for infection.
10. A patient who has had a cervical biopsy must be taught by the nurse to rest for _____ hours following the procedure.

## Learning Assessments

### NCLEX Examination Challenge #1

Which factor will the nurse assess in a male client who reports decreased libido? **Select all that apply.**

A. Diet
B. Tobacco use
C. Medication history
D. Consumption of alcohol
E. Use of illicit substances

### NCLEX Examination Challenge #2

Which information will the nurse teach a client who had a prostate biopsy to expect following the procedure?

A. Seminal fluid will appear normal within a day after the procedure.
B. A low-grade fever and bright red penile discharge are normal for several days.
C. Slight soreness and light rectal bleeding that is bright red are expected for a few days.
D. Swelling of the biopsy area and difficulty urinating are expected during the first week.

## NCLEX Examination Challenge #3

Which preprocedural teaching will the nurse provide to a client who is scheduled for a mammogram?

A.  Do not eat or drink anything 2 to 3 hours before the procedure.
B.  Abstain from sexual relations for 24 hours before the procedure.
C.  Wear a supportive bra, which will be worn during the diagnostic test.
D.  Do not use lotions, creams, or powder on the breasts on the day of the study.

# 62
CHAPTER

# Concepts of Care for Patients with Breast Conditions

## LEARNING OUTCOMES

1. Plan collaborative care with the interprofessional team to promote tissue integrity in patients with breast disorders.
2. Teach adults how to decrease the risk for breast disorders.
3. Teach the patient and caregiver(s) about common drugs and other management strategies used for breast disorders.
4. Plan patient- and family-centered nursing interventions to decrease the psychosocial impact caused by living with breast disorders.
5. Apply knowledge of anatomy, physiology, and pathophysiology to provide evidence-based care for patients with breast disorders.
6. Analyze assessment and diagnostic findings to generate solutions and prioritize nursing care for patients with breast disorders.
7. Organize care coordination and transition management for patients with breast disorders.
8. Use clinical judgment to plan evidence-based nursing care to promote favorable cellular regulation and prevent complications in patients with infection and pain in patient with breast conditions.
9. Incorporate factors that affect health equity into the plan of care for patients with breast disorders.

## Preliminary Reading

Read and review Chapter 62, pp. 1512–1536.

## Chapter Review

### Pathophysiology Review

#1. Match the type of condition in Column A with its description in Column B.

| Column A | Column B |
|---|---|
| ____1. Atypical hyperplasia | A. Changes in lobules, ducts, and stromal tissues |
| ____2. Ductal carcinoma in situ | B. Benign ridge of glandular tissue in male breast |
| ____3. Fibroadenoma | C. Most common type of invasive breast cancer |
| ____4. Fibrocystic changes | D. Noninvasive disease that is not a precursor of cancer |
| ____5. Fibrosis | E. Cancer without expression of estrogen, progesterone, and human epidermal growth factor receptors |
| ____6. Gynecomastia | F. Well-defined solid mass of connective tissue |
| ____7. Inflammatory breast cancer | G. Noncancerous change in cellular structure of cell |
| ____8. Invasive ductal carcinoma | H. Aggressive breast cancer with diffuse erythema and edema |
| ____9. Lobular ductal carcinoma | I. Normal cell replacement with connective tissue and collagen |
| ___10. Triple-negative breast cancer | J. Noninvasive type of breast cancer |

#2. Fill in the blank to explain how each nonmodifiable risk factor for breast cancer is significant.

| Risk Factor | How Risk Factor is Significant |
|---|---|
| Gender | Most breast cancer occurs in _____. |
| Age | Risk increases with aging, especially after the age of _____. |
| Genetic factors | Inherited mutations of _____ and/or _____ increase risk. |
| Race | Overall, _____ women are more likely to develop breast cancer than _____ women; however, in women younger than _____ years old, breast cancer is more common in _____ women. |
| Heritage | Women of _____ heritage have higher incidences of *BRCA1* and *BRCA2* genetic mutations, which raises the risk. |
| Personal history of certain benign breast conditions | Two benign breast conditions that slightly raise the risk for breast cancer:<br>• _____<br>• _____<br><br>One benign breast condition that significantly raises the risk for breast cancer:<br>• _____ |
| Breast density | Dense breasts contain more _____ and _____ tissue, which increases the risk for developing breast cancer. |
| Family history of breast cancer | Having a _____-degree relative with breast or ovarian cancer increases risk. |
| Menstrual history | The risk for breast cancer rises if the patient had early menstruation (younger than _____ years old) or late menopause (at the age of _____ or older), or both. |

## Activities

### Activity #1

For each statement, specify if the statement is **true (T)** or **false (F)**.

_____1.   Breast augmentation is most commonly done with saline-filled prostheses.

_____2.   Teach women that self-breast examination is preferred over clinical breast examination.

_____3.   Mastitis only occurs in women who are breastfeeding.

_____4.   Patients with ductal carcinoma in situ have metastasis to distant places in the body.

_____5.   Peau d'orange is characterized by edematous thickening and pitting of breast skin.

_____6.   All individuals who are positive for *BRCA1* and *BRCA2* will develop breast cancer.

_____7.   Lymphedema is a condition that is easily reversible.

_____8.   Aromatase inhibitors are used in premenopausal women whose estrogen is in the ovaries.

_____9.   The final step in breast reconstruction is the nipple–areola complex.

____10.   Teach women that postmastectomy exercises are discouraged to preserve tissue.

**Activity #2**
List five things the nurse will teach to a male client diagnosed with gynecomastia.

1. _____

2. _____

3. _____

4. _____

5. _____

**Activity #3**
Describe the population that each type of breast disorder often affects.

1. Fibroadenoma _____

2. Fibrocystic changes (FCCs) _____

3. Ductal ectasia _____

4. Intraductal papilloma _____

**Activity #4**
Indicate which Complementary and Integrative Therapy is *most* commonly used for each symptom that patients with breast cancer may experience. Some symptoms may support the use of more than one type of therapy.

| Type of Therapy |
| --- |
| Aromatherapy |
| Black cohosh |
| Ginger |
| Flaxseed |
| Massage |
| Progressive muscle relaxation |
| Yoga |

1. Pain_____

2. Nausea/vomiting_____

3. Fatigue_____

4. Hot flashes _____

5. Anxiety_____

6. Depression _____

Learning Assessments

## NCLEX Examination Challenge #1

When will the nurse expect a client with breast cancer to receive neoadjuvant therapy?

A. After surgery to ensure that all cancer cells have been destroyed

B. Before surgery to shrink the tumor and make it easier to remove

C. With radiation therapy to treat any metastasis that may occur

D. During surgery to make sure that all of the tumor cells are removed

## NCLEX Examination Challenge #2

Which finding is likely for the nurse to observe when assessing a client with very large breasts?

A. Presence of peau d'orange

B. Drainage from one or both nipples

C. Fungal infection underneath the breasts

D. Multiple instances of fibrocystic changes

## NCLEX Examination Challenge #3

Which teaching will the nurse provide to a client following mastectomy surgery?

A. Ambulation is discouraged until 1 week later.

B. Resume a regular diet 3 days following the procedure.

C. Check the surgical site for signs of infection or bleeding.

D. Rest the affected arm below heart level to promote drainage.

## NGN Challenge #1

A 59-year-old client is admitted to the postsurgical unit following mastectomy. The nurse reviews and analyzes the vital sign flow sheet data since admission to the unit after surgery.

| | 48 Hours After Surgery (0958) | 24 Hours After Surgery (0953) | Admission Postsurgery (0955) |
|---|---|---|---|
| T | 100.6°F (38.1°C) | 98.4°F (36.9°C) | 98.4°F (36.9°C) |
| HR | 90 beats/min | 78 beats/min | 62 beats/min |
| RR | 18 breaths/min | 18 breaths/min | 16 breaths/min |
| BP | 102/60 mm Hg | 112/62 mm Hg | 128/74 mm Hg |
| $SpO_2$ | 98% (on RA) | 97% (on $O_2$ 2 L/min) | 99% (on $O_2$ 2 L/min) |
| Urinary output | 998 mL | 860 mL | 950 mL |
| Level of consciousness | Drowsy but more difficult to arouse; oriented ×2 (person and place); restless when awakened | Drowsy but easily awakened; oriented ×3 | Drowsy but easily awakened; oriented ×3 |

Complete the following sentence by filling in the blanks using the lists of options.

The nurse analyzes the assessment data and determines that the client is most likely experiencing _____ 1 [Select]_____ as evidenced by _____ 2 [Select]_____ and _____3 [Select]_____.

| Options for 1 | Options for 2 | Options for 3 |
|---|---|---|
| Sepsis | Decreasing blood pressure | Variance in $SpO_2$ |
| Transient ischemic stroke | Orientation ×3 | Respiratory rate |
| Hypotension | Urinary output | Decreased level of consciousness |

## NGN Challenge #2

The nurse has recorded nursing notes for a 33-year-old client who has come to the primary health care provider reporting two new lumps in her breast.

| Vital Signs | Nurses Notes | Health Care Provider's Orders | Laboratory Results | |
|---|---|---|---|---|

**1302:** Client presents reporting finding two small lumps in her breast earlier this week when putting on lotion. She describes them as moveable and well-defined. Her main concern is that she has tumors indicating breast cancer. Denies breast pain or tenderness, nipple drainage, and unusual warmth on palpation. Denies any other significant ongoing health care problems or recent health changes. Health history positive for COVID-19 9 months prior; she recovered without intervention aside from quarantine and symptomatic management. Personal and family history negative for breast cancer. Lives at home with her partner; occasionally drinks a glass of wine. Denies use of tobacco or illicit drugs. Alert and oriented × 4. Somewhat tearful when providing history. Breasts appear symmetrical; no visible abnormalities noted. Two small, oval-shaped nodules located at 2:00 p.m. in the left breast. No other palpable nodules noted in left breast; none in right breast. No nipple drainage observed. Current VS: T 98.4°F (36.9°C); HR 70 beats/min and regular; RR 18 breaths/min; BP 128/728 mm Hg; SpO$_2$ 98%.

Complete the diagram by selecting from the choices to specify what **one** potential condition the client is at risk for, **two** priority actions the nurse would take to help prevent that condition, and **two** parameters the nurse would monitor to assess the client's progress.

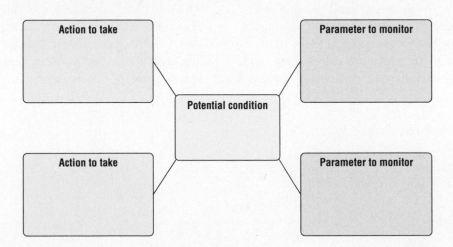

| Priority Actions to Take | Potential Condition | Parameters to Monitor |
|---|---|---|
| Assess if client is taking spironolactone | Atypical hyperplasia | Onset of back pain |
| Teach about benign breast tumors | Gynecomastia | Adherence to tamoxifen therapy |
| Assist with scheduling breast ultrasound | Ductal carcinoma in situ | Presence of future nodules that may arise |
| Explain that gynecomastia can occur in women | Fibroadenoma | Outcome of diagnostic testing |
| Arrange for prophylactic mastectomy | ///////////////////////////// | Lymphatic metastasis |

# 63

CHAPTER

# *Concepts of Care for Patients with Gynecologic Conditions*

## LEARNING OUTCOMES

1. Plan collaborative care with the interprofessional team to promote gynecologic health in patients with gynecologic disorders.
2. Teach adults how to decrease the risk for gynecologic disorders.
3. Teach the patient and caregiver(s) about common drugs and other management strategies used for gynecologic disorders.
4. Plan patient- and family-centered nursing interventions to decrease the psychosocial impact caused by living with a gynecologic disorder.
5. Apply knowledge of anatomy, physiology, and pathophysiology to provide evidence-based care

for patients with a gynecologic disorder affecting sexuality and reproduction.
6. Analyze assessment and diagnostic findings to generate solutions and prioritize nursing care for patients with a gynecologic disorder.
7. Organize care coordination and transition management for patients with a gynecologic disorder.
8. Use clinical judgment to plan evidence-based nursing care to promote sexuality and reproduction and prevent pain and complications in patients with a gynecologic disorder.
9. Incorporate factors that affect health equity into the plan of care for patients with gynecologic disorders.

## Preliminary Reading

Read and review Chapter 63, pp. 1537–1555.

## Chapter Review

### Pathophysiology Review

#1. Match the Key Term in Column A with its definition in Column B.

| Column A | Column B |
|---|---|
| ___1. Concurrent chemoradiation | A. Rectal protrusion through vaginal wall |
| ___2. Dyspareunia | B. Lower genital tract inflammation |
| ___3. Leiomyoma | C. Displacement from normal position |
| ___4. Prolapse | D. Benign uterine myometrium tumor |
| ___5. Rectocele | E. Use of chemotherapy and radiation together |
| ___6. Vulvovaginitis | F. Pain experienced with sexual intercourse |

#2. For each statement, specify if the statement is **true (T)** or **false (F)**.
_____1. Intramural leiomyomas protrude into the uterine cavity.
_____2. In utero exposure to diethylstilbestrol (DES) reduces the risk for leiomyoma development.
_____3. A small amount of bleeding at the site of laparoscopic incision is expected.
_____4. Following hysterectomy, patients must avoid use of tampons for 12 weeks.

____5.　Endometrial cancer is a rare and fast-growing type of cancer.
____6.　Brachytherapy can be used to prevent recurrence of endometrial cancer.
____7.　A *CA 125* test result is elevated only when a patient has cancer.
____8.　Human papillomavirus virus infection is the cause of most types of cervical cancer.
____9.　Gardasil 9 is available in the United States and Canada as an HPV vaccine.
___10.　Pediculicides are used to treat vulvovaginitis that is caused by a yeast infection.

## Activities

### Activity #1
Match the procedure in Column A with its description in Column B.

| **Column A** | **Column B** |
| --- | --- |
| ____1. Anterior colporrhaphy | A. Rectocele repair |
| ____2. Bilateral salpingo-oophorectomy | B. Cutting away of cervical cancer tissue |
| ____3. Colposcopy | C. Procedure to starve tumor of circulation |
| ____4. Loop electrosurgical excision procedure | D. Tightening of pelvic muscles for bladder support |
| ____5. Myomectomy | E. Removal of the fallopian tubes and ovaries |
| ____6. Posterior colporrhaphy | F. Examination of cervix and vagina to locate lesion |
| ____7. Total hysterectomy | G. Removal of leiomyomas from uterus |
| ____8. Uterine artery embolization | H. Removal of uterus and cervix |

### Activity #2
List five things the nurse will assess and monitor for a client who has had a hysterectomy.

1. _____

2. _____

3. _____

4. _____

5. _____

### Activity #3
Circle the correct word from the underlined choices to complete each sentence about the prevention of toxic shock syndrome.
1.　Do not use superabsorbent/regular/slim tampons.
2.　Change the tampon every 1-2/3-6/6-9 hours.
3.　Use perineal pads/tampons at night.
4.　Avoid use of birth control pills/condoms/insertable contraceptive devices.
5.　If you experience the sudden onset of a high temperature, take acetaminophen/wait 1-2 hours to see if it subsides/contact your primary health care provider.

**Activity #4**

List five important things the nurse will teach a patient about ways to prevent vulvovaginitis.

1. _____

2. _____

3. _____

4. _____

5. _____

## Learning Assessments

### NCLEX Examination Challenge #1

Which symptom does the nurse anticipate will be present for a client admitted with uterine leiomyomas?
A. Heavy vaginal bleeding
B. Intermittent abdominal pain
C. Urinary stress incontinence
D. Foul-smelling vaginal discharge

### NCLEX Examination Challenge #2

The nurse is caring for a client who had an anterior colporrhaphy. Which client statement indicates that the procedure achieved the desired therapeutic outcome?
A. "That constipated feeling has resolved."
B. "The abdominal pain is almost gone."
C. "I have good control over my urination."
D. "My vaginal bleeding has completely stopped."

### NCLEX Examination Challenge #3

Which client does the nurse identify that should be evaluated for possible endometrial cancer?
A. A 22-year-old with no menstrual period for 3 months
B. A 37-year-old with report of multiple sexual partners
C. A 50-year-old with irregular menses over the past 6 months
D. A 64-year-old with reports of bleeding after menopause

## NGN Challenge #1

The nurse has recorded notes for a 44-year-old client at the gynecologic health care provider's office for an annual examination.

| Vital Signs | Nurses Notes | Health Care Provider's Orders | Laboratory Results | |
|---|---|---|---|---|

**0800:** Client here for annual examination. Most recent examination last year was unremarkable. Mammogram was performed last week; evaluation shows no evidence of cancer. Reports she has been feeling very tired over the past few months. Says she doesn't have much of an appetite and gets full quickly when eating. Attributes the fatigue and lack of appetite to an increasing amount of stress because one of her children is getting married in 3 months and the other is graduating from college. Denies pain anywhere but does report occasional discomfort abdominally and some intermittent vaginal bleeding that she states "may be related to premenopause." Denies urinary frequency or incontinence. No weight loss noted. Sexual history reveals monogamy with one partner for 21 years. Medical history of elevated cholesterol managed with 20 mg lovastatin nightly. Surgical history of breast reduction 8 years ago with no subsequent complications. Alert and oriented × 4. Breath sounds clear in all lung fields. No wheezes, crackles, or dyspnea. $S_1$ and $S_2$ present; no murmurs. Bowel sounds present × 4. Abdomen nontender to touch. Current VS: T 98.4°F (36.9°C); HR 82 beats/min and regular; RR 16 breaths/min; BP 128/90 mm Hg; SpO$_2$ 98%.

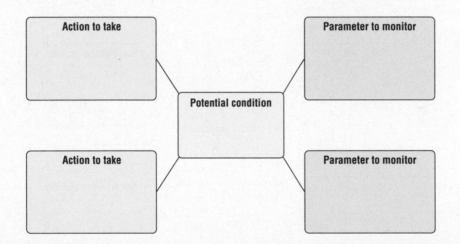

| Priority Actions to Take | Potential Condition | Parameters to Monitor |
|---|---|---|
| Prepare to assist with pelvic examination. | Vulvar cancer | Adherence to antibiotic therapy |
| Discuss the need for Gardasil 9 vaccination. | Cervical cancer | Weight |
| Arrange for appointment for abdominal CT. | Endometrial cancer | Nutrition status |
| Teach to use perineal pads instead of tampons. | Ovarian cancer | Results from cone biopsy |
| Administer calcium carbonate as prescribed. | ///////////////////////////////// | Outcome of loop electrosurgical excision procedure |

**NGN Challenge #2**

The nurse has recorded notes for a 19-year-old client who has come to the urgent care reporting unusual vaginal discharge.

| Vital Signs | Nurses Notes | Health Care Provider's Orders | Laboratory Results | |
|---|---|---|---|---|

**1404:** Client presents reporting 1 week of unusual vaginal discharge that began following her last menstrual cycle. She states she normally has scant clear discharge, yet this is different because it is yellowish, thick, and has a foul odor. Confirms that she has persistent vaginal itching despite bathing regularly and keeping the area dry. Denies chills, abdominal pain, changes in bowel or bladder habits. Sexual history includes one partner; they use a vaginal sponge and condoms with spermicide for contraceptive purposes. No remarkable medical history. Current on immunizations. Alert and oriented × 4. Bowel sounds present × 4; no abdominal tenderness noted upon palpation. Current VS: T 98.4°F (36.9°C); HR 80 beats/min and regular; RR 14 breaths/min; BP 116/72 mm Hg; SpO$_2$ 99%.

Complete the diagram by selecting from the choices to specify what **one** potential condition the client is at risk for, **two** priority actions the nurse would take to help prevent that condition, and **two** parameters the nurse would monitor to assess the client's progress.

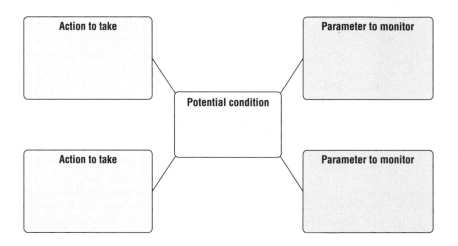

| Priority Actions to Take | Potential Condition | Parameters to Monitor |
|---|---|---|
| Recommend Gardasil 9 vaccination. | Toxic shock syndrome | Perineal tissue integrity |
| Assist health care provider with vaginal smear collection. | Vulvovaginitis | Development of fever |
| Teach to clean vagina and perineum with mild soap and warm water. | Leiomyoma | Onset of macular rash |
| Encourage douching after intercourse. | Cervical cancer | Avoidance of fragranced detergent, body wash, and lotion |
| Confirm that nylon underwear minimizes vaginal moisture. | ///////////////////////////////// | Attendance at follow-up appointment for endometrial cancer screening |

# 64 CHAPTER

# *Concepts of Care for Patients with Male Reproductive Conditions*

## LEARNING OUTCOMES

1. Plan collaborative care with the interprofessional team to promote elimination and cellular regulation in patients with male reproductive disorders.
2. Teach adults how to decrease the risk for male reproductive disorders.
3. Teach the patient and caregiver(s) about common drugs and other management strategies used for male reproductive disorders.
4. Plan patient- and family-centered nursing interventions to decrease the psychosocial impact caused by living with a male reproductive disorder.
5. Apply knowledge of anatomy, physiology, and pathophysiology to provide evidence-based care for patients with a male reproductive disorder affecting elimination or cellular regulation.
6. Analyze assessment and diagnostic findings to generate solutions and prioritize nursing care for patients with a male reproductive disorder.
7. Organize care coordination and transition management for patients with a male reproductive disorder.
8. Use clinical judgment to plan evidence-based nursing care to promote elimination and cellular regulation and prevent complications in patients with a male reproductive disorder.
9. Incorporate factors that affect health equity into the plan of care for patients with male reproductive disorders.

## Preliminary Reading

Read and review Chapter 64, pp. 1556–1582.

## Chapter Review

### Pathophysiology Review

#1. Match the Key Term in Column A with its definition in Column B.

| Column A | | Column B | |
|---|---|---|---|
| ___1. | Azoospermia | A. | Absence of living sperm in the semen |
| ___2. | Cryptorchidism | B. | Abnormal ureter distention |
| ___3. | Gynecomastia | C. | Low sperm count |
| ___4. | Hydroureter | D. | Abnormal enlargement of breasts in men |
| ___5. | Oligospermia | E. | Surgical procedure for prostate removal |
| ___6. | Prostate-specific antigen | F. | Failure of testes to descend into scrotum |
| ___7. | Transurethral resection of the prostate (TURP) | G. | Glycoprotein made by the prostate |

#2. For each statement, specify if the statement is **true (T)** or **false (F).**

\_\_\_\_1. Active surveillance involves monitoring treatment outcomes for someone with cancer.

\_\_\_\_2. Lower urinary tract symptoms (LUTS) can arise if a patient has urinary retention.

\_\_\_\_3. Both testes must be removed when an orchiectomy is performed.

\_\_\_\_4. Retrograde ejaculation is a condition in which semen flows backward into the kidney.

\_\_\_\_5. An enlarged prostate can cause bladder outlet obstruction.

\_\_\_\_6. Acute urinary retention is a medical emergency.

\_\_\_\_7. The nurse should teach patients at risk for BPH to minimize coffee and caffeine intake.

\_\_\_\_8. Prostate cancer occurs in young men as often as it does in older men.

\_\_\_\_9. The seminoma type of testicular cancer is localized, metastasizes late, and responds to treatment.

\_\_\_10. Erectile dysfunction is always physiological in nature.

## Activities

### Activity #1

List four nonmodifiable risk factors associated with the development of benign prostatic hyperplasia (BPH).

1. _____

2. _____

3. _____

4. _____

### Activity #2

For each statement, specify if the statement is **true (T)** or **false (F).**

\_\_\_\_1. The first-line treatment for benign prostatic hyperplasia (BPH) is TURP surgery.

\_\_\_\_2. Anticholinergic drugs can contribute to urinary retention in patients with BPH.

\_\_\_\_3. The nurse must teach patients taking finasteride that gynecomastia is a possible side effect.

\_\_\_\_4. Grapefruit juice can minimize the amount of tadalafil in the body.

\_\_\_\_5. Orthostatic hypotension can occur if a patient is taking alfuzosin.

\_\_\_\_6. The nurse will teach patients to take tamsulosin 30 minutes before meals at the same time daily.

\_\_\_\_7. Tadalafil is used to treat erectile dysfunction and lower urinary tract symptoms.

\_\_\_\_8. Patients prescribed dutasteride should open the capsule and sprinkle the contents onto applesauce.

\_\_\_\_9. The nurse will teach patients taking finasteride and dutasteride that these drugs are highly teratogenic.

\_\_\_10. Silodosin is an $alpha_1$-adrenergic antagonist.

## Activity #3
Match the procedure used to treat benign prostatic hyperplasia in Column A with its description in Column B.

**Column A**

____1. Aquablation
____2. Photoselective vaporization
____3. Transurethral needle ablation
____4. Transurethral microwave thermotherapy
____5. Transurethral electro vaporization of the prostate
____6. Transurethral water vapor therapy
____7. Urolift

**Column B**

A. Heated ball or wire loop inserted through the urethra to heat prostate tissue, which is reduced to vapor
B. Device placed in the obstructed urethra; implants placed to lift enlarged prostate
C. Low radiofrequency energy that shrinks the prostate
D. Use of a heat-free waterjet and cystoscope to remove prostate tissue
E. Sterile heated water vaporizes; vapor given by needle to targeted tissue as ablative therapy
F. Laser energy used to vaporize prostate tissue
G. Antennae placed through the penis toward the prostate to deliver electromagnetic waves that heat and destroy prostate tissue

## Activity #4
Explain how item works in the treatment of erectile dysfunction.

1. Phosphodiesterase-5 (PDE5) inhibitors (e.g., avanafil, sildenafil, tadalafil, vardenafil)

_____

_____

_____

2. Intraurethral alprostadil injections

_____

_____

_____

3. Penile injections

_____

_____

_____

4. Penile prosthesis

_____

_____

_____

5. Vacuum-assisted erection device

_____

_____

_____

## Activity #5
Identify five potential treatment measures for erectile dysfunction (ED) the nurse could share with a patient.

1. _____

2. _____

3. _____

4. _____

5. _____

## Activity #6
In a few words, describe each condition and list several signs/symptoms.

1. Hydrocele

   a. Description _____

   b. Signs/symptoms _____

2. Spermatocele

   a. Description _____

   b. Signs/symptoms _____

3. Varicocele

   a. Description _____

   b. Signs/symptoms _____

4. Paraphimosis

   a. Description _____

   b. Signs/symptoms _____

5. Priapism

   a. Description _____

   b. Signs/symptoms _____

6. Hydrocele

   a. Description _____

   b. Signs/symptoms _____

7. Epididymitis

   a. Description _____

   b. Signs/symptoms _____

8. Phimosis

   a. Description _____

   b. Signs/symptoms _____

## Learning Assessments

### NCLEX Examination Challenge #1
A client has continuous bladder irrigation after surgery yesterday. The amount of bladder irrigating solution that has infused over the past 12 hours is 1100 mL. The amount of fluid in the urinary drainage bag is 2240 mL. The nurse records that the client had _____ mL urinary output in the past 12 hours. **Fill in the blank.**

### NCLEX Examination Challenge #2
Which criteria will the nurse assess in a client with benign prostatic hyperplasia that may indicate the need for surgical intervention? **Select all that apply.**
A. Hematuria
B. Hydronephrosis
C. Acute urinary retention resulting from obstruction
D. Acute urinary infection unresponsive to first-line antibiotics
E. Chronic urinary tract infection secondary to residual urine in bladder

### NCLEX Examination Challenge #3
Which symptom does the nurse expect will be present when admitting a client diagnosed with benign prostatic hyperplasia?
A. Constipation
B. Scrotal discomfort
C. Erectile dysfunction
D. Difficulty urinating

**NGN Challenge #1**

The nurse reviews the Nurses Notes for a 72-year-old client who has come to the provider reporting difficulty urinating.

| Vital Signs | Nurses Notes | Health Care Provider's Orders | Laboratory Results |
|---|---|---|---|

**0902:** Client here to see provider. Reports has been having difficulty with urinating since last visit 4 months prior. Describes symptoms as "not being able to get started" when he needs to urinate, and "dribbling instead of peeing." Denies other changes such as bowel problems, different eating or drinking habits, or other symptoms. No remarkable weight loss noted. Denies new sexual partners; no penile discharge or pain reported. VS: T 98.0°F (37.6°C); HR 76 beats/min; RR 14 breaths/min; BP 134/72 mm Hg; SpO$_2$ 99% on RA.

Complete the diagram by selecting from the choices to specify what **one** potential condition the client may be experiencing, **two** actions the nurse would take to address that condition, and **two** parameters the nurse would monitor to assess the client's progress.

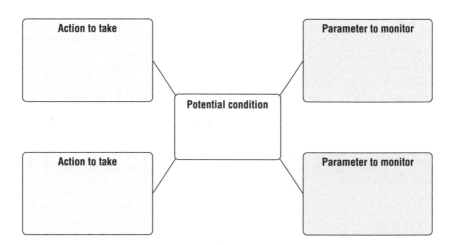

| Actions to Take | Potential Condition | Parameters to Monitor |
|---|---|---|
| Explain prostate artery embolization. | Urinary tract infection | Ability to create a urinary stream |
| Prepare for external beam radiation therapy. | Benign prostatic hypertrophy | Adherence to alpha$_1$-adrenergic antagonists |
| Assess for urinary retention. | Erectile dysfunction | Completion of antibiotic therapy |
| Teach that a digital rectal examination may be done. | Prostate cancer | Temperature |
| Anticipate the need for an antibiotic. | /////////////////////////////////// | Results of culture and sensitivity |

## NGN Challenge #2

The nurse reviews the Nurses Notes for a 40-year-old client admitted to the emergency department.

| Vital Signs | Nurses Notes | Orders | Laboratory Results |
|---|---|---|---|

**2244:** Client brought to emergency department by partner. Client appears to be in distress; states he has had an erection that has not resolved in the past 2 hours. Reports penile pain; states he was circumcised as an infant. Diaphoresis noted. Denies other symptoms such as chest or abdominal pain. Lung sounds clear; heart rate regular and tachycardic. History of sickle cell disease. VS: T 98.9°F (37.2°C); HR 112 beats/min; RR 22 breaths/min; BP 190/90 mm Hg; SpO₂ 98% on RA.

Complete the diagram by selecting from the choices to specify what **one** potential condition the client may be experiencing, **two** actions the nurse would take to address that condition, and **two** parameters the nurse would monitor to assess the client's progress.

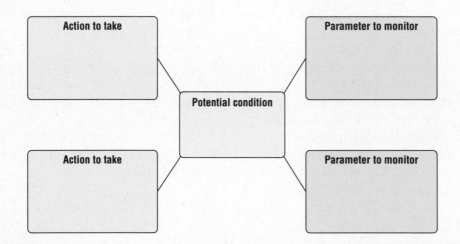

| Actions to Take | Potential Condition | Parameters to Monitor |
|---|---|---|
| Reassure that symptoms will resolve without intervention. | Paraphimosis | Resolution of erection |
| Elevate the scrotum. | Epididymitis | Adherence to full course of antibiotic therapy |
| Prepare for automated red blood cell exchange transfusion. | Spermatocele | Maintenance of proper hygiene |
| Give antibiotics intravenously. | Priapism | Subjective report of pain level on 0-10 scale |
| Administer phenylephrine by injection. | ///////////////////////////////// | Appearance of purulent penile drainage |

# 65 CHAPTER

# Concepts of Care for Patients with Sexually Transmitted Infections

## LEARNING OUTCOMES

1. Plan collaborative care with the interprofessional team to promote health in patients with a sexually transmitted infection.
2. Teach adults how to decrease the risk for sexually transmitted infections.
3. Teach the patient and caregiver(s) about common drugs and other management strategies used for sexually transmitted infections.
4. Plan patient- and family-centered nursing interventions to decrease the psychosocial impact caused by living with a sexually transmitted infection.
5. Apply knowledge of anatomy, physiology, and pathophysiology to provide evidence-based care for patients with a sexually transmitted infection.
6. Analyze assessment and diagnostic findings to generate solutions and prioritize nursing care for patients with a sexually transmitted infection.
7. Organize care coordination and transition management for patients with a sexually transmitted infection.
8. Use clinical judgment to plan evidence-based nursing care to promote health and prevent complications in patients with a sexually transmitted infection.
9. Incorporate factors that affect health equity into the plan of care for patients with a sexually transmitted infection.

## Preliminary Reading

Read and review Chapter 65, pp. 1583–1602.

## Chapter Review

### Pathophysiology Review

#1. Match the Key Term in Column A with its definition in Column B.

| Column A | Column B |
|---|---|
| ____1. Chancre | A. Acute syndrome involving gynecologic pain |
| ____2. Dyspareunia | B. Incurable viral disease of the genitalia |
| ____3. Dysuria | C. Treatment of sexual partners without a visit with a health care provider |
| ____4. Expedited partner therapy | |
| ____5. Genital herpes | D. Infection of the fallopian tube(s) |
| ____6. Pelvic inflammatory disease | E. Initial sign of syphilis infection |
| ____7. Salpingitis | F. Pain experienced with sexual intercourse |
| ____8. Sexually transmitted infection | G. Complex sexually transmitted infection that can become systemic |
| ____9. Syphilis | H. Passing of infectious organisms via intimacy |
| | I. Painful urination |

**Review of Nursing Care for Patients with Sexually Transmitted Infections**

#2.  For each statement, specify if the statement is **true (T)** or **false (F)**.

_____1.   It is possible for patients to not know that they have a sexually transmitted infection.

_____2.   Someone who has a history of a sexually transmitted infection is at risk for acquiring another sexually transmitted infection.

_____3.   Substance use has decreased the incidence and prevalence of sexually transmitted infections.

_____4.   Chancroid is a naturally notifiable condition.

_____5.   Women who have sex with women (WSW) have more sexually transmitted infections than other populations.

_____6.   Practicing mutual monogamy is considered a safer sex practice.

_____7.   The incubation period of genital herpes is 2 to 10 days.

_____8.   People with genital herpes are not contagious between outbreaks.

_____9.   Patients with pelvic inflammatory disease should rest in the supine position.

____10.   Douching is recommended for women who wish to avoid sexually transmitted infections.

**Activities**

**Activity #1**

Match the sexually transmitted infection in Column A with its primary initial symptom in Column B.

**Column A**

___1.   Genital herpes

___2.   Syphilis

___3.   Genital warts

___4.   *Chlamydia trachomatis*

___5.   Gonorrhea

___6.   Mpox

___7.   Pelvic inflammatory disease

**Column B**

A.   Small papillary growths

B.   Fever, myalgias, lymphadenopathy

C.   Clustered vesicles

D.   Yellowish-green penile or vaginal discharge

E.   Dull to acute pelvic pain

F.   Frequently asymptomatic

G.   Chancre ulcer

**Activity #2**

Construct five questions the nurse would ask when taking a history of a patient who may have a sexually transmitted infection.

1.   _____

2.   _____

3.   _____

4.   _____

5.   _____

**Activity #3**

From this list, indicate the sexually transmitted infections that are **nationally** notifiable.

1. HIV
2. Syphilis
3. Chancroid
4. Gonorrhea
5. Chlamydia
6. Genital herpes
7. Condylomata acuminata
8. Pelvic inflammatory disease

**Activity #4**

List five important things the nurse will teach a patient about the proper use of condoms.

1. _____

2. _____

3. _____

4. _____

5. _____

**Learning Assessments**

**NCLEX Examination Challenge #1**

The nurse is caring for a client with pelvic inflammatory disease (PID) who was just started on antibiotics and pain medication. Which assessment finding will the nurse report to the health care provider?

A. Yellowish vaginal discharge
B. Temperature 101.2°F (38.4°C)
C. RUQ and right shoulder pain
D. Spotting 2 weeks after a period

**NCLEX Examination Challenge #2**

The nurse has completed teaching for a client newly diagnosed with syphilis. Which client statement indicates that further nursing teaching is required?

A. "When the chancre goes away, this condition is resolved."
B. "Neurosyphilis can involve the loss of hearing or vision."
C. "Even if I don't have symptoms, this disease can still be contagious."
D. "If I develop a rash on the palms of my hands, I will notify the health care provider."

### NGN Challenge #1

The nurse has recorded nursing notes for a 23-year-old female client admitted to the medical surgical floor after being seen for abdominal pain and fever in the emergency department.

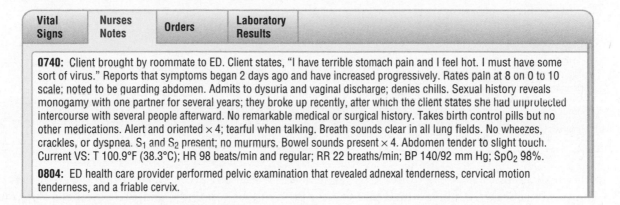

| Vital Signs | Nurses Notes | Orders | Laboratory Results |

**0740:** Client brought by roommate to ED. Client states, "I have terrible stomach pain and I feel hot. I must have some sort of virus." Reports that symptoms began 2 days ago and have increased progressively. Rates pain at 8 on 0 to 10 scale; noted to be guarding abdomen. Admits to dysuria and vaginal discharge; denies chills. Sexual history reveals monogamy with one partner for several years; they broke up recently, after which the client states she had unprotected intercourse with several people afterward. No remarkable medical or surgical history. Takes birth control pills but no other medications. Alert and oriented × 4; tearful when talking. Breath sounds clear in all lung fields. No wheezes, crackles, or dyspnea. $S_1$ and $S_2$ present; no murmurs. Bowel sounds present × 4. Abdomen tender to slight touch. Current VS: T 100.9°F (38.3°C); HR 98 beats/min and regular; RR 22 breaths/min; BP 140/92 mm Hg; $SpO_2$ 98%.

**0804:** ED health care provider performed pelvic examination that revealed adnexal tenderness, cervical motion tenderness, and a friable cervix.

Complete the diagram by selecting from the choices to specify what **one** potential condition the client is at risk for, **two** priority actions the nurse would take to help prevent that condition, and **two** parameters the nurse would monitor to assess the client's progress.

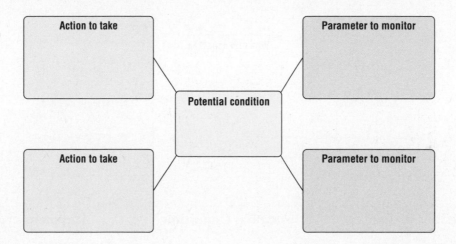

| Priority Actions to Take | Potential Condition | Parameters to Monitor |
| --- | --- | --- |
| Place client in the prone position. | Syphilis | Pain level |
| Teach about antiviral medication. | Mpox | Temperature |
| Insert a nasogastric tube. | Gonorrhea | ALT/AST |
| Administer antibiotics as ordered. | Pelvic inflammatory disease | Abdominal girth |
| Provide nonpharmacologic interventions for pain. | ///////////////////////////////// | Capillary refill |

**NGN Challenge #2**

The nurse has recorded nursing notes for a 28-year-old client who has come to the urgent care today after feeling fatigued.

| Vital Signs | Nurses Notes | Orders | Laboratory Results | |
|---|---|---|---|---|

**1000:** Client presents with reports of being fatigued for a week and waking up today with a low-grade fever. Denies chills, abdominal pain, changes in breathing or heart rate. Denies recent travel. Sexual history reveals intimate unprotected contact with another individual about 10 days prior. No remarkable medical history. Current on immunizations. Physical assessment reveals that client is alert and oriented × 4. Cervical and submental lymphadenopathy noted on palpation. Breath sounds clear in all lung fields. $S_1$ and $S_2$ present; no murmurs. Bowel sounds present × 4; no abdominal tenderness noted. Current VS: T 100.2°F (37.9°C); HR 70 beats/min and regular; RR 16 breaths/min; BP 122/70 mm Hg; $SpO_2$ 97%.

Complete the diagram by selecting from the choices to specify what **one** potential condition the client is at risk for, **two** priority actions the nurse would take to help prevent that condition, and **two** parameters the nurse would monitor to assess the client's progress.

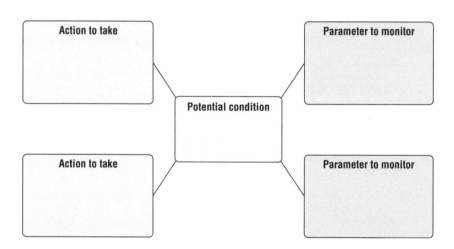

| Priority Actions to Take | Potential Condition | Parameters to Monitor |
|---|---|---|
| Discuss how to isolate at home. | Influenza | Temperature |
| Administer antibiotics as ordered. | Condylomata acuminata | Skin |
| Teach about potential rash that can arise. | Mpox | Anus for development of genital warts |
| Recommend vaccination for human papillomavirus (HPV). | Syphilis | Adherence to application of topical antifungal therapy |
| Obtain sputum specimen. | ///////////////////////////// | Culture and sensitivity for bacterial result |

# ANSWERS

## Chapter 1

### Answer Key

**Activity #1**

1. C
2. B
3. A
4. D

**Activity #2**

Any three of these common errors by nurses can jeopardize patient care:

- Lack of clear or adequate communication among patient, family, and members of the interprofessional health care team
- Lack of attentiveness and patient monitoring
- Lack of ability to make safe **clinical judgment**
- Inadequate measures to prevent health complications
- Errors in medication administration
- Errors in interpreting authorized provider prescriptions
- Lack of professional accountability and patient advocacy
- Inability to carry out interventions in an appropriate and timely manner
- Lack of mandatory reporting

**Activity #3**

1. F
2. I
3. J
4. C
5. E
6. G
7. A
8. D
9. H
10. B

**Activity #4**

Any three of these veteran health issues can be listed:

- Mental health issues
  - Posttraumatic stress disorder
  - Substance use disorder
  - Military sexual trauma
  - Suicide
  - Homelessness
- Medical-surgical health issues
  - Amputations
  - Environmental/chemical exposures
  - Traumatic brain injury (including blast concussions)
  - Hearing loss

**Activity #5**

1. Autonomy
2. Nonmaleficence
3. Fidelity
4. Veracity

**Activity #6**

Any four of these social determinants of health can be listed:

- Poverty (may not be able to afford healthy food, housing, and quality health care)
- Difficulty finding job (if disabled or physically limited by disorders such as arthritis)
- Low graduation rate (people with higher education levels are heathier and live longer)
- Poor-performing neighborhood schools
- Social discrimination and bullying
- No health insurance
- No primary health care provider
- No transportation to health care or live far away from health care settings
- High rates of violence, unsafe water, and other health risks in neighborhood

- Exposure to second-hand smoke and other risk factors
- Unsafe neighborhoods
- Racial/ethnic discrimination
- Lack of community support and positive relationships

## Learning Assessment
### NCLEX Examination Challenge #1
<u>Answer</u>: D
<u>Rationale</u>: The nurse in the test question is advocating for a client to do good by recognizing the client's need for pain medication. **Beneficence** is about promoting positive actions to help others or do good for others. Therefore, Choice D is the correct response. Autonomy is related to self-determination and management. Even though the nurse is functioning as an advocate in this situation, the client could act as one's own advocate because this client is alert and oriented. Therefore, Choice C is not correct. The situation has nothing to do with following through on obligations (Choice A) or being truthful (Choice B).

### NCLEX Examination Challenge #2
<u>Answer</u>: B
<u>Rationale</u>: Sources of evidence have various strengths, and large meta-analysis or synthesis studies are the strongest and therefore best sources of evidence (Choice B). Policies and procedures and expert opinion are low levels of evidence (Choices A and C). Data from the facility are not sources of evidence to determine best practices but instead are the information supporting a need for change (Choice D).

### NCLEX Examination Challenge #3
<u>Answer</u>: C
<u>Rationale</u>: There are five rights of delegation. The nurse is following up in this situation to determine if the assistive personnel carried out the delegated task correctly. This action is an example of the Right Supervision (Choice C). The task has already been communicated with an explanation of circumstances (Choices A, B, and D).

## Chapter 2
### Answer Key
#### Activity #1
1. clinical reasoning;
   critical thinking;
   clinical judgment
2. Evidence-Based Practice
3. Teamwork and Collaboration
4. Informatics;
   Quality Improvement
5. systems thinking

#### Activity #2
1. B
2. A
3. E
4. F
5. D
6. C

#### Activity #3

| Factors that Influence Health Equity/Patient Outcomes | Answer |
|---|---|
| Behavioral and social determinants of health | F |
| Evolving approaches to population health management | C |
| Policy and health care reform | E |
| Available and emerging technologies | A |
| Interprofessional practice with an emphasis on patient-centered care | B |
| Shift toward systems thinking | D |

#### Activity #4
1. B
2. C
3. D
4. A

## Learning Assessment

### NCLEX Examination Challenge #1
Answer: A, B, D, E
Rationale: Financial barriers, such as having insufficient personal finances for health care, are well-understood in the United States (Choice D). Other key barriers to implementation of care for communities include discrimination based on personal characteristics (Choice B), the need to correct workforce shortages (Choice A), and understanding and amelioration of social determinants of health (Choice E). Insurance coverage varies significantly from carrier to carrier; benefits are not always maximized (Choice C).

### NCLEX Examination Challenge #2
Answer: D
Rationale: Certified nurse practitioners, certified nurse midwives, clinical nurse specialists, and certified registered nurse anesthetists are all recognized as advanced practice nurses (APRNs) (Choice D). Registered nurses, clinical nurse educators, and licensed practical nurses are not APRNs (Choices A, B, and C).

## Chapter 3

### Answer Key
*Activity #1*

<2———3————————————1————————————4————————————5——>

**Adequate Cognition**                                    **Severe Impaired Cognition**

1. Older adult who has moderate-stage Alzheimer's disease and lives in an assisted living facility
2. Four-week-old full-term healthy newborn baby living at home with parents
3. Adolescent who was recently diagnosed with depression and anxiety and lives with grandparents
4. Middle-aged adult who had a severe hemorrhagic stroke and is unable to communicate
5. Young adult who experienced a severe traumatic brain injury from a motorcycle crash

*Activity #2*
Any five of these complications of immobility may be listed.

- Pressure injuries (pressure on skin over bony prominences)
- Disuse osteoporosis (increased bone resorption)
- Constipation (decreased GI motility)
- Weight loss or gain (decreased appetite and movement)
- Muscle atrophy (catabolism)
- Atelectasis/hypostatic pneumonia (decreased lung expansion)
- Venous thromboembolism (e.g., deep venous thrombosis and pulmonary embolus [decreased blood circulation])
- Urinary system calculi (stones) (urinary stasis)

*Activity #3*
**R** = Rest; **I** = Ice; **C** = Compression; **E** = Elevation

*Activity #4*
Any three of these factors that place individuals at risk for decreased immunity should be listed.

- Older adults (diminished immunity because of normal aging changes)
- Low socioeconomic groups (inability to obtain proper immunizations)
- Nonimmunized adults
- Adults with chronic illnesses (comorbidities) that weaken the immune system, including obesity
- Adults taking chronic drug therapy such as corticosteroids and chemotherapeutic agents
- Adults experiencing substance use disorder
- Adults who do not practice a healthy lifestyle
- Adults who have a genetic or familial risk for decreased or excessive immunity

## Activity #5

Any three of these physical assessment techniques that help to identify a patient's gas exchange status should be listed.

- Patient's breathing effort and rate
- Oxygen saturation ($SpO_2$)
- Capillary refill
- Thoracic expansion
- Lung sounds anteriorly and posteriorly

## Activity #6

| | | | |
|---|---|---|---|
| _C_ 1. | Immune compromise | A. | Pain |
| _D_ 2. | Food insecurity | B. | Tissue integrity |
| _A_ 3. | Osteoarthritis | C. | Infection |
| _E_ 4. | Diabetes mellitus | D. | Nutrition |
| _B_ 5. | Urinary incontinence | E. | Perfusion |

## Learning Assessment

### NCLEX Examination Challenge #1

Answer: A, B, C, D

Rationale: Smoking, advanced age, and immobility slow venous blood flow to the heart and can result in venous stasis and venous thromboembolism (VTE) because of increased clotting (Choices A, C, and D). Diabetes mellitus also affects blood vessels and decreases blood flow leading to clot formation (Choice B). Pressure injuries occur on bony prominences and do not contribute to increased clotting (Choice E).

### NCLEX Examination Challenge #2

Answer: B

Rationale: The client was alert and oriented before surgery, meaning that the client had adequate cognition. However, following surgery, the client had impaired cognition, indicating an acute change in cognitive status. Delirium is a cognitive impairment that has a sudden onset from a number of risk factors, including surgery (Choice B). Depression and dementia have a slower onset (Choices A and C). A delusion is a psychotic behavior, not an example of a cognitive decline.

### NCLEX Examination Challenge #3

Answer: A

Rationale: Adults experience many expected physiologic changes as they age, including changes in their sensory perception. Two of the most common changes include presbyopia (nearsightedness) and presbycusis (decreased hearing loss of the sensorineural type) (Choice A). Choices B, C, and D are not expected or normal physiologic changes associated with aging.

## Chapter 4

## Answer Key

### Activity #1

Any four of these SDOH:

- Lower or limited income
- Lower formal educational attainments
- Poor health resulting from inadequate access to care
- More chronic health conditions
- Residing in multigenerational households
- Residing in households with essential workers
- Working in institutions like nursing homes where COVID-19 incidence was high

### Activity #2

1. T
2. F
3. F
4. T
5. T
6. T
7. T
8. T
9. T
10. T
11. F
12. T

## Activity #3

Any three of these questions:

- Do you take five or more prescription medications?
- Do you take herbs, vitamins, other dietary supplements, or over-the-counter medications?
- Do you have your prescriptions filled at more than one pharmacy?
- Is more than one health care practitioner prescribing your medications?
- Do you take your medications more than once a day?
- Do you have trouble opening your medication bottles?
- Do you have poor eyesight or hearing?
- Do you live alone?
- Do you have a hard time remembering to take your medications?

## Activity #4

1. C
2. B
3. F
4. D
5. A
6. E

## Activity #5

1. What Matters
2. Medication
3. Mentation
4. Mobility

## Activity #6

Any five of these eight evidence-based risk factors:

- Altered mental status (confusion, disorientation, impulsivity)
- Symptomatic depression
- Altered elimination
- Dizziness or vertigo
- Two medication categories (antiepileptics and benzodiazepines)
- Gender (male)
- Decreased ability to rise from a chair (as measured by the Timed Up and Go-Test)

## Learning Assessment

### NCLEX Examination Challenge #1

Answer: C

Rationale: The nurse would be able to formulate a patient-centered plan of care if the factors that currently place the client at risk for falls could be determined. Therefore, this is the most appropriate nursing action (Choice C). Choice B would likely result in overstimulation of the client because the nurses' station is usually a very noisy and busy part of the unit. At times, the nurse may need to ask the family to stay with the client or obtain a sitter to prevent the client from getting out of bed without assistance (Choice A). However, at this time, it is not known if the client is able to climb out of the bed. Reorienting any older adult is appropriate but is not the most important action to help reduce fall risk.

### NCLEX Examination Challenge #2

Answer: A

Rationale: Many medications are inappropriate for older adults because of their risk for serious or harmful adverse drug events. Benzodiazepines like lorazepam are on the Beers list of inappropriate medications because of their anticholinergic effects (Choice A). As a result, the nurse would notify the provider to request a change in this drug. The other medications are not on the Beers list and are safe for older adults under medical supervision.

### NCLEX Examination Challenge #3

Answer: D

Rationale: The CAM is a tool used to screen for the presence of delirium in an older adult (Choice D). If the criteria are met, the client would have an acute onset of confusion and fluctuating mental status, inattention, and either disorganized thinking *or* altered level of consciousness. This tool is not useful to screen for any other mental health conditions (Choices A, B, and C).

## Chapter 5

### Answer Key
#### *Terminology Review*

#1

1. E
2. A
3. K
4. G
5. C
6. I
7. J
8. H
9. F
10. B
11. D

#### *Review of Nursing Care for Transgender and Nonbinary Patients*

#2

1. T
2. F
3. F
4. T
5. T
6. T
7. F
8. T
9. T
10. F

## Activities

### Activity #1

Examples of ways that the nurse can provide a safe environment of care for a patient who is transgender or nonbinary include (but are not limited to):

- Remind patients that they are safe in your care.
- Advocate for patients.
- Support the gender identity of all patients.
- Respect the right to dignity of all patients.
- Refer patients to agencies that hire LGBTQ staff and advertise LGBTQ friendliness.
- Provide comprehensive culturally appropriate resources.
- Ask patients which name and pronouns they use.

### Activity #2

Examples of client statements that indicate an understanding of these include:

1. Estrogen
   a. Estrogen can increase the risks for venous thrombophlebitis, elevated blood glucose, hypertension, estrogen-dependent cancers, and fluid retention.
   b. Estrogen is used with other interventions to achieve feminizing effects.
   c. Estrogen can cause a decrease in libido, erectile function, muscle mass, body hair growth, testicular size, ejaculatory fluid, and sperm count.
   d. Estrogen can cause an increase in breast tissue development and skin softening.

2. Spironolactone
   a. Spironolactone is a diuretic, so I might urinate more than usual.
   b. Spironolactone inhibits testosterone secretion and androgen binding to androgen receptors.

3. Cyproterone acetate
   a. Cyproterone acetate is a synthetic progesterone.
   b. Cyproterone acetate lowers endogenous total testosterone.

4. Finasteride
   a. Finasteride is a 5-alpha-reductase inhibitor.
   b. Finasteride is often used to treat benign prostatic hypertrophy (BPH).
   c. Finasteride blocks the conversion of testosterone to a more active ingredient that decreases hair loss associated with estrogen therapy and shrinks prostate tissue.

## Activity #3

1. K
2. B
3. G
4. L
5. M
6. C
7. F
8. D
9. E
10. A
11. I
12. J
13. H

## Activity #4

1. J
2. A or I
3. F
4. H
5. D

## Learning Assessments

### NCLEX Examination Challenge #1
Answer: A
Rationale: The nurse will greet the client by the name the client provided (Choice A). The nurse can then go on to determine if an update to the health record needs to be made. It is inappropriate to use the name on the chart because the client may not use this name anymore (Choice B). Expressing confusion about the name change may embarrass the client (Choice C). Asking why the client changed their name is nontherapeutic and inappropriate (Choice D).

### NCLEX Examination Challenge #2
Answer: B, C, D, E
Rationale: The MtF client will still have health needs based on their sex assigned at birth, if they have not undergone surgical intervention. The nurse will recommend Pap examinations to assess for cervical cancer or other abnormalities (Choice B) and mammograms (Choice D) as preventive health maintenance. The nurse will also provide teaching about the use of condoms when having sexual intercourse (Choice C); this is information all clients need to protect themselves from sexually transmitted infections, not just clients who are MtF. The nurse will provide information about oocyte freezing if the client is interested, especially before consideration of surgical intervention (Choice E). There is no need to teach about scheduling a prostate examination (Choice A) because a MtF client does not have a prostate.

### NCLEX Examination Challenge #3
Answer: C, D, E
Rationale: It is critical for the nurse to assess the client who has returned from vaginoplasty surgery for neurovascular status; capillary refill is appropriate for this assessment (Choice C). Following anesthesia, it is important to monitor for return of movement in the legs (Choice D). The nurse will also assess for bleeding, especially at the surgical site via looking at the dressing. If it is saturated with bright red blood, there is a concern for postsurgical bleeding or hemorrhage (Choice E). Dilation therapy does not begin until a week following the surgical procedure (Choice A). Although early catheter removal is evidence-based best practice, the urinary catheter will not be removed immediately following surgery (Choice A).

### NCLEX Examination Challenge #4
Answer: B, E
Rationale: The nurse will provide information that nullifying surgery can be done for clients who are nonbinary (Choice B). This procedure flattens the chest but not to the degree of masculinization. The nurse will also provide information about modified genital surgery available (Choice E). The nurse will refrain from asking the client why they want to have surgery (Choice A); this is nontherapeutic and may place the patient in a defensive position. It is inaccurate to state that there are no procedures available for a client who is nonbinary (Choice C). A phalloplasty is the creation of a penis; clients that choose nullification are unlikely to ask for a procedure that creates genitalia that is associated with a specific sex assigned at birth (Choice D).

## Chapter 6

### Answer Key

#### Activity #1

1.  Acute pain is the unpleasant sensory and emotional experience associated with tissue damage that results from acute injury, disease, or surgery.
2.  Breakthrough pain is additional pain that "breaks through" the pain being managed by the mainstay analgesic drugs.
3.  Nociceptive pain is pain that is the result of actual or potential tissue damage or inflammation and is often categorized as being somatic or visceral.
4.  Persistent pain is also called chronic pain; it is pain that persists or recurs for an indefinite period, usually for more than 3 months, often involves deep body structures, is poorly localized, and is difficult to describe.

#### Activity #2

1.  C
2.  A
3.  B
4.  A
5.  C
6.  A
7.  B
8.  A
9.  A
10. C

#### Activity #3

Ways in which the nurse can minimize bias when assessing a client's pain include, but are not limited to:

1.  Accept the patient's report of pain
2.  Respect preferences and values of patients
3.  Recognize personal bias or prejudice that can influence management of a patient's pain
4.  Establish a plan to set personal bias aside to meet the ethical responsibility of providing pain management
5.  Do not make judgments when a patient expresses symptoms of pain (verbally or nonverbally)
6.  Read, respect, and uphold the American Nurses Association (ANA) position statement regarding the ethical responsibility of nurses to manage pain
7.  Collaborate with other health care providers to help manage a patient's pain

#### Activity #4

1.  A
2.  C
3.  B
4.  C
5.  A
6.  D
7.  D

#### Activity #5

Examples of ways that unrelieved pain can affect a patient include, but are not limited to, include:

1.  Prolongs stress rate
2.  Increases heart rate, blood pressure, and oxygen demand
3.  Decreases GI motility
4.  Causes immobility
5.  Decreases immune response
6.  Delays healing
7.  Increases risk for development of chronic pain (if unrelieved pain is acute)
8.  Interferes with ADLs
9.  Causes anxiety, depression, hopelessness, fear, anger, and sleeplessness
10. Impairs family, work, and social relationships
11. Increases length of hospital stay
12. Contributes to loss of income and productivity

*Activity #6*

1. **S**
   a. Finding: Sleep, easy to arouse
   b. Acceptable
      i. No action necessary; may increase opioid dose if needed.

2. **1**
   a. Finding: Awake and alert
   b. Acceptable
      i. No action necessary; may increase opioid dose if needed.

3. **2**
   a. Finding: Slightly drowsy, easily aroused
   b. Acceptable
      i. No action necessary; may increase opioid dose if needed.

4. **3**
   a. Finding: Frequently drowsy, arousable, drifts off to sleep during conversation
   b. Unacceptable
      i. Monitor respiratory status and sedation level closely until sedation level is stable at less than 3 and respiratory status is satisfactory.
      ii. Decrease opioid dose 25% to 50%, or notify primary or anesthesia provider for orders.
      iii. Consider administering a nonsedating, opioid-sparing nonopioid such as acetaminophen or an NSAID if not contraindicated.
      iv. Ask patient to take deep breaths every 15 to 30 minutes.

5. **4**
   a. Finding: Somnolent, minimal or no response to verbal and physical stimulation
   b. Unacceptable
      i. Stop opioid.
      ii. Consider administering naloxone.
      iii. Call Rapid Response Team (code blue)
      iv. Stay with patient and stimulate and support respiration as indicated by patient status.
      v. Notify primary or anesthesia provider.
      vi. Monitor respiratory status and sedation level closely until sedation level is stable at less than 3 and respiratory status is satisfactory.

## Learning Assessment

### NCLEX Examination Challenge #1
Answer: A, D
Rationale: The nurse will document that the client has somatic (Choice A) and nociceptive (Choice D) pain. Somatic pain is reflected in the client's incisional pain from the surgical procedure. It is well-localized. The client's low back pain is also nociceptive and somatic in nature because it is a chronic, ongoing pain syndrome that is well localized in the back. There is no evidence of visceral pain (Choice B), which is characterized by pain in the organs or linings of the body cavities. There is also no evidence of radiating pain (Choice C), which is felt along a specific nerve or nerves. Neuropathic pain is characterized by shooting, burning, fiery, shock-like, tingling, or painfully numb sensations. The client has not reported any of these sensations, so neuropathic pain (Choice E) will not be documented.

### NCLEX Examination Challenge #2
Answer: A, C, D
Rationale: Pain holds unique meaning for the person experiencing it. The nurse must set aside bias and personal interpretations of a client's pain and fully assess and advocate for pain control (Choice A). It is critical to assess the pain of all clients, so the nurse will perform a full assessment, which includes asking the client to describe the pain and rate its intensity (Choice C). It is very likely that this client has new and different pain given the fall from the ladder (Choice D), and it is important for the nurse to know how that feels. Pharmaceutical therapy for the ongoing chronic back pain may not be sufficient to address acute pain that is occurring in response to the client's fall. The nurse must always refrain from assuming how a client is experiencing pain (Choice B), whether it is new or ongoing pain. The nurse will collaborate with the health care provider but not to convey that the client is overreacting to pain (Choice E). This is judgmental and inappropriate. Rather, the nurse will collaborate with the health care provider to manage the pain the client is currently experiencing.

*NCLEX Examination Challenge #3*
<u>Answer</u>: B, C, D, E
<u>Rationale</u>: The nurse will provide comprehensive assessment interventions to determine if a client who is nonverbal is experiencing pain. This includes using an evidence-based pain assessment tool, such as the Pain Assessment Checklist for Seniors with Limited Ability to Communicate-II (PACSLAC-II), when examining the client (Choice B). The nurse will also review the electronic health record where documentation about potential causes of pain (e.g., recent fall, urinary tract infection) can be identified (Choice C). It is important for the nurse to collaborate with other nursing staff who have recently cared for the client (Choice D) so trends or changes in behavior can be identified. The nurse will also look for trended behaviors during the shift such as grimacing, moaning, or guarding that could indicate the presence of pain (Choice E). The nurse will not assume there is no pain unless the client cries or attempts to vocalize (Choice A); people who are nonverbal are at high risk for untreated pain, and it is the nurse's responsibility to assess and advocate for the client.

## Chapter 7

### Answer Key

#### Activity #1
Conditions that can contribute to the need for rehabilitative care include, but are not limited to:
- Asthma
- Arthritis
- Cancer
- Chronic obstructive pulmonary disease (COPD)
- COVID-19
- Diabetes
- Heart disease
- Spinal cord injury (SCI)
- Stroke
- Trauma events
- Traumatic brain injury (TBI)
- Other chronic diseases or conditions

#### Activity #2
1. F
2. T
3. T
4. T
5. F
6. F
7. F
8. F
9. T
10. F

#### Activity #3
1. Physical therapists (PTs) intervene to help the patient achieve self-management by focusing on gross mobility skills (e.g., by facilitating ambulation and teaching the patient to use an assistive device such as a walker). They may also teach techniques for performing activities such as transferring (e.g., moving into and out of bed), ambulating, and toileting. In some settings, PTs play a major role in providing wound care.
2. Occupational therapists (OTs) work to develop the patient's fine motor skills used for ADL self-management such as those required for eating, bathing, grooming, and dressing. They also teach patients how to perform independent living skills such as cooking and shopping. To accomplish these outcomes, OTs teach skills related to coordination (e.g., hand movements) and cognitive retraining.
3. Recreational therapists work to help patients continue or develop recreation or leisure interests to bring meaning to the person's life. These activities may also contribute to strengthening fine motor skills.
4. Cognitive therapists work primarily with patients who have experienced a stroke, brain injury, brain tumor, or other conditions resulting in cognitive impairment. They may use computer programs to assist with cognitive retraining.

## Activity #4

1. G
2. C
3. B
4. A
5. E
6. D
7. H
8. F

## Activity #5

Examples of rights that a resident has while living in an assisted-living facility include, but are not limited to:

1. Wearing street clothes instead of hospital gowns
2. Deciding what they want to eat
3. Planning how to spend their day
4. Determining who they wish to spend time with
5. Organizing how they would like to decorate their room

## Activity #6

Members of the interprofessional health care team in a rehabilitation setting include:

1. Nurses and nursing assistants
2. Rehabilitation nurse case managers
3. Physicians and physician assistants (PAs)
4. Advanced practice nurses (APNs) such as nurse practitioners and clinical nurse specialists
5. Physical therapists and assistants
6. Occupational therapists (OTs) and assistants
7. Speech-language pathologists and assistants
8. Rehabilitation assistants/restorative aides
9. Recreational or activity therapists
10. Cognitive therapists or neuropsychologists
11. Social workers
12. Clinical psychologists
13. Vocational counselors
14. Spiritual care counselors
15. Registered dietitian nutritionists (RDNs)
16. Pharmacists

## Learning Assessment

### NCLEX Examination Challenge #1

Answer: A, B, C, D, E

Rationale: The nurse will include all of these foods in the plan of care for avoiding constipation in a client. At least eight glasses of water daily, and 20 to 35 g of fiber in the diet are recommended. Apples (Choice A), green peas (Choice B), baked beans (Choice C), bran muffins (Choice D), and whole grain bread (Choice E) all contain fiber.

### NCLEX Examination Challenge #2

Answer: D

Rationale: Short-term antibiotics such as trimethoprim (Choice D) or trimethoprim/sulfamethoxazole are often used to treat clients with symptomatic urinary tract infections. Oxybutynin (Choice A), solifenacin (Choice B), and tolterodine (Choice C) are antispasmodic drugs used to treat mild overactive bladder problems.

### NCLEX Examination Challenge #3

Answer: B, D

Rationale: The FIM developed by Granger and Gresham (1984) is commonly used when clients are in a rehabilitation or residential living environment. This tool is intended to measure the burden of care for a patient, not what a person should do or how the person would perform under different circumstances. Categories for assessment are self-care, sphincter control, mobility and locomotion, communication, and cognition. Scoring is on a 1 to 7 scale in which 1 is dependent and 7 is independent. A score of 6 demonstrates that the client is fairly independent. The nurse will encourage self-dressing (Choice B) to promote continued independence and assure there is a clear path from the bed to the bathroom (Choice D) as part of general safety measures. The nurse will not raise all bed rails at night (Choice A) because this could be considered a form of restraint; also, the client's FIM score indicates the ability to be quite independent. There is no need to have assistive personnel bathe the client (Choice C) or to have full-time care (Choice E) because of the client's high FIM score.

## Chapter 8
### Answer Key
#### Activity #1
1. H
2. E
3. G
4. I
5. C
6. F
7. D
8. B
9. A

#### Activity #2
1. F
2. T
3. T
4. T
5. T
6. T
7. F
8. T
9. F
10. T

#### Activity #3
Examples of signs and symptoms that may be noted or that a patient may experience when they are near death include, but are not limited to:
1. Decline in physical function
2. Weakness
3. Increased sleep
4. Anorexia
5. Cardiovascular function changes
6. Breathing pattern changes (e.g., periods of apnea, Cheyne-Stokes respirations)
7. Genitourinary changes
8. Decreased level of consciousness
9. Cold, mottled, cyanotic extremities
10. Decreased blood pressure
11. Increased heart rate (usually before becoming irregular, gradually decreasing, then stopping)
12. Loss of ability to speak
13. Incontinence
14. Congestion
15. Restlessness

#### Activity #4
Ways in which the nurse intervenes to contribute to a patient's "good death" include, but are not limited to:
1. Provides an atmosphere where the patient can die with dignity
2. Provides interventions that reduce distress and suffering for patients and families
3. Follows the patient's and family's wishes
4. Observes clinical practice standards
5. Provides meticulous physiological care (e.g., suctioning secretions, keeping lips moist, maintaining hygiene)
6. Affirms the patient's experience, even if they are seeing or hearing things the nurse and others cannot see or hear
7. Encourages family to say important things like "it's okay to go," "we'll be alright," "I love you," "thank you," "I'm sorry," etc.
8. Offers to place the patient and/or family in touch with clergy, a spiritual leader, or a grief counselor (only if the patient or family wishes)
9. Explains physical signs of approaching death
10. Stays with the patient and family throughout the dying process

#### Activity #5
1. Massage, when given with light pressure and only in the areas of intact skin, can improve circulation and promote relaxation, which can reduce pain.
2. Music therapy promotes relaxation, which can reduce pain; it is most effective when music the patient enjoys is played.
3. Guided imagery is the use of mental images through guided imagination or memory that helps promote relaxation, which can reduce pain.
4. Aromatherapy/use of essential oils can promote relaxation, which contributes to pain reduction. These are often used in addition to other treatments in end-of-life care. The most researched essential oil is lavender; chamomile, sweet marjoram, dwarf pine, rosemary, and ginger have also been shown to be effective in pain management.

*Activity #6*

Ways in which hospice care differs from palliative care include, but are not limited to:

| Hospice Care | Palliative Care |
|---|---|
| Patients have a prognosis of 6 months or less to live. | Patients can be in any stage of serious illness. |
| Care is provided when curative treatment such as chemotherapy has been stopped. | A consultation is provided that is concurrent with curative therapies or therapies that prolong life. |
| Care is provided in 60- and 90-day periods with an opportunity to continue if eligibility criteria are met. Medicare covers hospice services for 6 months. | Care is not limited by specific periods and may be covered by insurance, Medicare, or Medicaid. |

## Learning Assessment

### NCLEX Examination Challenge #1

Answer: A, B, E

Rationale: The nurse will provide oxygen via nasal cannula if dyspnea is noted (Choice A) because evidence shows that clients who are dying may feel more comfortable when their oxygen saturation is above 90%. The nurse will include the family in the caring process if the client and family desire for this to occur (Choice B). It is important for clients to be surrounded by people they want during the dying process, and it is important for family members to have the chance to say goodbye. The nurse will explain each nursing action to the client and family before they occur (Choice E); this can alleviate fear of what is taking place. The nurse will not discourage friends and family from using the terms "death" and "dying" (Choice C); it is important for them to be able to express feelings related to what is happening during the process of losing a loved one. The nurse will not withhold opioid drugs (Choice D); tolerance is not a concern at the end-of-life.

### NCLEX Examination Challenge #2

Answer: D

Rationale: The family member may have a difficult time using the actual word of "goodbye." It is important that the nurse provides reassurance that other terms such as "I love you" are still very effective ways of saying goodbye and expressing feeling (Choice D). It is nontherapeutic to ask the family member why they are feeling a certain way (Choice A); this places the family member on the defensive to have to explain feelings that they may not fully understand at this time. The nurse will not pressure the family member to say goodbye (Choice B); this is inappropriate and can place a burden of guilt onto the family member who is already struggling with words to say to their mother. The nurse will not state that the mother will not die in peace if they do not hear the family member say "goodbye" (Choice C); this is untrue and nontherapeutic.

### NCLEX Examination Challenge #3

Answer: A, B, C, D, E

Rationale: The nurse will use the HOPE mnemonic as a guide when assessing a patient's spirituality at the end-of-life. This includes determination of a client's:

- *H:* Sources of hope and strength (Choice A)
- *O:* Organized religion (if any) and role that it plays in the patient's life (Choices B and C)
- *P:* Personal spirituality, rituals, and practices (Choice D)
- *E:* Effects of religion and spirituality on care and end-of-life decisions (Choice E)

### NCLEX Examination Challenge #4

Answer: B

Rationale: When death is approaching, it is appropriate to cover the client who has cool and mottled extremities with a warm blanket (Choice B). The client's extremities are cool and mottled because of the normal process that occurs during end-of-life when peripheral circulation decreases and tissue is not well-perfused. Warmed IV fluids should not be used; this will not provide the client with any benefit and may cause discomfort (Choice A). Circulation will not improve with rubbing or massaging so this should be avoided (Choice C). Repositioning the client so that lower extremities are dependent will not benefit the client and could cause discomfort; this action should be avoided (Choice D).

## Chapter 9

### Answer Key

#### Activity #1

Definitions for each term should be close to the definition provided below.

1. **autologous donation:** Blood donation given by the patient before surgery for the purpose of reinfusing for self; reinfusing the patient's own blood during surgery
2. **carboxyhemoglobin:** Carbon monoxide on oxygen-binding sites of the hemoglobin molecule
3. **dehiscence:** Partial or complete separation of the outer wound layers
4. **evisceration:** Total separation of all wound layers and protrusion of internal organs through the open wound
5. **malignant hyperthermia (MH):** Inherited muscle disorder; an acute, life-threatening complication of certain drugs used for general anesthesia
6. **morbidity:** An illness or an abnormal condition or quality; number of serious diseases
7. **myoglobinuria:** Muscle proteins in the urine due to rhabdomyolysis
8. **perioperative:** Operative experience consisting of the preoperative, intraoperative, and postoperative time phases
9. **pulse deficit:** Difference between the apical and peripheral pulses
10. **sanguineous:** Bloody (as in drainage)
11. **serosanguineous:** Yellowish mixed with light red or pale pink (as in drainage)
12. **serous:** Serum-like, or yellow (as in drainage)

#### Activity #2

1. F
2. F
3. T
4. T
5. F
6. T
7. T
8. F
9. T
10. F

#### Activity #3

Order: A, B, C, E, F, D

#### Activity #4

1. A
2. C
3. A
4. B
5. B
6. C
7. B
8. B
9. C
10. C

#### Activity #5

Things the nurse will assess for when collecting a health history and general review of systems include, but are not limited to:

**General (constitutional)**
Fevers and/or chills
Generalized weakness

**Eyes**
Dryness or infection of conjunctiva and/or lids
Blurring or changes in vision

**Ears, nose, mouth, and throat**
Ear drainage or pain
Difficulty or changes in hearing or breathing through nose
Sinus tenderness
Oral lesions
Changes in dentition (e.g., cavities, dentures)
Difficulty in swallowing

**Cardiovascular**
Edema
Exercise intolerance
Pain
Palpitations
Venous thromboembolism
History of ischemic heart disease

**Respiratory**
Cough with sputum or blood
Pain or shortness of breath when breathing
Obstructive sleep apnea

## Gastrointestinal
New or unusual masses or tenderness
Bowel changes or difficulty

## Genitourinary
Pain or burning on urination
Frequency, urgency, or incontinence
Bladder changes or difficulty

## Musculoskeletal
Clubbing or cyanosis in digits or nails
Pain in joints
Symmetry of extremities
Loss of or change in range of motion

## Integumentary (including skin and breasts)
Dryness, rashes, lesions, or ulcerations

## Neurologic
Changes in memory or usual state of orientation
One-sided weakness
Numbness or tingling
Loss of balance
History of cerebrovascular disease

## Psychiatric
General mood
Depression over diagnosis or anxiety about surgery

## Endocrine
Increased thirst or urination
Unexplained weight loss or gain

## Hematologic and lymphatic
Swollen nodes
New or unusual bleeding
Nonhealing wounds

## Allergic and immunologic
Seasonal, food, chemical allergies
Changes in immune system

### *Activity #6*
1. B
2. E
3. C
4. G
5. D
6. A
7. F

## Learning Assessment

### NCLEX Examination Challenge #1
Answer: A
Rationale: Curative surgery is performed to resolve a health problem by repairing or removing the cause. Examples include removal of a portion of the colon (such as in a colectomy), removal of a cancerous tumor, or removal of the gallbladder (Choice A). Diagnostic surgery is performed to determine the origin and cause of a disorder (Choice B). Preventive surgery is performed with the intention that a condition will not develop (Choice C). Transplantation surgery is performed to replace a malfunctioning structure (Choice D).

### NCLEX Examination Challenge #2
Answer: B
Rationale: The nurse's role includes the ability to serve as witness that the surgeon fully informed the client about benefits and risks of a surgical procedure before it is done (Choice B). It is the surgeon's responsibility – not the nurse's role – to provide a complete explanation of the planned surgical procedure and to have the consent form signed before sedation is given and before surgery is performed (Choice A). The perioperative nurse is **not** responsible for providing detailed information about the surgical procedure. Informed consent is obtained before the surgery begins (Choice C), not afterward. The nurse's role is not limited to assuring that informed consent is in the health record (Choice D). It also includes verification that the consent form is signed, dated, and timed, serving as witness to the signature if needed, and clarifying facts and dispelling myths that the client or caregiver may have about surgery after the surgeon has provided information.

### NCLEX Examination Challenge #3
Answer: C
Rationale: The older adult has a slower metabolism than a younger adult. It takes longer to clear anesthesia and other drugs from the system, which can alter cognition. The client still knows the caregiver's identity, and that they have had surgery and it is not unusual to be confused about day and time in the early hours following surgery under general anesthesia (Choice C). There is no need to notify the surgeon, as this is an expected finding (Choice A). There is no need to perform a full mental status assessment (Choice B)

unless other signs or symptoms are present. There is no indication of dementia or Alzheimer's disease in this situation, given that the client was preoperatively healthy (Choice D). Asking the caregiver about it will only increase their concerns.

### NCLEX Examination Challenge #4
Answer: A
Rationale: Increased release of immature neutrophils (bands) (also known as a "*left shift*" or "*bandemia*")

is an indication of an infection that has outpaced the client's immune defenses (Choice A). It is not a normal white blood cell finding following surgery (Choice B) and has nothing to do with anemia (Choice C) or clotting factors (Choice D).

## Chapter 10
### Answer Key
#### Activity #1
1. C
2. D
3. J
4. I
5. A
6. H
7. G
8. B
9. F
10. E

#### Activity #2
1. T
2. F
3. T
4. T
5. F
6. F
7. F
8. T
9. T
10. T

#### Activity #3
Ways the nurse can intervene when receiving a patient in the ED who is unconscious and cannot provide identity or a health history include, but are not limited to:

A. Perform a two-person search of belongings looking for identification, medical alert jewelry, or belongings that may contain information.
   a. Look for a medical alert necklace or bracelet that indicates any health conditions.
   b. Look for a wallet in the patient's pocket; a bank card or driver's license may contain a name.
   c. If a phone is in the patient's pocket, see if it unlocks and has emergency contact information.
B. Search among belongings for the name of the client's health care provider or pharmacy, a medication list, and/or bottles or containers that may provide information.
C. Check patient's belongings for drugs or drug paraphernalia as well as weapons. If drugs or drug paraphernalia is present, this may be important information regarding what has affected the patient.
D. If any sources containing information are found, call numbers that are available to see if next of kin can be reached who can provide a health history.

### Activity #4
1. Level III
2. Level I
3. Level IV
4. Level II

### Activity #5
Specific actions the nurse will take before the family enters the room of a deceased client for which no forensic investigation is required include, but are not limited to:
1. Ensure the body is as clean as possible.
2. Remove IV lines and indwelling tubes.
3. Cover the body with a sheet or blanket leaving the patient's face exposed.
4. Dim the lights in the room.
5. Explain what the family can expect to see.

### Activity #6
Signs of human trafficking that require the nurse to assess further include, but are not limited to:
1. Burns
2. Bruises
3. Self-harm
4. Head injury
5. Jaw problems
6. Missing patches of hair
7. Requests for pregnancy tests
8. Suspected physical or sexual abuse
9. Unusual tattoos or "branding marks"
10. Inability to provide or verify a home address
11. Demonstration of shame, self-loathing, and fear
12. Recurrent sexually transmitted infections (STIs)
13. Deferral to a controlling individual accompanying them to the ED

## Learning Assessment
### NCLEX Examination Challenge #1
Answer: B, C
Rationale: EDs use several methods of ensuring safety. Strategically located panic buttons and remote door access controls allow staff to get help and secure major entrances and access points. The triage reception area—a particularly vulnerable access point into the ED—is often designed to serve as a security barrier with bulletproof glass and staff-controlled door entry into the treatment area. The nurse will activate the panic button when an emergency exists such as a possible infant abduction (Choice B) or a person entering the area and threatening staff with a weapon (Choice C). Frustrated clients in long lines (Choice A), emergency medical services bringing in a client in full arrest (Choice D), and clients who begin to complain (Choice E) are not emergent situations that require use of a panic button. These occurrences are expected parts of a day in an ED.

### NCLEX Examination Challenge #2
Answer: B
Rationale: The SBAR method (Situation, Background, Assessment, Recommendation/ Request) is used to ensure complete and clear communication. The nurse will begin by stating the Situation, which is that a 65-year-old client came to the ED with a severe headache (Choice B). Background is that the client has a history of hypertension and quit taking medication 3 months ago (Choice D). Assessment includes a report of the client's vital signs (Choice C) and current physical and psychosocial presentation. Recommendation/Request includes the action that needs to take place next, which is contacting the on-call hospitalist for admission (Choice A).

### NCLEX Examination Challenge #3
Answer: B
Rationale: The emergent triage category implies that a condition exists that poses an immediate threat to life or limb. The nurse will triage the client with potential internal injuries following a motor vehicle crash as emergent (Choice B); this client may have internal bleeding and needs to be seen right away. The clients with a dislocated shoulder (Choice C), back pain and hematuria with a history of kidney stones (Choice D), and generalized skin rash after eating shellfish for breakfast almost 24 hours prior (Choice E) will likely be identified as urgent; they do need to be seen and treated soon, but an immediate threat to life does not exist at the moment. The client from a long-term care facility with ongoing dysuria (Choice A) will be triaged as nonurgent unless other symptoms arise.

## Chapter 11

### Answer Key

#### Activity #1

1. C
2. I
3. A
4. J
5. H
6. B
7. G
8. D
9. F
10. E

#### Activity #2

1. T
2. F
3. T
4. F
5. T
6. F
7. T
8. T
9. F
10. T

#### Activity #3

Important teaching points the nurse will include when providing education to a community group about avoiding lightning injuries include, but are not limited to:

A. Check weather forecasts when planning to be outside.

B. A lightning strike is imminent if your hair stands on end, you see a blue halo around objects, or you hear high-pitched or crackling noises. If you cannot move away from the area immediately, crouch on the balls of your feet and tuck your head down to minimize the target size; do not lie on the ground or make contact with your hands to the ground.

C. Seek shelter when you hear thunder. Go inside the nearest building or an enclosed vehicle. Avoid isolated sheds and cave entrances. Do not stand under an isolated tall tree or structure (e.g., ski lift, flagpole, boat mast, power line) in an open area such as a field, ridge, or hilltop; lightning tends to strike high points. Instead, seek a low area under a thick growth of saplings or small trees.

D. Leave water immediately (including an indoor shower or bathtub) and move away from any open bodies of water.

E. Avoid metal objects such as chairs or bleachers; put down tools, fishing rods, garden equipment, golf clubs, and umbrellas; and stand clear of fences, exposed pipes, motorcycles, bicycles, tractors, and golf carts.

F. If inside a car with a solid hood, close the windows and stay inside. If in a convertible, leave the car at least 49 yards (45 meters) away and huddle on the ground.

G. If inside a tent, stay away from the metal tent poles and wet fabric of the tent walls.

H. If you are caught out in the open and cannot seek shelter, attempt to move to lower ground such as a ravine or valley; stay away from any tall trees or objects that could result in a lightning strike splashing over to you; place insulating material between you and the ground (e.g., sleeping pad, rain parka, or life jacket).

I. If inside a building, stay away from open doors, windows, fireplaces, metal fixtures, and plumbing.

J. Turn off electrical equipment, including computers, televisions, and stereos, to avoid damage.

K. Stay off land-line telephones. Lightning can enter through the telephone line and produce head and neck trauma, including cataracts and tympanic membrane disruption. Death can result. Avoid use of cellular phones, which can transmit loud static that can cause acoustic damage.

#### Activity #4

1. A
2. C
3. D
4. B
5. B
6. F
7. A
8. A
9. F
10. E

## Activity #5

Appropriate actions for the nurse to take when a client with heat stroke has been admitted to the ED include, but are not limited to:

1. Give oxygen by mask or nasal cannula; be prepared for endotracheal intubation.
2. Start at least one IV with a large-bore needle or cannula.
3. Support perfusion by administering fluids as prescribed, using cooled solutions if available.
4. Use a cooling blanket.
5. Obtain baseline laboratory tests as quickly as possible: urinalysis, serum electrolytes, cardiac enzymes, liver enzymes, and complete blood count (CBC).
6. Do not administer aspirin or any other antipyretics.
7. An esophageal probe offers the most accurate continuous temperature measurement (Lipman et al., 2019). However, if an esophageal probe is not used, insert a rectal probe to measure core body temperature continuously or use a rectal thermometer and assess temperature as clinically indicated.
8. Insert an indwelling urinary drainage catheter. If a bladder catheter with a thermistor for the continuous measurement of core body temperature is available, it may be used in lieu of a rectal probe.
9. Monitor vital signs frequently as clinically indicated.
10. Assess arterial blood gases.
11. Administer muscle relaxants or benzodiazepines as prescribed if the patient begins to shiver.
12. Measure and monitor urine output and specific gravity to determine fluid needs.
13. Stop cooling interventions when core body temperature is reduced to 102°F (39°C).

## Activity #6

Planetary health is an initiative that brings together environmental and health experts to better understand and act on ways in which the Earth and therefore health are affected by human use of the planet's natural systems. Nurses must recognize those people who are particularly vulnerable to these factors when considering the influence of the environment on health. This population includes children; pregnant women; older adults; those who work in certain occupations; those who have low income, chronic health conditions, or disabilities; as well as marginalized groups.

## Learning Assessment

### NCLEX Examination Challenge #1

Answer: B

Rationale: It is within the scope of assistive personnel's practice to obtain, report, and record vital signs (Choice B). Inserting the nasogastric tube (Choice A), advising the family of resuscitation efforts (Choice C), and assisting with the bag-valve-mask device (Choice D) require additional education and training and are within the scope of practice of the nurse.

### NCLEX Examination Challenge #2

Answer: C

Rationale: When a client has white, waxy appearing body parts, the indication is frostnip, a condition that may produce pain, numbness, and pallor but does not cause impaired tissue integrity. In this case, the appropriate action is to gently warm the affected body part with a body part that is already warm (e.g., hands) (Choice C) because frostnip is easily managed using body heat to warm the affected area(s). Warmed IV fluids are not necessary (Choice A). Massaging the affected area briskly can be uncomfortable and damage tissue integrity (Choice B). Cool water compresses should not be applied to the waxy areas (Choice D) because this will not alleviate the frostnip and may aggravate any pain or numbness that is present.

### NCLEX Examination Challenge #3

Answer: A

Rationale: Any client who has sustained multiple stings should be observed in an emergency care setting for several hours to monitor for the development of toxic venom effects (Choice A). This client needs to be transported to the ED, even if they are not having immediate symptoms, where a critical care admission may be prescribed. Anxiety alone does not require contacting 911 (Choice B). It is expected that bee stings are red, swollen, and painful (Choice C); this does not require contacting 911. That the provider gave the client cortisone cream the last two times a sting occurred indicates that there is a low likelihood that this sting will result in a more severe outcome (Choice D); this does not require contacting 911.

## Chapter 12

**Answer Key**

*Activity #1*

Definitions for each term should be close to the definition provided.

1. **community relations officer:** Person who serves as a liaison between the health care facility and the media. Also known as *public relations officer*.
2. **containment:** The act of limiting the expansion or spread of a contagion or toxic substance.
3. **emergency preparedness:** A goal or plan to meet an extraordinary need for hospital beds, staff, drugs, personal protective equipment, supplies, and medical devices such as mechanical ventilators.
4. **Hospital Incident Command System (HICS):** An organizational model for disaster management in which roles are formally structured under the hospital or long-term care facility incident commander, with clear lines of authority and accountability for specific resources.
5. **hospital incident commander:** As defined in a hospital's emergency response plan, the person (either an emergency physician or administrator) who assumes overall leadership for implementing the institutional plan at the onset of a mass casualty incident. This role can also be fulfilled by a nursing supervisor functioning as the on-site hospital administrator after usual business hours until hospital leadership personnel arrive. This person has a global view of the entire situation, facilitates patient movement through the system, and brings in resources to meet patient needs.
6. **medical command physician:** As defined in a hospital's emergency response plan, the person responsible for determining the number, acuity, and medical resource needs of victims arriving from the incident scene and for organizing the emergency health care team response to injured or ill patients.
7. **personal emergency preparedness plan:** An individual plan that outlines specific arrangements in the event of disaster, such as childcare, pet care, and older adult care.
8. **personal readiness supplies:** A preassembled disaster supply kit for the home and/or automobile that contains clothing and basic survival supplies. Also called a *go bag*.

9. **triage:** The process of sorting or classifying patients into priority levels depending on illness or injury severity, with the highest acuity needs receiving the quickest evaluation and treatment.
10. **triage officer:** In a hospital's emergency response plan, the person who rapidly evaluates each patient who arrives at the hospital. In a large hospital, this person is generally a physician who is assisted by triage nurses; however, a nurse may assume this role when physician resources are limited.

*Activity #2*

1. F
2. F
3. T
4. T
5. T
6. T
7. F
8. T
9. F
10. T

*Activity #3*

Order: B, D, C, E, F, A

*Activity #4*

1. B
2. A
3. B
4. D
5. A
6. C
7. D
8. B
9. A
10. D
11. B
12. A
13. C
14. C
15. B
16. C
17. D
18. A
19. D
20. C

## Activity #5

Ways in which the nurse who provided care during a mass casualty event can reduce the risk for developing PTSD include, but are not limited to:

1. Make and keep appointments with counseling services that are offered through the employer.
2. Meet regularly with a crisis intervention specialist.
3. Encourage and support coworkers.
4. Monitor the stress level and performance of yourself and coworkers.
5. Take breaks when needed.
6. Talk about feelings (while being mindful of HIPAA).
7. Drink plenty of water and eat healthy snacks for energy.
8. Keep in touch with family, friends, and significant others.
9. Do not work more than 12 hours per day.
10. Engage in regular physical exercise.
11. Recognize that feelings (guilt, anger, sadness, frustration, etc.) associated with the event are normal.

## Activity #6

The role of the nurse in responding when a fire breaks out in the work setting includes:

- Removing any patient or staff from immediate danger of the fire or smoke
- Discontinuing oxygen for all patients who can breathe without it
- Maintaining the respiratory status manually for patients on life support until removed from the fire area
- Directing ambulatory patients to walk to a safe location
- Asking ambulatory patients (if possible) to help push patients in wheelchairs out of danger
- Moving bed-bound patients from the fire area in bed, by stretcher, or in a wheelchair or by having one or two staff members move patients on blankets or carry them
- Seeking to contain the fire after everyone is out of danger by closing doors and windows and using an ABC extinguisher (which can put out any type of fire) if possible
- Refraining from risking injury to self or staff members while moving patients or attempting to extinguish the fire

## Learning Assessment

### NCLEX Examination Challenge #1

Answer: A

Rationale: This client self-transported to the ED. A danger of clients coming to the ED without having been screened by a decontamination team at the site of exposure is unknowingly carrying contaminants from nuclear, biologic, or chemical incidents into the hospital. The priority action for the nurse is to quarantine the client to stop the spread of the bioterrorism agent to others (Choice A). Then, other actions can take place including activation of the emergency preparedness plan (Choice B), calling the appropriate authorities (Choice C), and collecting a history while assessing for symptoms (Choice D).

### NCLEX Examination Challenge #2

Answer: D

Rationale: The medical command physician is in charge of deciding the number, acuity, and resource needs of patients. Of these choices, the nurse assisting the medical command physician will be assigned to assist with determining resources available, such as how many beds on nursing units are available for victims (Choice D). If assisting the triage officer, the nurse would likely provide triage (Choice A). The community relations or public information officer will be responsible for speaking with the media (Choice B). The hospital incident commander is responsible for implementation of the emergency plan (Choice C).

### NCLEX Examination Challenge #3

Answer: B

Rationale: DMATs are medical relief teams that are part of the National Disaster Medical System (NDMS) in the United States. A DMAT is made up of civilian medical, paraprofessional, and support personnel that deploy to a disaster area with enough medical equipment and supplies to sustain operations for 72 hours. They provide relief services ranging from primary health care and triage to evacuation and staffing to assist health care facilities that have become overwhelmed with casualties. Licensed health care providers such as nurses act as federal employees when they are deployed, so their professional licenses are recognized and valid in all states during the deployment (Choice B). There is no need to notify DMAT that Kentucky does not recognize Ohio nursing licenses (Choice A), to call the Ohio State Board of Nursing to ask if an Ohio license is valid in Kentucky (Choice C), or to apply for an emergency Kentucky nursing license (Choice D).

**NCLEX Examination Challenge #4**
Answer: A, B, C, D
Rationale: An external disaster is an event that occurs outside the health care facility or campus or somewhere in the community that requires the activation of the facility's emergency management plan. A violent shooter in a park (Choice A), a terrorist act at a shopping mall (Choice B), an Mpox outbreak in the community (Choice C), and a fire in a nearby long-term care agency (Choice D) are all examples of external disasters because they to not take place at the hospital. A broken hospital generator that interrupts power is considered an internal disaster (Choice E).

## Chapter 13
### Answer Key
#### Activity #1
1. E
2. I
3. H
4. F
5. J
6. D
7. A
8. G
9. B
10. C
11. K

#### Activity #2
1. T
2. T
3. F
4. F
5. T
6. F
7. F
8. T
9. F
10. T

#### Activity #3
1. Skin, lungs, GI tract, salivation, drainage from fistulas and drains
2. 9.0 mg/dL (2.25 mmol/L)
3. Hypermagnesemia, kidney disease, hypothyroidism, adrenal insufficiency
4. 0.9
5. Hyper
6. Iso
7. 0.45
8. Hyperkalemia
9. Hypocalcemia
10. Hypocalcemia, hypomagnesemia

#### Activity #4
1. C
2. B
3. A
4. A
5. B
6. A
7. B
8. C
9. C
10. A
11. C
12. C
13. A
14. B
15. A

## Activity #5

Foods that the nurse will teach a patient following a low-sodium diet to avoid include, but are not limited to:

1. Soy sauce
2. Smoked foods
3. Deli meats (e.g., bacon, bologna, lunch meat)
4. Pickled foods (e.g., herring, sardines)
5. Snack foods that have a high sodium content
6. Processed foods (e.g., boxed meals or mixes)
7. Condiments with high sodium content (e.g., salad dressings, barbecue sauce)
8. Canned foods that have high sodium content (e.g., canned vegetables)
9. Crackers
10. Potato chips
11. Certain seasonings

## Activity #6

Answers should resemble this process related to calcium in the body:

Calcium enters the body by dietary intake and absorption through the intestinal tract. Absorption of dietary calcium requires the active form of vitamin D. Most body calcium is stored in the bone matrix rather than in any fluid compartment. When more calcium is needed, parathyroid hormone (PTH) is released from the parathyroid glands. PTH increases serum calcium levels by:

- Releasing free calcium from bone storage sites (bone *resorption* of calcium)
- Stimulating vitamin D activation to help increase intestinal *absorption* of dietary calcium
- Inhibiting kidney calcium excretion
- Stimulating kidney calcium *reabsorption* into the blood

When excess calcium is present in plasma, PTH secretion is inhibited and the secretion of *thyrocalcitonin* (TCT), a hormone secreted by the thyroid gland, is increased. TCT causes the plasma calcium level to decrease by inhibiting bone resorption of calcium, inhibiting vitamin D–associated intestinal uptake of calcium, and increasing kidney excretion of calcium in the urine.

## Learning Assessment

### NCLEX Examination Challenge #1

Answer: A, B, C, E

Rationale: Fluid overload is an excess of body fluid. It is a clinical indication of a problem in which fluid intake or retention is greater than the body's fluid needs. The most common type of fluid overload is hypervolemia because the problems result from excessive fluid in the extracellular fluid (ECF) space. Most problems caused by fluid overload are related to excessive fluid in the vascular space or to dilution of specific electrolytes and blood components. The conditions leading to fluid overload are related to excessive intake or inadequate excretion of fluids. Assessment findings that are characteristic of fluid overload include liver enlargement (Choice A), increased pulse rate (Choice B), crackles in the lungs (Choice C), and pitting edema in dependent areas (Choice E). Fluid overload is characterized by an increase in the respiratory rate; not a decrease (Choice D).

### NCLEX Examination Challenge #2

Answer: C

Rationale: A normal sodium level is 136 to 145 mEq/L. The elevated value of 149 mEq/L prompts the nurse to further assess and intervene (Choice C). A normal potassium value is 3.5 to 5.0 mEq/L; a finding of 3.9 mEq/L is normal and does not indicate hypernatremia (Choice A). A normal chloride value is 98 to 106 mEq/L; a finding of 103 mEq/L is normal and does not indicate hypernatremia (Choice B). A normal magnesium value is 1.3 to 2.1 mEq/L; a finding of 1.8 mEq/L is normal and does not indicate hypernatremia (Choice D).

### NCLEX Examination Challenge #3

Answer: B

Rationale: The minimum amount of urine output per day needed to excrete toxic waste products is 400 to 600 mL. This minimum volume is called the obligatory urine output. If the 24-hour urine output falls below the obligatory output amount, wastes are retained and can cause lethal electrolyte imbalances, acidosis, and a toxic buildup of nitrogen. Therefore, when the nurse assesses that a client's output has fallen below this minimum, it is necessary to assess for electrolyte imbalances (Choice B). Fluid volume intake would not be decreased as this would lead to further impairment in output (Choice A). The finding is not normal, as the client's output has fallen below the obligatory urine output amount (Choice C). The Rapid Response Team is not indicated at this time (Choice D) because the nurse will need to further assess and determine appropriate interventions.

**NCLEX Examination Challenge #4**
Answer: A
Rationale: Cardiovascular changes associated with hypomagnesemia are serious, so the nurse will first assess the rhythm strip (Choice A). Low magnesium levels increase the risk for hypertension, atherosclerosis, hypertrophic left ventricle, and a variety of dysrhythmias including premature contractions, atrial fibrillation, ventricular fibrillation, and long QT intervals. The nurse will also assess the GI system (Choice B), the renal system (Choice C), and neuromuscular function (Choice D); however, assessment of the cardiac function must be done first.

## Chapter 14

### Answer Key

#### Activity #1
1. H
2. F
3. C
4. D
5. B
6. E
7. G
8. A
9. I

#### Activity #2
1. T
2. T
3. F
4. F
5. F
6. T
7. T
8. T
9. T
10. F

#### Activity #3
1. B
2. A
3. A
4. B
5. A
6. B
7. A
8. A
9. B
10. B
11. A
12. B
13. A
14. A
15. B

#### Activity #4
Key assessment points the nurse will complete to determine whether a patient has acid-base balance include, but are not limited to:
1. Comparing the patient's mental status with what the family, significant other, or health record states is the patient's baseline
2. Checking the rate and depth of respiration
3. Determining whether the patient can complete a sentence without stopping for breath
4. Examining the color of nail beds and mucous membranes

5. Examining skin turgor for dehydration. Attempt to pinch the skin to form a tent over the sternum and on the forehead. If a tent forms, record how long it remains
6. Measuring the rate and quality of the pulse
7. Monitoring clinical responses and laboratory values while the acid-base imbalance is being corrected

### Activity #5
Answers should resemble this process related to buffers in the body:

Buffers are substances that, when dissolved in fluid, can react as either an acid (releasing a hydrogen ion) or a base (binding a free hydrogen ion), depending on the pH of that fluid. Buffers always try to keep body fluid pH as close as possible in the range of 7.35 to 7.45. If a body fluid is basic (with few free hydrogen ions), the buffer releases hydrogen ions into the fluid. If a body fluid is acidic (with many free hydrogen ions), the buffer binds some of the excess hydrogen ions. In this way buffers act like hydrogen ion "sponges," soaking up hydrogen ions when too many are present and squeezing out hydrogen ions when too few are present. This flexibility allows buffers to help keep body fluid pH in the normal range.

## Learning Assessment

### NCLEX Examination Challenge #1
Answer: B
Rationale: The normal arterial pH range is 7.35 to 7.45. The normal $PaCO_2$ range is 35 to 45 mm Hg. The normal $PaO_2$ range is 80 to 100 mm Hg. The normal arterial bicarbonate range is 21 to 28 mEq/L (mmol/L). Choice B has the only set of values in which all findings are normal. In Choice A, the pH, $PaCO_2$, and bicarbonate are abnormal. In Choice C, the $PaCO_2$ and bicarbonate are abnormal. In Choice D, all values are abnormal.

### NCLEX Examination Challenge #2
Answer: C, E
Rationale: Higher concentration of hydrogen ions (reflected by a lower pH) reduces the function of hormones (Choice C) and decreases cardiac electrical conduction (Choice E). Higher concentrations of hydrogen ions increase the serum potassium levels rather than lowering them (Choice A), decrease the effectiveness of drugs instead of increasing them (Choice B), and reduce enzyme function instead of increasing it (Choice D).

### NCLEX Examination Challenge #3
Answer: A
Rationale: Base excesses are caused by excessive intake of bicarbonates, carbonates, acetates, and citrates. Citrates are products used to preserve blood components for transfusion therapy. A massive blood transfusion can increase citrate levels, resulting in a base excess alkalosis, so the nurse will monitor this client most closely for the development of this condition (Choice A). A decreasing $PaO_2$ coupled with a rising $PaCO_2$ (Choice B), hyperkalemia (Choice C), and a diminished respiratory rate (likely resulting from surgical anesthesia and/or opioid drugs following surgery) (Choice D) are associated with acidosis.

### NCLEX Examination Challenge #4
Answer: C
Rationale: During acidosis, the body attempts to bring the pH closer to normal by moving free hydrogen ions into cells in exchange for potassium ions. This exchange can cause hyperkalemia, which can block electrical conduction through the heart and cause severe bradycardia and even cardiac arrest. A hallmark of hyperkalemia is tall, peaked T waves on the ECG. For these reasons, the nurse will assess this laboratory value first (Choice C). Although serum glucose (Choice A), serum sodium (Choice B), and serum magnesium (Choice D) are affected to some degree, the most important one to assess is the serum potassium level.

## Chapter 15
**Answer Key**

### Activity #1

Infusion nurses may perform any or all of these activities:

- Develop evidence-based policies and procedures.
- Insert and maintain various types of peripheral, midline, and central venous catheters and subcutaneous and intraosseous accesses.
- Monitor patient outcomes of infusion therapy.
- Educate staff, patients, and families regarding infusion therapy.
- Consult on product selection and purchasing decisions.
- Provide therapies such as blood withdrawal, therapeutic phlebotomy, hypodermoclysis, intraosseous infusions, and administration of medications.

### Activity #2

1. T
2. F
3. T
4. F
5. F
6. F
7. T
8. F
9. T
10. T
11. F
12. T
13. F
14. F
15. F
16. T
17. F

### Activity #3

Nursing interventions that can be used to address each given complication of IV therapy include those listed in this chart.

| Complication | Interventions |
|---|---|
| Infiltration | <ul><li>Stop infusion and remove short peripheral catheter immediately after identification of problem.</li><li>Apply sterile dressing if weeping from tissue occurs.</li><li>Elevate extremity.</li><li>Warm or cold compresses may be used according to organizational policy.</li><li>Warm compresses increase circulation to the area and speed healing.</li><li>Cool compresses may be used to relieve discomfort and reduce swelling.</li><li>Insert a new catheter in the opposite extremity.</li></ul> |
| Extravasation | <ul><li>Stop infusion and disconnect administration set.</li><li>If possible, aspirate drug from short PIVC, CVC, or port access needle.</li><li>Leave short PIVC, CVC, or port access needle in place to deliver antidote if indicated by established policy.</li><li>Apply cold compresses for all drugs EXCEPT vinca alkaloids and epipodophyllotoxins.</li><li>Photograph site and assess the extremity (both above and below the insertion site).</li><li>Surgical interventions may be required.</li><li>Provide written instructions to patient and family.</li></ul> |

| Complication | Interventions |
|---|---|
| Phlebitis | • Remove short PIVC at the first sign of phlebitis; use warm compresses to relieve pain.<br>• Assess frequently.<br>• Document using Phlebitis Scale.<br>• Insert a new catheter using the opposite extremity.<br>• Phlebitis occurring in the first week after PICC insertion may be treated without catheter removal. Apply continuous heat; rest and elevate the extremity. Significant improvement is seen in 24 hours, and complete resolution is seen within 72 hours.<br>• Remove catheter if treatment is unsuccessful. |
| Thrombosis | • Stop infusion and remove short PIVC immediately.<br>• Apply cold compresses to decrease blood flow and stabilize the clot.<br>• Elevate extremity.<br>• Surgical intervention may be required.<br>• For CVCs, notify the health care provider for a diagnostic study. Low-dose thrombolytic agents may be used to lyse the clot. |
| Thrombophlebitis | • Same as for phlebitis and thrombosis.<br>• Apply cold pack initially followed by warm compress. |
| Ecchymosis and hematoma | • When removing device, apply light pressure; excessive pressure could cause other fragile veins in the area to rupture.<br>• For hematoma, apply direct pressure until bleeding has stopped. Elevate extremity, apply ice pack for first 24 hours, and then apply a warm compress for comfort. |
| Site infection | • Clean exit site with alcohol, expressing drainage if present.<br>• For short PIVC, midline catheter, or PICC, remove using sterile technique and avoid contact between skin and catheter.<br>• Send catheter tip for culture, if requested.<br>• Clean site with alcohol and cover with dry, sterile dressing; health care provider to evaluate for septic phlebitis; possible need for antimicrobial therapy or surgical intervention. |
| Venous spasm | • Temporarily slow infusion rate.<br>• Apply warm compress.<br>• Do not immediately remove short PIVC.<br>• If occurring during midline catheter or PICC removal, do not apply tension or attempt forceful removal.<br>• Reapply a dressing, apply heat, encourage patient to drink warm liquids and keep extremity covered and dry; 12 to 24 hours may be required before catheter can be removed. |

*Activity #4*
1. C
2. E
3. D
4. B
5. G
6. A
7. F

## Activity #5

Indications for the use of each gauge of catheter include:

| Catheter Gauge | Indications |
|---|---|
| 24–26 gauge<br>Smallest, shortest (¾- inch length) | Infants and small children |
| 22 gauge | Adequate for most therapies including blood |
| 20 gauge (1- to 1¼-inch length) | Adequate for all therapies (minimum size for use during surgery) |
| 18 gauge | Preferred size for surgery |
| 14–16 gauge | Trauma and surgical patients requiring rapid fluid resuscitation |

## Activity #6

1. checklist
2. Hand hygiene
3. "time-out"
4. sterile
5. mask
6. stop
7. chlorhexidine
8. upper arm; subclavian vein

## Learning Assessment

### NCLEX Examination Challenge #1

Answer: A, B, C, D, E

Rationale: The nurse may need to obtain vascular access in a client to administer medication (Choice A), correct fluid imbalance (Choice B), maintain acid-base balance (Choice C), provide chemotherapy (Choice D), or maintain an open line in case access is needed (Choice E).

### NCLEX Examination Challenge #2

Answer: B

Rationale: For short PIVCs, 3 mL normal saline is used to flush (Choice B). This maintains patency of the catheter without the risks associated with the use of heparin flushes. Heparin (Choice A), heparinized saline (Choice C), and bacteriostatic saline (Choice D) are not necessary to flush short PIVCs.

### NCLEX Examination Challenge #3

Answer: B

Rationale: A hypotonic solution has a lower than normal blood plasma osmolarity (fluids less than 270 mOsm/L). An example of a hypotonic solution is 0.45% NaCl (Choice B). Isotonic fluids have the same solute concentration as blood (between 270 and 300 mOsm/L) and include 0.9% saline (NS) (Choice A), Ringer's lactate solution (Choice C), and 5% dextrose in water ($D_5W$). Hypertonic solutions have a higher-than-normal blood plasma osmolarity (greater than 300 mOsm/L) and include 5% dextrose in 0.45% saline (D5 1/2) and 10% dextrose in water ($D_{10}W$).

# Chapter 16
## Answer Key
### Activity #1
Ways in which leukocytes provide protection through defensive actions include:

1. Recognition of self versus non-self for the initiation of defensive inflammation and immunity actions for protection
2. Destruction of foreign invaders, cellular debris, and unhealthy or abnormal self cells
3. Production of antibodies directed against invaders
4. Complement activation forming membrane attack complexes (MACs) to enhance phagocytosis
5. Maintenance of self-tolerance
6. Production of cytokines that stimulate increased formation of leukocytes in bone marrow and increase specific leukocyte activity

### Activity #2
1. T
2. T
3. T
4. F
5. T
6. T
7. F
8. F
9. F
10. T

### Activity #3
Actions that take place during each stage of the inflammation sequence should resemble this information:

**Stage I**
- Vascular response that starts changes in blood vessels.
- Injured tissues and the leukocytes and tissue mast cells in this area secrete histamine, serotonin, and kinins (especially bradykinin) that constrict small veins and dilate arterioles. These changes cause redness and warmth of the tissues. This increased blood flow increases delivery of nutrients to injured tissues.
- Blood flow to the area increases (hyperemia), and edema forms at the site of injury or invasion. Capillary leak also occurs, allowing blood plasma to leak into the tissues. This response causes swelling and pain. Edema protects the area from further injury by creating a cushion of fluid. The duration of these responses depends on the severity of the initiating event, but usually they subside within 24 to 72 hours.

**Stage II**
- Cellular exudate part of the response.
- Neutrophilia (an increased number of circulating neutrophils) occurs. Pus containing dead WBCs, necrotic tissue, and fluids that escape from damaged cells is formed as an exudate. Neutrophils, basophils, eosinophils, and tissue mast cells are active in this stage, with continuing activation triggered by the release of cytokines from macrophages in the area.
  - The eosinophils and mast cells promote a continued inflammatory response.
  - Under the influence of cytokines, the neutrophil count can increase hugely within 12 hours after inflammation starts. Neutrophils attack and destroy organisms and remove dead tissue through phagocytosis.
  - Basophils and tissue mast cells continue or sustain the initial responses.
  - In acute inflammation, the healthy adult produces enough mature segmented neutrophils to keep pace with invasion and prevent the organisms from growing. At the same time, the WBCs and inflamed tissues secrete cytokines, which allow tissue macrophages to increase and trigger bone marrow production of monocytes.
- During this phase, the arachidonic acid cascade starts to increase inflammation. This action begins with the conversion of fatty acids in plasma membranes of injured or infected cells into arachidonic acid (AA). The enzyme cyclooxygenase (COX) converts AA into chemicals that are further processed into the substances (mediators) that promote continued inflammation.

- When an infection-stimulating inflammation lasts longer than just a few days, the bone marrow begins to release immature neutrophils, reducing the number of circulating mature neutrophils. This problem limits helpful effects of inflammation and increases the risk for sepsis.

**Stage III**

- Involves tissue repair and replacement.
- WBCs involved in inflammation start the replacement of lost tissues or repair of damaged tissues by inducing the remaining healthy cells to divide.
- In tissues that cannot divide, WBCs trigger new blood vessel growth and scar tissue formation. Because scar tissue does not act like the tissue it replaces, function is lost wherever scar tissue forms as replacement for normal tissue.

*Activity #4*
1. D
2. B
3. F
4. E
5. A
6. C

*Activity #5*
1. Artificial active immunity
2. Artificial passive immunity
3. Natural active immunity
4. Natural passive immunity
5. Innate immunity

*Activity #6*
All of these cardinal symptoms of inflammation should be listed. They can be presented (for purposes of this activity) in any order.
1. Warmth
2. Redness
3. Swelling
4. Pain
5. Decreased function

## Learning Assessment

**NCLEX Examination Challenge #1**
Answer: A, B, C, D, E
Rationale: The nurse identifies a number of client conditions that reduce immunity. These include taking certain medications such as NSAIDs and corticosteroids daily (Choice A); having type 2 diabetes, regardless of whether it is well-controlled (Choice B); being an older adult (Choice C); using public facilities because of the exposure to pathogenic microorganisms (Choice D); and eating less than a balanced diet (Choice E) because this reduces immunity by limiting intake of substances critical for immune cell function.

**NCLEX Examination Challenge #2**
Answer: A
Rationale: The segmented neutrophils are normally the largest population of circulating leukocytes (55% to 70%) and provide immediate protection against infection. The percentage of circulating band neutrophils should be much lower (about 5%). The greatly increased band population with a decrease in the segmented neutrophil population indicates an ongoing infection in which bone marrow production of fully functional neutrophils is failing (Choice A). This is known as a *left shift*. The normal lymphocyte count is greatly higher than the basophil count (Choice B). The monocyte count (Choice C) and total WBC count (Choice D) are within the normal range.

**NCLEX Examination Challenge #3**
Answer: C
Rationale: Regulator T cells have the opposite action of helper T cells. For optimal cell-mediated immunity, a balance between helper T-cell activity and regulatory T-cell activity must be maintained. This balance occurs when the helper T cells outnumber the regulatory T cells by a ratio of 2:1. When this ratio increases, overreactions can occur. These include allergies to almost anything, including allergens and drugs (Choice C). Some of these overreactions are minimally bothersome, others damage tissue, and some can be dangerous. The client does not need extra vaccinations (Choice A), is not more susceptible to infections (Choice B), and does not have an increased risk for development of cancer (Choice D).

## Chapter 17
**Answer Key**
*Chapter Review*
**Pathophysiology Review**
#1

1. Type II
2. Type III
3. Type IV
4. Type I
5. Type IV
6. Type I
7. Type I
8. Type IV
9. Type III
10. Type II

#2 Onset should match exactly what is listed here. Signs and symptoms may include any of the information below.

| Type | Onset After Exposure | Signs and Symptoms |
|---|---|---|
| **Type I** **or** **Anaphylactic Reaction** **or** **Immediate Reaction** | Immediate reaction occurs in __30__ to _60___ minutes  Accelerated reaction occurs in _1__ to __72___ hours | Allergic asthma  Anaphylaxis  Angioedema  Bronchospasm  Difficulty breathing  Itchy, red, watery eyes  Rhinorrhea  Urticaria |
| **Type II** **or** **Cytotoxic-Mediated Response** | Can happen in minutes to hours | Specific symptoms are associated with the causative agent  (e.g., difficulty breathing, sense of anxiety, elevated pulse, and increased respiratory rate that arises during blood infusion) |
| **Type III** **or Immunocomplex Reaction** | Can happen in hours to ___days____ | Dependent on specific disorder(s) |
| **Type IV** **or** **Delayed Hypersensitivity Reaction** | __12___ to ___72__ hours | At site of exposure:  Edema  Induration  Ischemia  Tissue damage |

## Activities

### Activity #1

1. F
2. T
3. F
4. T
5. F
6. F
7. T
8. T
9. T
10. F

### Activity #2

Signs and symptoms of rejection can include any of the listed findings.

| Organ | Signs and Symptoms of Rejection |
|---|---|
| Heart | • Ankle edema<br>• Hypotension<br>• Decreased energy<br>• Tachycardia or arrythmias<br>• Diminished ability to exercise<br>• Shortness of breath at rest or with activity<br>• Weight gain of at least 2.2 lb (1 kg) daily |
| Kidney | • Fever >100°F (37.8°C) and chills<br>• Diminished or absent urinary output<br>• Notable swelling of hands, legs, or eyelids<br>• Tenderness or pain over area of transplantation<br>• Weight gain of 2–4 lb (1–2 kg) in a 24-hour period |
| Liver | • Fever >100°F (37.8°C) and chills<br>• Tenderness or pain in the abdomen |
| Lung | • Dry cough<br>• Decreased energy<br>• Decreased home spirometry<br>• Tenderness or pain in the chest<br>• Decreased appetite and/or nausea<br>• Fever >100°F (37.8°C) and chills<br>• Shortness of breath with light or moderate activity |
| Pancreas | • Decreased energy<br>• Glucose elevation<br>• Fever >100°F (37.8°C)<br>• Tenderness or pain over the area of transplantation |

**Activity #3**

1. E
2. D
3. A
4. B
5. F
6. G
7. C

**Activity #4**

Potential assessment findings should resemble the ones listed.

| System | Potential Assessment Findings |
|---|---|
| **Cardiovascular** | |
| Heart failure | Dysrhythmias |
| **Endocrine** | |
| Hormonal changes | Low testosterone, menstrual irregularity, lipodystrophy |
| **Gastrointestinal** | |
| Anorexia, malabsorption, weight loss | Change in intake, lack of appetite, unplanned weight loss |
| Diarrhea (can result in "AIDS wasting syndrome") | Diarrhea and electrolyte imbalances (can lose up to 10% of body weight) |
| Oral and esophageal lesions | Lesions in oral cavity |
| **Immune** | |
| *Candida albicans* | Difficulty swallowing, mouth and throat pain |
| Human papillomavirus (HPV) | Anal and cervical dysplasia |
| **Integumentary** | |
| Kaposi's sarcoma (KS) | Purplish lesions over the body |
| **Neurologic** | |
| HIV-associated dementia (HAD) | Decrease in cognitive domains with observable impairment in completing ADLs |
| **Renal** | |
| HIV-associated nephropathy (HIVAN) | Rapid deterioration in kidney function, proteinuria |
| **Respiratory** | |
| *Pneumocystis jiroveci* pneumonia (PCP) | Dry cough (ongoing), shortness of breath, tachypnea |
| Tuberculosis (TB) | Cough, dyspnea, chest pain, fever, chills, night sweats, weight loss |

**Activity #5**

Common autoimmune disorders can include any of these choices:

1. Ankylosing spondylitis (AS)
2. Autoimmune hemolytic anemia
3. Autoimmune thrombocytopenic purpura
4. Celiac disease
5. Crohn's disease
6. Dermatomyositis
7. Eczema
8. Goodpasture's syndrome
9. Graves' disease
10. Guillain-Barré syndrome
11. Hashimoto's thyroiditis
12. Multiple sclerosis (MS)
13. Myasthenia gravis
14. Pernicious anemia
15. Psoriasis
16. Psoriatic arthritis
17. Rheumatoid arthritis
18. Scleroderma
19. Sjögren syndrome (SS)
20. Systemic lupus erythematosus (SLE)
21. Type 1 diabetes
22. Vasculitis
23. Ulcerative colitis (UC)

**Learning Assessments**

**NCLEX Examination Challenge #1**

Answer: D

Rationale: The concern that requires the nurse to intervene is the potential hypersensitivity to contrast medium (Choice D). The client has clearly had some type of adverse reaction during a test using contrast dye previously and may be at great risk for a more severe reaction during the scheduled procedure. The nurse must notify the radiologist and primary health care provider to explore this potential risk immediately. Diabetes and high blood pressure that are in the client's family history are not risks associated with the procedure that is scheduled (Choice A). The sister's allergies are not relevant to the client's upcoming procedure because these are different types of dyes (Choice B). Although the client also has seasonal allergies, these are not associated with hypersensitivity to contrast medium (Choice C).

**NCLEX Examination Challenge #2**

Answer: C, D

Rationale: Wheezing on exhalation is an indication of bronchoconstriction, which occurs during anaphylaxis (Choice D). The bronchoconstriction is severe enough to result in some degree of hypoxia, which is consistent with the pulse oximetry of 88% (Choice C). Skin becomes cyanotic, not flushed, during anaphylaxis (Choice A). Bradycardia does not occur with anaphylaxis; clients become tachycardic with a weak and thready pulse because of sympathetic nervous system compensation for shock (Choice B). Increased deep tendon reflexes are not associated with anaphylaxis (Choice E).

**NCLEX Examination Challenge #3**

Answer: C

Rationale: In Stage I of Lyme disease, the client usually develops a "bull's-eye" rash known as *erythema migrans* and a low-grade fever (Choice C). Acute confusion is not present in Stage I but can be a part of Stages II and III (Choice A). Cardiac dysrhythmias are not present in Stage I but can be a part of Stages II and III (Choice B). Symptoms that occur in Stage II but not in Stage I include continued flu-like symptoms and pain in the knee, ankle, and wrist joints (Choice D).

**NGN Challenge #1**

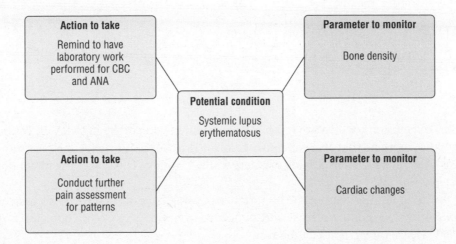

Rationale: The client's presenting concerns are consistent with the vague symptomology that often accompanies SLE. SLE is characterized by arthralgias, osteoporosis, discoid rash on the face, photosensitivity, chronic fatigue, generalized inflammation, and intermittent joint discomfort. Diagnosis can be challenging, and numerous diagnostic assessments are often performed before a firm diagnosis is made. The nurse will remind the client to have the required laboratory work done.

A CBC is usually ordered first with an (antinuclear antibody) ANA test. Although results from these two tests are not definitive, they are the foundation on which further assessment can be performed. The nurse will also further assess the patterns of pain the client experiences. In SLE, pain is often variable.

On exacerbation, organ damage occurs. Because organ damage can occur without treatment and may continue to occur albeit more slowly with treatment, the nurse will monitor for outcomes that are associated with SLE including changes in bone density that can lead to osteoporosis and cardiac changes because dysrhythmias can develop.

Lyme disease is associated with the bite of a tick; there is no indication that the client has been outside or been bitten by a tick. HIV is characterized in the early stage by more prominent flu-like symptoms (e.g., ongoing fever, night sweats) that usually fully resolve. There is no evidence of psoriasis, which is characterized by scaled lesions.

There is no need to arrange for a driver to take the client to receive HIV testing results because the symptoms are not consistent with this diagnosis. Therefore, this test is less likely to be ordered compared with others. Warm heat is used to relieve pain associated with inflammation; ice packs can damage tissue integrity. The discoid rash on the client's face is not infectious and does not need an antibiotic. This is a "butterfly rash" over the bridge of the nose and onto the cheeks that is characteristic of SLE.

There is no need to monitor for confusion, scaled lesions, or opportunistic lesions based on the client's presentation and most likely condition. Confusion is associated with later stages of Lyme disease and HIV-III, not SLE. Scaled lesions are associated with psoriasis, not SLE. Opportunistic infections develop in HIV-III, not SLE.

NGN Challenge #2

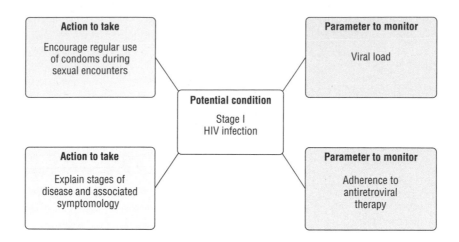

Rationale: The client's symptoms, which are resolving, are characteristic of Stage I HIV infection, which often involves flu-like symptoms that spontaneously resolve. The client reports feeling better and discusses unprotected sexual encounters with new male partners while drinking. This raises the likelihood of the client having been infected with HIV.

The nurse will provide education about the importance of using condoms consistently to avoid spreading the virus and will explain the stages of the disease and associated symptomology. With appropriate early treatment, HIV is a chronic disease that the client can manage.

The nurse will monitor the client's viral load, which is indicative of the actual amount of HIV viral RNA particles present in 1 mL of blood. This result is used to measure prognosis, disease progression, effectiveness of therapy, and need for prophylactic therapy and to determine survivability. The nurse will also monitor the client's adherence to antiretroviral therapy, which influences the viral load and helps to manage the condition as a chronic disease.

It is less likely that the client has COVID-19, mononucleosis, or influenza, given the additional information about the client's activities over the past couple of weeks that coincide with development of symptoms.

The nurse will not offer PrEP therapy. This practice involves the person who is HIV negative, yet at high risk for HIV infection, taking antiretroviral drugs *before* sexual activity or drug injection to avoid infection. Because the client's unprotected sexual activity is in the past, PrEP therapy is not appropriate. Monoclonal antibodies may be used to treat COVID-19, but they are not used to treat HIV infection. The Epstein-Barr virus is related to mononucleosis; it is unlikely that the client has this condition when all other data is analyzed.

Bedrest is unnecessary. There is no need for an antibiotic, so adherence to this therapy is unnecessary to monitor. The client does not need to be quarantined (which would have been appropriate for COVID-19 infection), but rather needs to enact safer sex practices.

## Chapter 18
### Answer Key
*Pathophysiology Review*
#1.

1. E
2. J
3. B
4. F
5. D
6. A
7. I
8. G
9. C
10. H

#2. Actions should resemble these below. **Key actions are bolded.**

| Step | Actions |
|------|---------|
| Initiation | • **Loss of cellular regulation influences normal cells to become cancer cells.**<br>• **Carcinogens change the activity of a normal cell.**<br>• Initiation is an irreversible event that can lead to cancer development. |
| Promotion | • **This step involves enhanced growth of an initiated cell by substances known as promoters.**<br>• **Once a normal cell has been initiated by a carcinogen and is a cancer cell, it can become a tumor if its growth is enhanced.**<br>• Many normal hormones and body proteins, such as insulin and estrogen, can act as promoters and make cells divide more frequently.<br>• The time between a cell's initiation and the development of an overt tumor is called the *latency period,* which can range from months to years. Exposure to promoters can shorten the latency period. |
| Progression | • **This step involves the continued change of a cancer cell, which makes it more malignant over time.**<br>• After cancer cells have grown to the point that a detectable tumor is formed, it starts to develop its own blood supply, ensuring its continued nourishment and growth.<br>• As tumor cells continue to divide, some of the new cells undergo genetic mutations that change features from the original cancer cell. Over time, the tumor cells have fewer normal cell features. |
| Metastasis | • **Metastasis occurs when cancer cells move from the primary location by breaking off from the original tumor and establishing remote tumors.** |

## Activities

### Activity #1

1. T
2. T
3. F
4. T
5. F
6. F
7. T
8. F
9. F
10. T

### Activity #2

Early and late sides effects of radiation therapy per body location should include any of these answers:

| Body Location | Early Effect | Late Effect |
|---|---|---|
| Central nervous system | • Alopecia and dermatitis of the scalp<br>• Ear and external auditory canal irritation<br>• Cerebral edema and increased intracranial pressure<br>• Nausea and vomiting<br>• Blurry vision | • Brain necrosis<br>• Leukoencephalopathy<br>• Cognitive and emotional dysfunction<br>• Pituitary and hypothalamic dysfunction<br>• Spinal cord myelopathies |
| Head and neck | • Oral mucositis<br>• Taste changes<br>• Oral candidiasis, herpes, or other infections<br>• Acute xerostomia<br>• Dental caries<br>• Esophagitis and pharyngitis | • Xerostomia and dental caries<br>• Trismus<br>• Osteoradionecrosis<br>• Hypothyroidism |
| Breast and chest wall | • Skin reactions<br>• Esophagitis | • Atrophy, fibrosis of breast tissue<br>• Lymphedema |
| Chest and lung | • Esophagitis and pharyngitis<br>• Taste changes<br>• Pneumonia<br>• Cough | XXXXXXXXXXXXXXXXXXXXXXXXXXXX |
| Abdomen and pelvis | • Anorexia<br>• Nausea and vomiting<br>• Diarrhea<br>• Cystitis or proctitis<br>• Vaginal dryness/vaginitis<br>• Sexual and fertility problems | • Small and large bowel injury<br>• Diarrhea |
| Eye | • Conjunctival edema and tearing | XXXXXXXXXXXXXXXXXXXXXXXXXXXX |

**Activity #3**

The Seven Warning Signs of Cancer should include:

| C | Changes in bowel or bladder habits |
|---|---|
| A | A sore that does not heal |
| U | Unusual bleeding or discharge |
| T | Thickening or lump in the breast or elsewhere |
| I | Indigestion or difficulty swallowing |
| O | Obvious change in a wart or mole |
| N | Nagging cough or hoarseness |

**Activity #4**

Methods the nurse would use when assessing an older adult for each type of cancer include (but are not limited to) these examples.

| Cancer Type | Assessment Methods |
|---|---|
| Colorectal cancer | Ask the patient whether bowel habits have changed over the past year (e.g., in consistency, frequency, color). Ask whether the patient has noticed any obvious blood in the stool. Test at least one stool specimen for occult blood during the patient's hospitalization. Review the results of a baseline colonoscopy with the health care provider. |
| Lung cancer | Observe the skin and mucous membranes for color. Ask the patient about whether they currently have or have experienced:<br>• Cough<br>• Hoarseness<br>• Smoking history (including use of electronic cigarettes or "vaping")<br>• Exposure to particulate matter (inhalation irritants) and/or asbestos<br>• Shortness of breath<br>• Activity tolerance<br>• Frothy or bloody sputum<br>• Pain in the arms, shoulders, or chest<br>• Difficulty swallowing |
| Prostate cancer | Ask the patient about whether they currently have or have experienced:<br>• Urinary hesitancy<br>• Change in the size of the urine stream<br>• New onset of pain in the lower back or legs<br>• History of persistent urinary tract infections |
| Skin cancer | Examine skin areas for moles or warts. Ask the patient about changes in moles (e.g., color, edges, sensation). |

| Cancer Type | Assessment Methods |
|---|---|
| Leukemia | Observe the skin for color, petechiae, or ecchymosis. Ask the patient about whether they currently have or have experienced: <br>• Fatigue<br>• Bruising<br>• Bleeding tendency<br>• History of infections and illnesses<br>• Night sweats and/or fevers |
| Bladder cancer | Ask the patient about whether they currently have or have experienced:<br>• Pain on urination<br>• Blood in the urine<br>• Cloudy urine<br>• Increased frequency or urgency |

**Activity #5**

Characteristics of each type of surgery that can be used to address a cancer diagnosis include:

*Prophylactic surgery*
- Removal of potentially cancerous tissue as a means of preventing cancer development
- Performed when a patient has a strong predisposition for development of a specific cancer

*Diagnostic surgery* (e.g., excisional biopsy)
- Removal of all or part of a suspected lesion for examination and testing to confirm or rule out a cancer diagnosis

*Curative surgery*
- Removal of all cancer tissue
- Surgery alone can result in a cure when all visible and microscopic tumor is removed
- Most effective for small, localized tumors or noninvasive skin cancers

*Debulking surgery*
- Removal of part of the tumor if removal of the entire mass is not possible
- Decreases the size of the tumor and the number of cancer cells, which may help alleviate symptoms, enhance the success of other types of cancer treatment, and increase survival time

*Palliative surgery*
- Surgery done to promote symptom relief and improve the quality of life
- Noncurative

*Reconstructive* or *restorative surgery*
- Surgery that increases function, enhances appearance, or both

Learning Assessments

### NCLEX Examination Challenge #1

Answer: A, B, C, E

Rationale: The skin in the path of radiation is injured by the treatment. The degree of injury is related to the intensity and duration of treatments. Six weeks of daily radiation treatment is a large dose and usually results in skin redness, tenderness, and peeling during the treatment period and for weeks afterward. If markings are present, they must remain in place through the treatment to appropriately direct the radiation beam (Choice A). The area remains sensitive to sun damage, heat damage, and direct contact damage for up to a year after therapy is complete; therefore, avoidance of sun during this time frame is important (Choice B). It is important for the client to avoid trauma to the area by using only mild soap and water, and to cleanse the area with hands rather than a cloth (Choice C). It is also important to wear loose clothing to avoid irritating the skin further (Choice E). Heat to the area will make the skin reaction worse, so heating pads should not be used (Choice D).

### NCLEX Examination Challenge #2

Answer: D

Rationale: Oral chemotherapy drugs should not be crushed, cut, or chewed; the nurse needs to provide further teaching to the patient who thinks they can do this or has been doing it (Choice D). Alternate actions that can make them easier to swallow include taking them with a spoonful of pudding or thick drink. These drugs can be more convenient than taking IV chemotherapy (Choice A). The client is correct that missed doses can reduce therapy outcomes (Choice B). These drugs can be absorbed through the skin and only the client should have direct contact with them (Choice C). These statements do not require further teaching.

### NCLEX Examination Challenge #3

Answer: A

Rationale: Excessive bleeding occurs when the platelet count is this low (thrombocytopenia). In addition to handling the client gently, pressure needs to be applied after injections, blood draws, and discontinuation of an IV (Choice A). The client who has thrombocytopenia (and no other symptoms) is not at increased risk for infection and does not have an infection, so a contact isolation room is not necessary (Choice B). Platelets do not carry oxygen, and low platelet counts do not cause hypoxia or dyspnea, so oxygen is not needed as dyspnea is not expected (Choice C). Edema formation is not a result of a low platelet count, so fluids do not need to be restricted (Choice D).

### NGN Challenge #1

The nurse documents assessment findings for a 58-year-old client who is seeing the primary health care provider for an annual checkup.

**Answer:**

| Health History | Nurses Notes | Vital Signs | Laboratory Results |
|---|---|---|---|

**1010:** Client is here to see primary care provider for an annual health checkup. Electronic health record shows it has been 16 months since his last annual evaluation. Denies any health changes other than a bit of blood in stool recently that he attributes to hemorrhoids. Quantifies that "recently" means that the blood in stool began about 2 months ago and occurs several times a week. States it is not profuse, noting about 1 tablespoon of bright red blood in toilet following some bowel movements. Denies pain with defecation. No changes in urinary habits. Medical history positive for GERD controlled by omeprazole 20 mg, three times daily before meals. Reports that this usually works most of the time, but has been experiencing some abdominal discomfort and reflux following meals over the last few months. States, "a couple of times I took a double dose of omeprazole but it didn't help".
Alert and oriented × 3. Breath sounds clear in all lung fields. No wheezes, crackles, or dyspnea. $S_1$ and $S_2$ present; no murmurs. Bowel sounds present × 4. Abdomen nontender upon gentle palpation. Current VS: T 98.4°F (36.9°C); HR 84 beats/min and regular; RR 18 breaths/min; BP 130/90 mm Hg; $SpO_2$ 99%.

Rationale: Abnormal findings include waiting 16 months to be seen for an annual checkup (annually is recommended at this age), finding blood in stool 2 months ago, having about 1 tablespoon of blood in the toilet as well as blood in stool several times weekly, having increased episodes of reflux, taking extra medication over what has been prescribed, and the slightly elevated blood pressure of 130/90 mm Hg.

The nurse analyzes the findings to determine the client's condition. **Select two findings that require immediate follow-up by the nurse.**
**Answer:**
☑  Blood in stool
☑  Bright red blood in toilet

Rationale: Although the nurse will follow up on all of these findings at some time during the visit, the two findings that require immediate follow-up are the blood in stool and the bright red blood in the toilet. Both of these are concerning signs.

**Answer:**

| Options for 1 | Options for 2 and 3 |
|---|---|
| Stomach | Increased reflux |
| Prostate | Blood in toilet |
| Colon | Taking extra GERD medication |
| Esophageal | Blood in stool |
| Throat | Hypertension |

Rationale: The client is at the highest risk for colon cancer, as evidenced by blood in the toilet and blood in the stool. Both are characteristic findings associated with colon cancer. The presenting symptoms are not characteristic of stomach, prostate, esophageal, or throat cancer. Although the client does have increased reflux and has taken some extra GERD medication, stomach or esophageal cancer is still less likely than colon cancer, given the magnitude of the symptoms associated with visible, frank blood. The client's blood pressure is slightly elevated, but it is not overwhelmingly concerning considering the other symptoms present.

**Answer:**
Which item will the nurse gather for the examination and remainder of the visit? **Select all that apply.**
A.  Hemoccult card
B.  Plastic speculum
C.  Handout on colonoscopies
D.  Information about a low-fat diet
E.  Brochure on high-fiber food choices
F.  Plate for gonorrhea and chlamydia smears

Rationale: The nurse will gather supplies that will be used for the examination and remainder of the visit. The health care provider will perform a hemoccult test to evaluate the blood in the stool, so a hemoccult card will be needed (Choice A). The health care provider will also likely order a colonoscopy, so a handout on this procedure will be necessary (Choice C). To decrease the risk for development or spread of colon cancer, the client will be taught by the nurse to eat a low-fat (Choice D), high-fiber diet (Choice E), so this information will be important. The client can take home brochures and use them for dietary planning purposes. A plastic speculum would be used to examine a person who was assigned female at birth during a pelvic examination (Choice B). There is no indication the client will need to have smears done for gonorrhea and chlamydia (Choice F), which are sexually transmitted infections.

**Answer:**

A.  Chemotherapy can be immunosuppressive.
B.  It is normal to have a fever and rash during chemotherapy.
C.  Certain chemotherapy side effects can be life-threatening.
D.  If oral chemotherapy drugs expire, flush them down the toilet.
E.  Oral chemotherapy drugs are less toxic than intravenous chemotherapy.
F.  Chemotherapeutic agents kill only the cancer cells that are present in the body.
G.  If children are desired in the future, a sperm bank representative can provide options.

Rationale: The nurse will teach that chemotherapy can be immunosuppressive (Choice A), so any sign of infection (such as a fever or rash) can be life-threatening and should be reported to the health care provider right away (Choice C). Chemotherapy can cause fertility issues, so if biological children are desired in the future, the nurse will refer the client to a sperm bank representative who can discuss options (Choice G). Fever and rash can indicate infection and must be reported immediately to the health care provider (Choice B). Oral chemotherapeutic agents are just as toxic as intravenous agents (Choice E), so they should not be disposed of in a toilet (Choice D). Chemotherapy can kill healthy cells as well as cancer cells (Choice F).

**Answer:**

| Previous Client Finding | Current Client Finding | Effective | Not Effective |
|---|---|---|---|
| Blood in stool | No further blood in stool reported | X | |
| Blood in toilet | States no blood has been found in the toilet since surgery and chemotherapy | X | |
| Platelet count 225,000/mm$^3$ (225 × 10$^9$/L) (Reference range 150,000–400,000/mm$^3$ or 150–400 × 10$^9$/L [SI units]) | Platelet count 176,000/mm$^3$ (176 × 10$^9$/L) | X | |
| White blood cell count 6500/mm$^3$ (6.5 × 10$^9$/L) (Reference range 5000–10,000/mm$^3$ or 5–10 × 10$^9$/L [SI units]) | White blood cell count 5300/mm$^3$ (5.3 × 10$^9$/L) | X | |

Rationale: Interventions have been effective when the nurse assesses that there is no further blood in the stool or toilet. This is a favorable sign that colon cancer has likely been treated effectively. Interventions have also been successful when platelet counts and white blood cell counts are still within normal limits. This demonstrates that the client has not developed thrombocytopenia or neutropenia during chemotherapy.

## Chapter 19

### Answer Key

#### Activity #1

Any two of these physiologic body defenses:

- Intact skin and mucous membranes
- Respiratory tract filtration, humidification, and/or cough
- GI tract gastric acid, peristalsis, and/or enzymes
- Low urinary pH
- Phagocytosis by neutrophils
- Inflammatory enzymes
- Antibody-mediated immunity
- Cell-mediated immunity

#### Activity #2

1. D
2. E
3. A
4. G
5. C
6. B
7. H
8. F

#### Activity #3

Any four of these physiologic changes of aging or other factors:

- Decreased immune system (decreased antibodies, lymphocytes, and fever response)
- Thinning skin and decreased subcutaneous tissue
- Decreased cough and gag reflexes
- Decreased gastric acid and GI motility
- Chronic diseases such as diabetes mellitus
- Functional and cognitive impairments
- Invasive devices
- Institutionalization

#### Activity #4

1. C
2. D
3. A
4. B

#### Activity #5

Any three of these interventions:

- Acetaminophen as needed
- Cooling blanket
- Increased oral or IV fluids
- Antimicrobial therapy
- Frequent vital sign monitoring
- Monitoring for dehydration, especially in older adults

#### Activity #6

1. T
2. T
3. F
4. T
5. F
6. T

### Learning Assessment

#### NCLEX Examination Challenge #1

Answer: B

Rationale: OSHA is the national organization that develops regulations that all employers must follow. Regulations are law (Choice B). The CDC develops voluntary guidelines on preventing and controlling infections (Choice A). The FDA protects the public by ensuring the safety of food and medications used for people and animals (Choice C). The NIH conducts research to identify the standard of care for a variety of client conditions (Choice D).

#### NCLEX Examination Challenge #2

Answer: A, B, C, E

Rationale: The client could have been exposed to particulate matter at the workplace or at home. The nurse would include questions about each setting to determine the type of particulate matter exposure (Choices A, B, C, E). All of the questions are, therefore, important to include except for Choice D. It is not useful to determine if the client's workplace is part of a corporation or if it is a private company because that information does not help with identifying exposure to particulate matter.

**NCLEX Examination Challenge #3**

<u>Answer</u>: A

<u>Rationale</u>: This client likely acquired a systemic infection from the GSW that became locally infected. Therefore, a positive wound culture would be expected to confirm a local infection (Choice D). The client's local infection progressed to a systemic infection, which would typically cause an increased WBC count, an increased ESR, and increased neutrophil count because of a shift to the left (Choices A, B, C). Therefore, Choice A is the correct response.

## Chapter 20

**Answer Key**
*Chapter Review*
**Anatomy & Physiology Review**
#1.

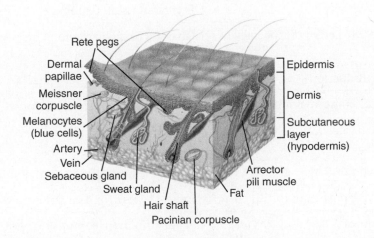

#2.
1. Stratum corneum
2. Purpura
3. Keratin
4. Nits
5. Ecchymoses
6. Hirsutism
7. Keratin
8. Dandruff
9. Primary lesion
10. Rete pegs

## Activities

### Activity #1

Answers may include five of these common integumentary system changes associated with aging:

| Physical Changes | Clinical Findings |
|---|---|
| Epidermis | |
| Decreased epidermal thickness | Skin transparency and fragility |
| Decreased cell division | Delayed wound healing |
| Decreased epidermal mitotic homeostasis | Skin hyperplasia and skin cancers (especially in sun-exposed areas) |
| Increased epidermal permeability | Increased risk for irritation |
| Decreased immune system cells | Decreased skin inflammatory response |
| Decreased melanocyte activity | Increased risk for sunburn |
| Hyperplasia of melanocyte activity (especially in sun-exposed areas) | Changes in pigmentation (e.g., liver spots, age spots) |
| Decreased vitamin D production | Increased risk for osteomalacia |
| Flattening of the dermal-epidermal junction | Increased risk for shearing forces, resulting in blisters, purpura, skin tears, and pressure-related injuries |
| Dermis | |
| Decreased dermal blood flow | Increased susceptibility to dry skin |
| Decreased vasomotor responsiveness | Increased risk for heat stroke and hypothermia |
| Decreased dermal thickness | Paper-thin, transparent skin with an increased susceptibility to trauma |
| Degeneration of elastic fibers | Decreased tone and elasticity |
| Benign proliferation of capillaries | Cherry hemangiomas |
| Reduced number and function of nerve endings | Reduced sensory perception |
| Subcutaneous layer | |
| Thinning subcutaneous layer | Increased risk for hypothermia |
| | Increased risk for pressure injury |

### Activity #2

1. Body temperature, fluid and electrolyte balance
2. Capillaries, lymph vessels
3. Melanin production
4. The sun, tanning booths
5. Secondary lesions
6. Serpiginous
7. Cardiac insufficiency
8. Hypoxia, lung cancer
9. Punch biopsy
10. Wood

## Activity #3

1. T
2. F
3. T
4. T
5. F
6. F
7. T
8. F
9. T
10. F

## Activity #4

Pertinent questions the nurse will ask about the current concerns of a patient with a skin condition include, but are not limited to:

- Can you describe the problem (e.g., is it associated with itching, burning, stinging, numbness, pain)?
- Have you had any accompanying symptoms (e.g., fever, nausea, vomiting, diarrhea, sore throat, chills, stiff neck)?
- When did you first notice the problem?
- Where on the body did the problem begin?

- Has the problem gotten better or worse? If yes:
  - o What has made the problem better?
  - o What has made the problem worse?
- Has a similar skin condition ever occurred before? If yes:
  - o Can you describe it, and how was it treated?
- Have you recently consumed any new foods? If yes:
  - o Please list which new food(s) you have consumed, and when it/they were last eaten.
- Have you recently applied new bed linens, worn new unwashed clothing, used new unwashed towels, and/or used new soaps or cosmetics? If yes:
  - o Please list which new item(s) you've used and when you had your last exposure.
- Have you encountered any significantly stressful situations recently? If yes:
  - o Did the skin condition appear around the time you began experiencing stress?

## Learning Assessments

### NCLEX Examination Challenge #1

Answer: B, C, D, E

Rationale: The nurse assesses each lesion on a client for these ABCDE features that are associated with skin cancer: **A**symmetry of shape; **B**order irregularity; **C**olor variation within one lesion; **D**iameter greater than 1/4 of an inch or 6 mm; and **E**volving or changing in any feature (shape, size, color, elevation, itching, bleeding, or crusting). The nurse will notify the health care provider of signs that are associated with melanoma, which include lesion asymmetry (Choice B), bleeding from a lesion (Choice C), diameter of a lesion exceeding 6 mm (Choice D), and a variation in lesion's color (Choice E). Border regularity (Choice A) is a normal finding that does not require notification of the health care provider unless other signs are also present.

### NCLEX Examination Challenge #2

Answer: A

Rationale: Ecchymoses (bruises) are larger areas of hemorrhage. In older adults, bruising is common after minor trauma to the skin. Certain drugs (e.g., aspirin, warfarin, corticosteroids) and low platelet counts lead to easy or excessive bruising. Although the nurse will always review all laboratory results, the nurse will check the platelet count as the priority because it is directly connected to the presence of ecchymoses (Choice A). The hemoglobin level (Choice B), white blood cell count (Choice C), and INR (Choice D) can be reviewed after the platelet level has been observed.

**NCLEX Examination Challenge #3**

Answer: D

Rationale: Erythematous refers to redness of the skin; diffuse is widespread over most of the body; and pruritic refers to itching (Choice D). Although the rash is red, macular implies that the rash is flat when it is actually raised; also, the rash is over most of the body, so it is not lichenified, which implies that it is leathery in nature (Choice A). A cyanotic appearance would be blue; the rash is not ringlike so it cannot be described as annular; it is also not circular, so it cannot be described as circinate (Choice B). Linear implies that the rash occurs in a straight line, which is not true because it is over most of the body; universal means that the entire body is involved, which is inaccurate because only most of the body is affected; nummular means coinlike, which is inaccurate, as the shape of the lesions are not identified as round (Choice C).

## Chapter 21

**Answer Key**

*Pathophysiology Review*

#1.

1. H
2. C
3. J
4. D
5. A
6. I
7. B
8. E
9. G
10. F

#2.

| Lesion Type | Flat or Raised? | Description | Primary Location |
|---|---|---|---|
| Actinic (solar) keratosis (premalignant) | Flat or raised | Macule or papule Indurated | Cheeks Ears Forearms Forehead Hands – back |
| Squamous cell carcinoma | Raised | Crust Indurated Nodule | Burns Head Lip Neck Scars |
| Basal cell carcinoma | Raised | Central crater Papule Pigmented (flecks) | Head Neck |
| Melanoma | Raised | Indurated Papule or plaque Pigmented | Back – upper Feet – soles Hands – palms Legs – lower Nevi (nearby) |

#3.

| Test | Normal Ranges (SI Units) | Significance of Changes From Normal |
|---|---|---|
| **Blood studies** | | |
| Hemoglobin, total | *Females:* 12–16 g/dL (7.4–9.9 mmol/L)<br>*Males:* 14–18 g/dL (8.7–11.2 mmol/L) | Elevated because of fluid volume loss |
| Hematocrit | *Females:* 37%–47% (0.37–0.47 volume fraction)<br>*Males:* 40%–52% (0.40–0.52 volume fraction) | Elevated because of fluid volume loss |
| Urea nitrogen | *Adult:* 10–20 mg/dL or 3.6–7.1 mmol/L (SI units)<br>*Older adult:* May be slightly higher than adult | Elevated because of fluid volume loss |
| Glucose | *Adult:* 74–106 mg/dL or 4.1–5.9 mmol/L<br>*Older adult aged 60-90 years:* 82–115 mg/dL or 4.6–6.4 mmol/L<br>*Older adult aged >90 years:* 75–121 mg/dL or 4.2–6.7 mmol/L | Elevated because of the stress response and altered uptake across injured tissues |
| **Electrolytes** | | |
| Sodium | *Adult and older adults:* 136–145 mEq/L or 136–145 mmol/L (SI units) | Decreased because of sodium being trapped in edema fluid and lost through plasma leakage |
| Potassium | *Adult and older adults:* 3.5–5.0 mEq/L or 3.5–5.0 mmol/L (SI units) | Elevated because of disruption of the sodium-potassium pump, tissue destruction, and red blood cell hemolysis |
| Chloride | *Adult and older adults:* 98–106 mEq/L or 98–106 mmol/L (SI units) | Elevated because of fluid volume loss and reabsorption of chloride in urine |
| **Arterial blood gases** | | |
| $Po_2$ | 80–100 mm Hg<br>*Older adults:* values may be lower | Slightly decreased or decreased from respiratory injury |
| $Pco_2$ | 35–45 mm Hg | Slightly increased from respiratory injury |
| pH | 7.35–7.45 | Low as a result of metabolic acidosis |

| Test | Normal Ranges (SI Units) | Significance of Changes From Normal |
|---|---|---|
| Carboxyhemoglobin (COHb, carbon monoxide) | Saturation of hemoglobin<br>Nonsmoker: <3%<br>Smoker: 12% | Elevated because of inhalation of smoke and carbon monoxide |
| **Other** | | |
| Total protein | *Adult/older adult:*<br>6.4–8.3 g/dL or 64–83 g/L (SI units) | Low because protein exudate is lost through wounds |
| Albumin | 3.5–5 g/dL or 35–50 g/L (SI units) | Low because protein is lost through the wound and vascular membranes from increased permeability |

## Activities

### Activity #1

1. T
2. T
3. F
4. T
5. T
6. F
7. F
8. F
9. F
10. T

### Activity #2

| | Finding | Local Indicator | Systemic Indicator |
|---|---|---|---|
| 1 | Excessive burn wound drainage | X | |
| 2 | Oliguria | | X |
| 3 | Hypoxemia | | X |
| 4 | Graft sloughing | X | |
| 5 | Wound odor | X | |
| 6 | Heart rate 122 beats/min | | X |
| 7 | Crusting of granulation tissue | X | |
| 8 | Edema arising around burn wound | X | |
| 9 | Glucose 362 mg/dL | | X |
| 10 | Body temperature instability | | X |
| 11 | Eruption of vesicular lesions in healed skin | X | |

| | Finding | Local Indicator | Systemic Indicator |
|---|---|---|---|
| 12 | Blood pressure 90/60 mm Hg | | X |
| 13 | Change in level of consciousness | | X |
| 14 | Ulceration of skin surrounding burn site | X | |
| 15 | Respiratory rate 32 breaths/min | | X |

## Activity #3

Expected findings that the nurse would anticipate in a client with <u>no</u>, <u>mild</u>, <u>moderate</u>, or <u>severe</u> carbon monoxide poisoning include:

| Carbon Monoxide Level | Physiologic Effects |
|---|---|
| 1%–10% (normal) | Increased threshold to visual stimuli<br>Increased blood flow to vital organs |
| 11%–20% (mild poisoning) | Headache<br>Decreased cerebral function<br>Decreased visual acuity<br>Slight breathlessness |
| 21%–40% (moderate poisoning) | Headache<br>Tinnitus<br>Nausea<br>Drowsiness<br>Vertigo<br>Altered mental state<br>Confusion<br>Stupor<br>Irritability<br>Decreased blood pressure, increased and irregular heart rate<br>Depressed ST segment on ECG and dysrhythmias<br>Pale to reddish-purple skin |
| 41%–60% (severe poisoning) | Coma<br>Convulsions<br>Cardiopulmonary instability |

## Activity #4

| Burn Description | Burn Depth |
|---|---|
| 1. Extends to dermis<br>2. Moderate edema<br>3. Pain rated at 8 on 0-10 scale<br>4. No eschar | Superficial second degree |
| 1. Extends to tendon<br>2. Black in color<br>3. No blistering<br>4. Eschar present | Fourth degree |

| Burn Description | Burn Depth |
|---|---|
| 1. Yellow in color<br>2. Severe edema<br>3. No pain<br>4. Inelastic eschar | Third degree |
| 1. Dry appearance<br>2. No edema<br>3. Pain rated 4 on 0-10 scale<br>4. New epidermis noted | Superficial first degree |
| 1. Extends into dermis<br>2. Moderate edema<br>3. No blistering<br>4. Soft eschar | Deep second degree |

**Activity #5**

Characteristics of each type of pressure injury can include any of these descriptions:

Stage 1—nonblanchable erythema of intact skin usually over bony prominences
- Color (not purple or maroon)
  - Light skin: nonblanchable redness
  - Dark skin: may not have visible blanching; color of pressure injury site will differ from surrounding tissue
- May be preceded by changes in sensation, temperature, or firmness

Stage 2—partial-thickness loss with exposed dermis
- Color:
  - Light skin: wound bed is viable, pink or red, and moist
  - Dark skin: wound bed may be red or pink without slough, or area may be shiny without slough or bruising
- May look like intact or ruptured serum-filled blister
- Adipose (fat), granulation tissue, slough, and eschar are not visible

Stage 3—full-thickness skin loss
- Adipose (fat) visible in the ulcer
- Granulation tissue and rolled wound edges are often present
- Slough and/or eschar may be present
- Undermining and tunneling may be present
- Fascia, muscle, tendon, ligament, cartilage, or bone are not exposed

Stage 4—full-thickness loss of skin and tissue
- Full-thickness skin loss with exposed or palpable fascia, muscle, tendon, ligament, cartilage, or bone
- May have slough or eschar
- Rolled edges, undermining, or tunneling are often present

Unstageable—obscured full-thickness skin and tissue loss
- Full-thickness skin and tissue loss
- Extent of damage cannot be confirmed because of being obscured by eschar or slough

Deep-tissue pressure injury—persistent nonblanchable deep red, maroon, or purple discoloration
- Intact or nonintact skin
- Localized area of persistent nonblanchable deep red, maroon, or purple discoloration (discoloration may appear differently in skin with dark pigmentation)
- Epidermal separation reveals a dark wound bed or blood-filled blister

## Learning Assessments

### NCLEX Examination Challenge #1

<u>Answer</u>: A, C, D, E

<u>Rationale</u>: Factors that increase the risk for development of pressure injuries include lack of mobility (Choice A), malnourishment (Choice C), sitting for long periods of time (Choice C), obesity (Choice D), and aging skin (Choice E). Clients with cognitive decline or impairment are at risk if they are unable to fully participate in care (Choice E). The client who is ambulatory with *occasional* urinary incontinence is not at increased risk (Choice B). Exposure of skin to *ongoing* and *excessive* moisture (e.g., chronic urinary or fecal incontinence) increases the risk for development of pressure injuries.

### NCLEX Examination Challenge #2

<u>Answer</u>: A, C, D, E

<u>Rationale</u>: With a suspected inhalation injury, the nurse assesses the mouth, throat, and nose. The nurse listens for coughing (Choice A), shortness of breath (Choice C), or hoarseness of the voice (Choice D), which may indicate smoke inhalation. Another sign of inhalation injury includes singed nasal hairs (Choice E). Cherry red skin is a sign of carbon monoxide poisoning, not inhalation injury (Choice B).

### NCLEX Examination Challenge #3

<u>Answer</u>: A, B, D

<u>Rationale</u>: The nurse will teach the adult client to avoid sun exposure when the sun is at its brightest point (Choice A) because this is when burning is most likely. The nurse will also teach to wear a hat and sunglasses (Choice B) for protection. It is important for the nurse to teach to take pictures of lesions and compare them monthly for changes (Choice D) because early intervention is important if skin changes are noted. Tanning beds should be completely avoided (Choice C), not used in moderation. Sunscreen should be used all of the time when someone is outside (Choice E), not just when outside in the sun for more than an hour.

## NGN Challenge #1

The nurse documents assessment findings for a 32-year-old client brought to the ED with multiple first- and second-degree burns.

| Health History | Nurses Notes | Vital Signs | Laboratory Results |
|---|---|---|---|

**1644:** Brought to emergency department by squad after experiencing first- and second-degree burns. Client was at work when a fire broke out; client returned to primary work station to obtain sketches of a building that was being worked on and was burned in the process when attempting to escape. Client has obesity. Other health history unremarkable. Multiple first- and second-degree burns noted on arms. Height: 74 in (188 cm); weight: 298 lb (135.2 kg). VS: T 99.0°F (37.2°C); HR 110 beats/min/ RR 22 breaths/min; BP 180/98 mm Hg. SpO$_2$ 96% on RA. Reports pain of 4 on 0 to 10 scale.

**Highlight the client findings in the note that are abnormal.**
Rationale: The client is noted to have first- and second-degree burns on the arms after reentering a burning building. The client's weight reflects obesity, and the heart rate, respiratory rate, and blood pressure are all high.

Answer:
The client is at high risk for **infection** as evidenced by **18% TBSA burned**.
Rationale: The client is at risk for infection because of the percentage of total body surface area burned. This is a large area, and microorganisms could easily invade and cause infection. At this time, there is no evidence for shock, hyperosmolar hyperglycemia state, or fluid volume deficit. Although the respiratory rate, blood pressure, and temperature are all somewhat elevated, they are not critical and are most likely the result of the fight or flight response that was activated when the client experienced the fire.

Answer:
The *priority* for the client at this time is to manage **open wounds** to prevent **infection**.
Rationale: At this time, the client is not in crisis. Therefore, the nurse will prioritize management of the open wounds to prevent infection. There is no indication that the client will spike a fever, nor is there evidence of a fluid balance problem. Disfigurement is not a priority; keeping the client free from infection is more important.

Answer:
A. Gauze
B. Foam sheets
C. Cotton 4 × 4s
D. Normal saline
E. Sterile maggots
F. Hydrogel sheets
G. Alginate dressing
H. Sharp instrument for débridement
I. 3M Tegaderm superabsorbent dressing

Rationale: The nurse will gather gauze, cotton 4 × 4s, and normal saline to bring into the client's room. These items will be used to cleanse and gently dress the first- and second-degree burns. There is no need for foam sheets, hydrogel sheets, alginate dressings, or 3M Tegaderm dressings; these are used primarily in the treatment of pressure injuries. There is no need for débridement based on the information received; therefore, a sharp instrument for débridement nor sterile maggots are needed.

Answer:
A.  Change dressings at least twice daily.
B.  Use acetaminophen or ibuprofen to manage pain.
C.  Apply ice packs directly to the skin to cool the wounds.
D.  Take antiviral medication to minimize the chance for infection.
E.  Clean wounds with normal saline each time dressings are changed.
F.  An over-the-counter topical triple antibiotic can be used on the burns.
G.  If any purulent or odorous drainage arises, report this to the health care provider.

Rationale: It is important to teach the client to change dressings at least twice daily and to clean the wounds with normal saline on each dressing change because this minimizes the chance for infection. An OTC triple antibiotic can be used also to minimize the chance for infection. Purulent or odorous drainage could indicate infection, so this needs to be reported to the health care provider. Acetaminophen or ibuprofen is generally enough to manage pain for these types of wounds. Ice packs should be placed over a washcloth or towel; never directly on the skin because this can impair tissue integrity. Antiviral medications will not reduce the chance for infection.

Answer:

| Previous Client Finding | Current Client Finding | Effective | Not Effective |
|---|---|---|---|
| Multiple first- and second-degree burns noted | Several first-degree burns appear to be healed over | X | |
| Multiple first- and second-degree burns noted | Greenish-yellow drainage is noted from two second-degree burns | | X |
| Reported pain of 4 on 0 to 10 scale | Reports that pain is 2 on 0 to 10 scale and some areas are "itchy" | X | |
| Temperature = 99.0°F (37.2°C) | Temperature = 101.0°F (38.3°C) | | X |

Rationale: Interventions have been effective when the nurse assesses that several first-degree burns are healed, and the client reports that pain is decreased to 2 on a 0 to 10 scale. It is normal for healing wounds to somewhat itch. Interventions were not effective when greenish-yellow drainage is noted from two second-degree burns, and there is a 2-degree increase in temperature because this is likely indicative of infection.

**Chapter 22**
**Answer Key**
*Chapter Review*
**Anatomy & Physiology Review**
#1.

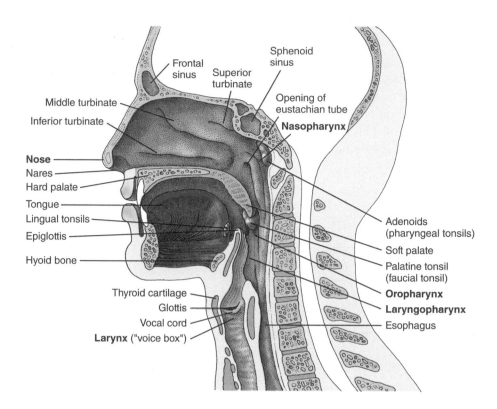

Frontal sinus
Superior turbinate
Sphenoid sinus
Middle turbinate
Inferior turbinate
Opening of eustachian tube
**Nasopharynx**
**Nose**
Nares
Hard palate
Tongue
Lingual tonsils
Epiglottis
Hyoid bone
Adenoids (pharyngeal tonsils)
Soft palate
Palatine tonsil (faucial tonsil)
**Oropharynx**
Thyroid cartilage
**Laryngopharynx**
Glottis
Vocal cord
Esophagus
**Larynx** ("voice box")

#2.
1. Fremitus
2. Hemoptysis
3. Surfactant
4. Crepitus
5. Thoracentesis
6. Pack-years
7. Bronchoscopy
8. Orthopnea

## Activities

### Activity #1

Answers should resemble these characteristics of adventitious lung sounds:

| Adventitious Sound | Characteristics |
|---|---|
| Fine rales | Popping, discontinuous sounds caused by air moving into previously deflated airways; sounds like hair being rolled between fingers near the ear<br>"Velcro" sounds late in inspiration usually associated with restrictive disorders |
| Coarse crackles | Lower-pitched, coarse, rattling sounds caused by fluid or secretions in large airways; likely to change with coughing or suctioning |
| Rhonchi | Lower-pitched, coarse, continuous snoring sounds<br>Arise from the large airways |
| Pleural friction rub | Loud, rough, grating, scratching sounds caused by the inflamed surfaces of the pleura rubbing together; often associated with pain on deep inspirations<br>Heard in lateral lung fields |

### Activity #2

1. wheezes (or wheezing)
2. 60
3. calcium
4. thyroid cartilage
5. Any of these items can be used: cigarettes, cigars, pipes, hookah pipes, water-pipes, electronic cigarettes, vape pens, e-cigarettes.

### Activity #3

1. F
2. T
3. F
4. T
5. T
6. F
7. F
8. F
9. T
10. T

### Activity #4

Answers should resemble these age-related changes:

- Alveolar surface area decreases.
- Diffusion capacity decreases.
- Elastic recoil decreases.
- Bronchioles and alveolar ducts dilate.
- Ability to cough decreases.
- Airways close early.
- Residual volume increases.
- Vital capacity decreases.
- Efficiency of oxygen and carbon dioxide exchange decreases.
- Elasticity decreases.
- Muscles atrophy.
- Vocal cords become slack.
- Laryngeal muscles lose elasticity and airways lose cartilage.
- Vascular resistance to blood flow through pulmonary vascular system increases.
- Pulmonary capillary blood volume decreases.
- Risk for hypoxia increases.
- Body's response to hypoxia and hypercarbia decreases.
- Respiratory muscle strength, especially the diaphragm and the intercostals, decreases.
- Effectiveness of the cilia decreases.
- Immunoglobulin A decreases.
- Alveolar macrophages are altered.
- Anteroposterior diameter increases.
- Thorax becomes shorter.
- Progressive kyphoscoliosis occurs.
- Chest wall compliance (elasticity) decreases.
- Mobility of chest wall may decrease.
- Osteoporosis is possible, leading to chest wall abnormalities.

**Activity #5**

Answers regarding nursing interventions should resemble these listed. The specific nursing interventions are located next to the changes that they address.

| Change | Nursing Interventions |
|---|---|
| Alveolar surface area decreases. Diffusion capacity decreases. Elastic recoil decreases. Bronchioles and alveolar ducts dilate. Ability to cough decreases. Airways close early. | Encourage vigorous pulmonary hygiene (i.e., encourage patient to turn, cough, and deep breathe) and use of incentive spirometry, especially if they are confined to bed or have had surgery to reduce the risk for infectious respiratory or mechanical complications. Encourage upright position to minimize ventilation-perfusion mismatching. |
| Residual volume increases. Vital capacity decreases. Efficiency of oxygen and carbon dioxide exchange decreases. Elasticity decreases. | Include inspection, palpation, percussion, and auscultation in lung assessments to detect normal age-related changes. Help patient actively maintain health and fitness to keep losses in respiratory functioning to a minimum. Assess patient's respirations for abnormal breathing patterns, such as Cheyne-Stokes, which can occur in older adults without pathology. Encourage frequent oral hygiene to aid in the removal of secretions. |
| Muscles atrophy. Vocal cords become slack. Laryngeal muscles lose elasticity, and airways lose cartilage. | Have face-to-face conversations with patient when possible because the patient's voice may be soft and difficult to understand. |
| Vascular resistance to blood flow through pulmonary vascular system increases. Pulmonary capillary blood volume decreases. Risk for hypoxia increases. | Assess patient's level of consciousness and cognition because hypoxia from acute respiratory conditions can cause confusion. |
| Body's response to hypoxia and hypercarbia decreases. | Assess for subtle manifestations of hypoxia to prevent complications. |
| Respiratory muscle strength, especially the diaphragm and the intercostals, decreases. | Encourage pulmonary hygiene and help patient actively maintain health and fitness to promote maximal functioning of the respiratory system and prevent respiratory illnesses. |
| Effectiveness of the cilia decreases. Immunoglobulin A decreases. Alveolar macrophages are altered. | Encourage pulmonary hygiene and help patient actively maintain health and fitness to promote maximal functioning of the respiratory system and prevent respiratory illnesses. |
| Anteroposterior diameter increases. Thorax becomes shorter. Progressive kyphoscoliosis occurs. Chest wall compliance (elasticity) decreases. Mobility of chest wall may decrease. | Discuss the normal changes of aging to help reduce anxiety about changes that occur. Discuss the need for increased rest periods during exercise because exercise tolerance decreases with age. |
| Osteoporosis is possible, leading to chest wall abnormalities. | Encourage adequate calcium intake to help prevent or reduce later osteoporosis. |

## Learning Assessments

### NCLEX Examination Challenge #1

Answer: A, C

Rationale: The nurse will intervene to provide further education when the client thinks they will not have lung problems because of occasional smoking (Choice A). Even infrequent smoking can damage lung tissue. The nurse will also provide further education about vaping being just as dangerous as smoking cigarettes (Choice C); serious lung injuries have occurred in people who have vaped less than 2 years. Recognizing that cigarette smoking can cause lung and heart problems (Choice B), admitting to having a problem with smoking (Choice D), and deciding to refrain from using a hookah (Choice E) all show that the client understood the nurse's teaching.

### NCLEX Examination Challenge #2

Answer: A

Rationale: Varenicline interferes with nicotine receptors, so the pleasure derived from smoking is reduced while taking this drug (Choice A). Varenicline does not reduce cravings like bupropion (Choice B); it does not cause the taste of smoking to make the client ill (Choice C); and it is not a chewable drug that releases nicotine (Choice D).

### NCLEX Examination Challenge #3

Answer: B, E

Rationale: Pursed-lip breathing is abnormal and generally used only by clients who have obstructive disease with air trapping; this finding needs to be reported to the health care provider (Choice B). Rough scratching sounds heard over the right lower lobe are an abnormal sound known as a pleural friction rub; this must be reported to the health care provider (Choice E). The trachea should be midline and slightly moveable (Choice A). No breath sounds are heard below the diaphragm because the lungs are located above the diaphragm (Choice C). A flat percussive sound is expected in the upper center of the chest because the sternum is located there (Choice D). These findings do not need to be reported to the health care provider.

## Chapter 23

### Answer Key

#### *Chapter Review*

#### Pathophysiology Review

#1  Any four of these warning signs of head and neck cancer:
- Throat pain
- Lump in the mouth, throat, or neck
- Difficulty swallowing
- Color changes in the mouth or tongue to red, white, gray, dark brown, or black
- Oral lesion or sore that does not heal in 2 weeks
- Persistent or unexplained oral bleeding
- Numbness of the mouth, lips, or face
- Change in the fit of dentures
- Burning sensation when drinking citrus juices or hot liquids
- Persistent, unilateral ear pain
- Hoarseness or change in voice quality
- Persistent or recurrent sore throat
- Shortness of breath
- Anorexia and weight loss

#2
1. T
2. T
3. F
4. T
5. T
6. F
7. T

## Activities

### Activity #1

Any four of these risk factors for head and neck cancer that the nurse would include in health teaching:

- Tobacco use
- Alcohol use
- Voice abuse
- Chronic laryngitis
- Exposure to chemicals or dusts
- Poor oral hygiene
- Long-term gastroesophageal reflux disease (GERD)
- Oral infection with HPV

### Activity #2

1. T
2. T
3. T
4. T
5. T
6. F
7. T
8. F
9. T
10. T

### Activity #3

Any three of these actions the nurse would implement as part of emergency care for a client who has an anterior nosebleed:

- Maintain Standard Precautions or Body Substance Precautions.
- Position the patient upright and leaning forward to prevent blood from entering the larynx and possible aspiration.
- Reassure the patient and attempt to keep the patient quiet to reduce anxiety and blood pressure.
- Apply direct lateral pressure to the nose for 15-20 minutes, and apply ice or cool compresses to the nose and face if possible.
- If nasal packing is necessary, loosely pack both nares with gauze or nasal tampons.
- To prevent rebleeding from dislodging clots, instruct the patient to not blow the nose for 24 hours after the bleeding stops.
- Instruct the patient to seek medical assistance if these measures are ineffective or if the bleeding occurs frequently.

### Activity #4

Any three discharge teaching points the nurse would include about home laryngectomy care:

- Avoid swimming and use care when showering or shaving.
- Lean slightly forward and cover the stoma when coughing or sneezing.
- Wear a stoma guard or loose clothing to cover the stoma.
- Clean the stoma with mild soap and water. Lubricate the stoma with a non–oil-based ointment as needed.
- Increase humidity by using a bedside humidifier, houseplants, and using saline in the stoma as instructed.
- Obtain and wear a MedicAlert bracelet and emergency care card for life-threatening situations.

## Learning Assessments

### NCLEX Examination Challenge #1

Answer: A

Rationale: All of these expected outcomes are appropriate for the client who has reconstructive surgery for OSAS. However, the priority outcome is for the client to maintain a patent airway (Choice A). If this outcome is not met, the client would be in a potentially life-threatening situation, which would not be true if other outcomes are not met (Choices B, C, and D).

### NCLEX Examination Challenge #2

Answer: D

Rationale: All of these statements would be part of discharge teaching for the client who has an IMF for a fractured jaw. However, Choice D is essential to avoid aspiration, which causes pneumonia and could result in death. The other choices do not involve potential life-threatening situations (Choices A, B, and C).

### NCLEX Examination Challenge #3

Answer: A, B, C, E

Rationale: All of these health teaching statements are important to protect the skin that is radiated except for Choice D. Although the skin usually becomes reddened and peels, the dead skin should not be removed to prevent infection. The skin is the primary barrier to prevent infection in the body.

### NGN Challenge #1

Answer:

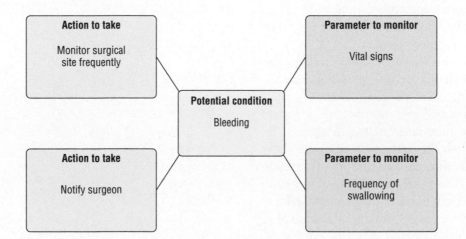

Rationale: The oropharynx is very vascular and has been traumatized by the reconstructive surgery. Therefore, bleeding is a common postoperative complication. The client has tachycardia and is swallowing frequently either from oral secretions or blood. The client is not hypoxic and does have a partial airway obstruction as evidenced by a normal $SpO_2$, normal RR, and no stridor or adventitious breath sounds. The client is also oriented. There is no foul odor from the surgical drainage or fever, suggesting that the client likely does not have an infection. If bleeding is suspected, the nurse would notify the surgeon to examine the client and monitor the surgical site frequently for signs of new bleeding. The nurse would also administer analgesia, but this action does not address the client's major potential problem. There is no need at this point to increase oxygen flow rate or administer antibiotics. To assess for effectiveness of nursing and collaborative actions, the nurse would monitor vital signs, especially the HR and blood pressure, to determine the extent of bleeding. In the presence of bleeding, the client would likely continue to frequently swallow and possibly have belching. Other parameters would be monitored for additional potential postoperative complications, but they would not be useful in assessing postoperative bleeding.

## Chapter 24
### Answer Key
#### *Chapter Review*
**Pathophysiology Review**

#1
1. D
2. F
3. H
4. A
5. G
6. C
7. I
8. E
9. B

#2
1. T
2. T
3. T
4. F
5. T
6. F
7. T
8. F
9. T
10. T

## Activities

### Activity #1
Any three of these nursing considerations when caring for older adults who have a respiratory condition:
- Provide rest periods between activities such as bathing, meals, and ambulation.
- Have the patient sit in an upright position for meals to prevent aspiration.
- Encourage nutritional fluid intake after a meal to prevent an early sensation of fullness and promote increased calorie intake.
- Schedule medications around routine activities to increase adherence to drug therapy.
- Arrange chairs in strategic locations to allow the patient with dyspnea to stop and rest while walking.
- Urge the patient to notify the primary health care provider promptly for any symptoms of infection.
- Encourage the patient to receive the pneumococcal vaccines and to have an annual influenza vaccination.
- For patients who are prescribed home oxygen, instruct them to keep tubing coiled when walking to reduce the risk for tripping.

### Activity #2
1. T
2. T
3. T
4. F
5. T
6. T
7. T
8. T
9. T
10. F

### Activity #3
1. L
2. G
3. D
4. J
5. K
6. C
7. H
8. F
9. A
10. I
11. B
12. E

## Activity #4
Any four of these home health considerations for clients who have COPD:
Assess respiratory status and adequacy of gas exchange:
- Measure rate, depth, and rhythm of respirations.
- Examine mucous membranes and nail beds for evidence of hypoxia.
- Determine use of accessory muscles.
- Examine chest and abdomen for paradoxical breathing.
- Count number of words patient can speak between breaths.
- Determine need and use of supplemental oxygen. (Identify how many liters per minute the patient is using.)
- Determine level of consciousness and presence/absence of confusion.
- Auscultate lungs for abnormal breath sounds.
- Measure oxygen saturation by pulse oximetry.
- Determine sputum production, color, and amount.
- Ask about activity level.
- Observe general hygiene.
- Measure body temperature.

Assess cardiac status for adequate perfusion:
- Measure rate, quality, and rhythm of pulse.
- Check dependent areas for edema.
- Check neck veins for distention with the patient in a sitting position.
- Measure capillary refill.

Assess nutrition status:
- Check weight maintenance, loss, or gain.
- Determine food and fluid intake.
- Determine use of nutritional supplements.
- Observe general condition of the skin.

Assess the patient's and caregiver's understanding of disease and adherence to management, including:
- Correct use of supplemental oxygen
- Correct technique and dosing schedule for use of inhalers
- Symptoms to report to the primary health care provider indicating the need for acute care
- Increasing severity of resting dyspnea
- Increasing severity of usual symptoms
- Development of new symptoms associated with poor gas exchange
- Respiratory infection
- Failure to obtain the usual degree of relief with prescribed therapies
- Use of pursed-lip and diaphragmatic breathing techniques
- Scheduling of rest periods and priority activities
- Participation in pulmonary rehabilitation activities

## Activity #5
1. barrel
2. pulmonary function tests
3. control
4. metered-dose inhalers
5. protein, calories
6. pneumonia
7. lower than
8. thoracentesis

## Learning Assessments

### NCLEX Examination Challenge #1
Answer: A
Rationale: All of these expected outcomes are appropriate for the client who has reconstructive surgery for OSAS. However, the priority outcome is for the client to maintain a patent airway (Choice A). If this outcome is not met, the client would be in a potentially life-threatening situation, which would not be true if other outcomes are not met (Choices B, C, and D).

### NCLEX Examination Challenge #2
Answer: D
Rationale: All of these statements would be part of discharge teaching for the client who has an IMF for a fractured jaw. However, Choice D is essential to avoid aspiration, which causes pneumonia and could result in death. The other choices do not involve potential life-threatening situations (Choices A, B, and C).

**NCLEX Examination Challenge #3**
Answer: A, B, C, E
Rationale: All of these health teaching statements are important to protect the skin that is radiated except for Choice D. Although the skin usually becomes reddened and peels, the dead skin should not be removed to prevent infection. The skin is the primary barrier to prevent infection in the body.

**NGN Challenge #1**
Answer:

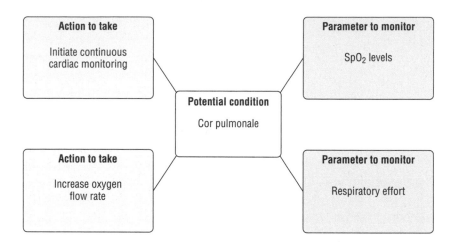

| Action to take | | Parameter to monitor |
|---|---|---|
| Initiate continuous cardiac monitoring | | SpO$_2$ levels |
| | **Potential condition**<br>Cor pulmonale | |
| **Action to take** | | **Parameter to monitor** |
| Increase oxygen flow rate | | Respiratory effort |

Rationale: The client has long-term, advanced COPD with symptoms that reflect heart failure, such as jugular distention, bilateral pedal edema, cyanosis, and a bounding, irregular HR. In addition, the client's SpO$_2$ is well below the normal of 95% even with supplemental oxygen of 3 L/min. Clients who have heart failure resulting from chronic lung disease is right-sided failure known as cor pulmonale. The client's symptoms arc not associated with respiratory failure, such as fatigue of respiratory muscles, unresponsive hypoxemia, and respiratory acidosis or pulmonary arterial hypertension in which some clients experience chest pain with dyspnea and fatigue. The client does not have a moist chronic cough, which is very common in clients who have chronic bronchitis. Because the client has right-sided heart failure and an irregular heart rate, the nurse would place the client on continuous cardiac monitoring. The nurse would also increase the client's oxygen rate from 3 L to 4 L/min because of a low SpO$_2$. At this point, the client does not have the symptoms of respiratory failure and, therefore, does not require intubation. There is no indication that antibiotic therapy or an analgesic mediation is needed. The nurse would monitor the SpO$_2$ for improvement. The goal for this client is an SpO$_2$ of between 88% and 92%. Although this goal is below the typical normal range, it is an appropriate range for a client with advanced COPD. The nurse would also monitor respiratory rate and effort for improvement or worsening.

**NGN Challenge #2**
Answer: The nurse determines that the client is experiencing **respiratory acidosis** as evidenced by **low arterial pH** and **high carbon dioxide level**.
Rationale: The client has acidosis because the arterial pH is below the minimum of 7.35 normal pH. In respiratory acidosis, the client's low pH is due to an increase in carbon dioxide (hypercarbia). This client has an elevated PaCO$_2$ level. To help compensate for the low pH, the kidneys retain increased amounts of bicarbonate (base) to increase the arterial pH. This client's bicarbonate level is above normal. If the client had metabolic acidosis, the cause would be a low bicarbonate level, which is not the case. The client does not have hypocarbia, which is a low level of carbon dioxide. If the client had respiratory failure, the client would have severe hypoxemia. A PaO$_2$ of 69 mm Hg is not uncommon for a client with long-term COPD, and is, therefore, not considered severe hypoxemia.

## Chapter 25
### Answer Key
*Chapter Review*
**Pathophysiology Review**

#1

1. G
2. D
3. J
4. E
5. H
6. A
7. I
8. C
9. F
10. B

#2

1. F
2. T
3. T
4. T
5. T
6. T
7. F
8. T
9. T
10. F

## Activities

### Activity #1
Any four of these activities or lifestyle habits that nurses would include in health teaching about how to prevent respiratory infection in the community:

- Wash hands frequently or use sanitizer.
- If sick, stay home from work, school, or crowded places.
- Use proper cough/sneeze etiquette.
- Avoid close contact with other people if sick.
- Obtain recommended respiratory infection vaccines, including influenza, pneumonia, and COVID-19.
- Obtain annual screenings for tuberculosis if high risk.
- Maintain adequate immunity by practicing healthy habits, such as eating a well-balanced diet, getting adequate rest and sleep, effectively coping with stress, and engaging in regular exercise.

### Activity #2
1. F
2. T
3. T
4. T
5. T
6. T
7. T
8. T
9. T
10. T

### Activity #3
1. B
2. C
3. A
4. B
5. C
6. B
7. A
8. B

### Activity #4
Any four nursing interventions that can help prevent transmission of COVID-19 in an inpatient setting (for patient and staff safety):

1. Don standard PPE for patients with suspected or confirmed COVID-19, which includes:
   - Gown
   - Gloves
   - Respirator: N95 or equivalent
   - Eye protection: Goggles or face shield; eyeglasses are not sufficient.
2. While inside the patient's room by the door or in anteroom:
   - Remove gloves using a gloved hand to remove the first glove, then slide your fingers of the ungloved hand under the remaining glove to remove the glove without touching the exterior of the glove. Discard the gloves in a waste container.

- Remove the gown by touching the inside of the gown only and rolling the gown inside out and away from your body. Discard in a waste container.
- You may now exit the patient's room.
- Remove the goggles or the face shield by touching the headband or earpieces. If reusable, place in container for processing.

- Remove the respirator. Do not remove the respirator until you are outside the room. Follow agency policy on reuse or extended use of the respirator. Remember, the outside of the respirator is contaminated. If you touch the outside of the respirator, you must wash your hands immediately with soap and water.
- Wash your hands immediately.

*If hands become contaminated between steps, stop and perform hand hygiene.

## Learning Assessments

### NCLEX Examination Challenge #1
Answer: A, B, C, D
Rationale: All of these comorbidities except for E are risk factors that predispose individuals to severe COVID-19, usually leading to hospitalization and possibly intubation and mechanical ventilation (Choices A, B, C, D). Individuals who are aged 65 years or older are most at risk but not those younger than 60 years of age (Choice E).

### NCLEX Examination Challenge #2
Answer: B, C, E, F
Rationale: All of these choices for PPE care are appropriate but only gowns, gloves, N95 mask, and eyewear are essential to protect health care workers from becoming infected when caring for clients who have COVID-19 (Choices B, C, E, F). Shoe and hair coverings are optional but are used in some settings (Choices A and D).

### NCLEX Examination Challenge #3
Answer: C
Rationale: The client who does not adhere to prescribed drug therapy for TB still needs the medications to treat the infectious organism. The best way to ensure adherence is directly observed therapy such that the client must take the drugs with a health care professional present (Choice C). A change of drugs would likely not increase adherence, and admission to acute care is not realistic for a drug regimen that must continue for months (Choices A and B). Determining why the client is not adherent does not ensure that the client will continue taking the medications (Choice D).

**NGN Challenge #1**

<u>Answer:</u>

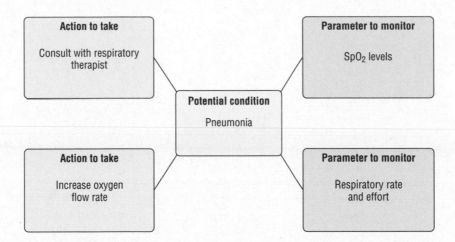

<u>Rationale:</u> The client experienced new symptoms today of chest pain and increased dyspnea with cough. These changes added to 2 days of anorexia, fatigue, and acute confusion suggests that the client may have pneumonia. Additionally, the client has not been vaccinated for any of the common respiratory infections, including pneumonia, making the client susceptible to this condition. Fever is not common in older adults who have pneumonia, but hypoxemia usually occurs. This client would be expected to have a low peripheral oxygen saturation level, but the recommended range for a client who has COPD is between 88% and 92%. The client has not had symptoms over a long period, does not have a chronic cough, and has not had anorexia for more than 2 days, indicating that the client likely does not have tuberculosis. A chronic moist cough is also a major symptom of chronic bronchitis. The client who has COVID-19 usually has a variety of symptoms including fever, chills, and other flu-like symptoms. Many clients also lose their sense of smell and/or taste. A rapid test could rule out this infection rather quickly.

The nurse would increase the client's oxygen to increase the $SpO_2$ and consult a respiratory therapist to determine the best treatment to improve breathing. It is not known whether the client has a more localized pneumonia with consolidation versus a more diffuse infection, but an x-ray would likely verify the pathology. To determine if these interventions are effective, the nurse would continue to monitor the $SpO_2$, RR, and dyspnea level or respiratory effort. If the pneumonia is caused by a virus, antibiotic therapy would be ineffective. Cardiac monitoring is not indicated at this point, although the client has tachycardia, which is consistent with pneumonia, possibly resulting from dehydration. The client is not experiencing symptoms of impending or actual respiratory failure, so intubation is not indicated.

## NGN Challenge #2
Answer:

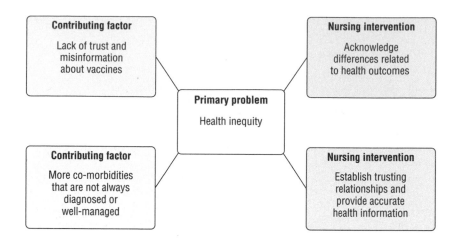

Rationale: As defined in Chapter 1 of the textbook, health equity is the ability to recognize differences in the resources and/or knowledge needed for individuals to fully participate in health care and achieve optimal outcomes. The clinical outcomes of clients who were hospitalized with COVID-19 during the pandemic were distinctly different when comparing White clients with other groups, especially Black/African American, Hispanic/Latino, American Indian, and Alaska native adults. The incidence of COVID-19 illness and rate of death was much greater for minority groups when compared with Whites. Research has since determined that social determinants of health and other factors contribute to this health inequity, even when health care quality is the same for all groups. One of these factors is the prevalence of chronic disease and other comorbidities, such as obesity and overweight, in people of color when compared with White clients. Lack of access to health care and mistrust further contribute to these factors. Misinformation about COVID-19 vaccines is very common and exacerbates mistrust of health care professionals. Nurses need to respect all clients and treat them with dignity and respect. Priority nursing interventions include acknowledging that health outcome differences exist and establishing trusting relationships before providing client education and correcting misinformation, especially about vaccines.

## Chapter 26
### Answer Key
*Pathophysiology Review*

#1.
1. G
2. D
3. J
4. L
5. B
6. K
7. F
8. I
9. A
10. E
11. H
12. C

#2.
1. T
2. T
3. T
4. F
5. T
6. F
7. T
8. T
9. T
10. T

## Activities

### Activity #1

Any four of these risk factors for the development of venous thromboembolism that can lead to pulmonary embolism:

- Prolonged immobility
- Central venous catheters
- Surgery within the past 3 months
- Pregnancy and within 3 months postpartum
- Obesity
- Advancing age
- General and genetic conditions that increase blood clotting
- History of thromboembolism
- COVID-19 infection
- Infection
- Smoking
- Estrogen therapy

### Activity #2

1. T
2. T
3. T
4. T
5. F
6. T
7. F
8. T
9. T
10. T

### Activity #3

1. greater than 4
2. protamine sulfate; vitamin K
3. respiratory acidosis
4. 60
5. 100% oxygen is given
6. tension pneumothorax
7. prone
8. ET
9. neuromuscular-blocking
10. end-tidal carbon dioxide
11. patent airway
12. pneumonia

### Activity #4

1. C
2. G
3. D
4. F
5. A
6. E
7. B

## Learning Assessments

### NCLEX Examination Challenge #1

Answer: A, C, D, E

Rationale: The client who has surgery is a high risk for venous thromboembolism. All of the choices for nursing actions are appropriate and essential except for Choice B. Pillows should not be placed under the client's knees because they may hinder venous blood flow. Additionally, placing pillows under the popliteal spaces would position the client's lower extremities below the level of the heart and reduce venous return. Ambulation and movement by exercising the extremities would increase blood flow to the lower extremities (Choices A and C). The legs should not be crossed to prevent inhibition of venous flow (Choice D). Legs should not be massaged because a clot could become dislodged and travel as an embolus to another organ, including the lungs (Choice E).

### NCLEX Examination Challenge #2

Answer: D

Rationale: The high-pressure alarm sounds when peak inspiratory pressure (PIP) reaches the set alarm limit (usually set 10–20 mm Hg above the client's baseline PIP). One of the major reasons why PIP increases is excessive secretions or mucous plugs, and, therefore, suctioning is needed to remove the cause (Choice D). It is not necessary at this time to call the Rapid Response Team (Choice A) or request a chest x-ray (Choice C). Tubing connections would be checked if the low-exhaled volume (low-pressure) alarm sounded (Choice D).

**NCLEX Examination Challenge #3**
Answer: A, B, C, E
Rationale: All of these laboratory abnormalities are common in clients who have severe COVID-19 infection with the exception of Choice D. The CPK level is usually increased, not decreased. Inflammatory markers and muscle enzymes are usually increased because COVID-19 can cause systemic inflammation.

**NGN Challenge**
*Item #1*
Answer: A, B, D, F, G, H
Rationale: The nurse would be most concerned about the client's COVID-19 lung involvement, which is evidenced by a fever, frequent cough, crackles, and worsening shortness of breath (Choices A, B, F, and H). The nurse would also be very concerned that the client has 50% of the lungs affected by infiltrates with a subsequent low $SpO_2$ level of 92% (normal range is 95% or greater) (Choices D and G). The client's history of hypertension and BMI over 24.9 are risk factors for COVID-19, but the client already tested positive for this infection. Therefore, these findings are not of concern at this time for the nurse (Choices C and E).

*Item #2*
Answer: Based on analysis of relevant client findings, the nurse determines that the client has **viral pneumonia** as a result of COVID-19 infection.
Rationale: The client has chest infiltrates, fever, crackles, shortness of breath, low $SpO_2$, and lung infiltrates, which support the client's condition of pneumonia resulting from the virus that causes COVID-19 infection. The client's cues do not support that the client has acute respiratory failure, acute respiratory distress syndrome, or pulmonary embolism at this time.

*Item #3*
Answer: The nurse's priority for the client's care would be to implement interventions to prevent **acute lung injury,** which could result from **inflammation** caused by COVID-19 pneumonia.
Rationale: COVID-19 and other types of pneumonia are causes of acute lung injury (ALI) because inflammation occurs as a pathologic response. If not responsive to treatment, ALI can lead to acute respiratory distress syndrome, which is a life-threatening complication. Therefore, the priority for care is to implement interventions that can possibly prevent this problem. There is no evidence that the client has asthma, atelectasis, or pulmonary embolism. The client has infiltrates rather than consolidation in the lungs per the chest x-ray findings.

*Item #4*
Answers:

| Potential Nursing Action | Appropriate | Not Appropriate |
|---|---|---|
| Initiate high-flow nasal cannula oxygen at 60 L/min | X | |
| Assess respiratory status every 4 hours | | X |
| Schedule awake pronation periods | X | |
| Prepare for possible intubation and mechanical ventilation | | X |

Rationale: The client's $SpO_2$ is decreasing even though the oxygen flow has been increased. Arterial blood gases were drawn to determine if the client has hypoxemia, which was confirmed. The client also has respiratory acidosis. High-flow nasal cannula (HFNC) is a noninvasive, preferred method of providing high levels of oxygen without placing a client on mechanical ventilation. A special nasal cannula is used to provide 60 or more liters of warmed and humidified supplemental oxygen and is an appropriate action for this client. Additionally, research supports that awake pronation can improve the client's oxygenation. The client's respiratory status should be assessed every 1 to 2 hours rather than every 4 hours. Frequent assessment is essential because changes in the lung can occur quickly.

## Item #5
Answer: A, B, D, F

Rationale: All of these choices are appropriate except for C and E. The client should not be intubated at this time until noninvasive methods like HFNC are used and IV antibiotic therapy would be ineffective for a viral lung infection (Choices C and E). Antibiotics are used for bacterial infections.

## Item #6
Answer:

| Current Client Findings | Client Findings on Admission | Effective | Not Effective |
| --- | --- | --- | --- |
| Bilateral crackles in both lung bases | Bilateral crackles throughout lung fields | X | |
| Respiratory rate 20 breaths/min | Respiratory rate 32 breaths/min | X | |
| SpO$_2$ 90% on RA | SpO$_2$ 96% on RA | X | |
| Heart rate 98 beats/min | Heart rate 96 beats/min | | X |
| Chest x-ray shows 50% of lung fields with diffuse infiltrates | Chest x-ray shows 20% of lung fields with few infiltrates | X | |

Rationale: The current client findings show that the client has improved in all areas except for heart rate. Therefore, the nursing and collaborative actions to manage this client were likely effective to meet optimal clinical outcomes. The client's heart rate remains in the upper 90s, which may require follow up to rule out any cardiac pathology.

Chapter 27
**Answer Key**
*Chapter Review*
**Anatomy & Physiology Review**
#1.

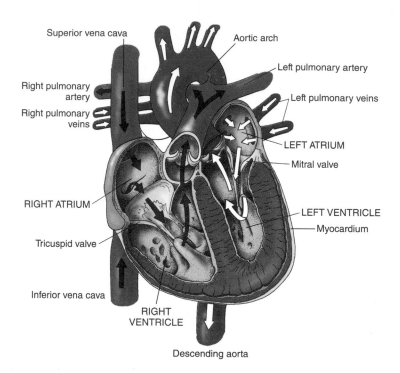

#2.
1. Stroke volume
2. venous
3. aorta
4. 60 to 70
5. Cardiac output
6. Baroreceptors
7. arterial
8. afterload

## Activities

### Activity #1
Any four of these common physiologic cardiovascular system changes associated with aging:
- Calcification and mucoid degeneration, especially in mitral and aortic valves
- Decrease in number of pacemaker cells
- Increase in fibrous tissue and fat in the sinoatrial node
- Few muscle fibers in the atrial myocardium and bundle of His
- Increase in conduction time
- Increase in the size of the left ventricle
- Stiffened left ventricle with fibrotic changes that decrease the speed of early diastolic filling by about 50%
- Less sensitive baroreceptors
- Thickened and stiffer aorta and other large arteries causing increased systolic blood pressure
- Increase in systemic vascular resistance, contributing to left ventricular hypertrophy

## Activity #2
1. Heart disease
2. pack-years
3. palpitations
4. syncope
5. orthostatic (postural) hypotension
6. pulse pressure
7. Bruits
8. 200
9. Cardiac catheterization
10. Echocardiography

## Activity #3
1. T
2. T
3. F
4. T
5. T
6. F
7. T
8. T
9. T
10. F

## Activity #4
1. B
2. G
3. D
4. J
5. F
6. A
7. I
8. E
9. H
10. C

## Learning Assessments

### NCLEX Examination Challenge #1
Answer: C
Rationale: A swishing sound heard over an artery is called a bruit. Bruits are caused my blood turbulence as it tries to flow through a narrowed artery, not a vein (Choice D). Therefore, Choice C is the correct response. A murmur is heard over the heart (Choices A and B).

### NCLEX Examination Challenge #2
Answer: A
Rationale: All of the laboratory test results are abnormal except for Choice A. High-density lipoproteins provide protection for a client and ideally are in a high range. Elevated lipoproteins, triglycerides, and total cholesterol are not desired and indicate an increased risk of cardiovascular disease or event (Choices B, C, and D).

### NCLEX Examination Challenge #3
Answer: D
Rationale: The nurse would frequently monitor the client's vital signs and perform cardiovascular assessments to detect dysrhythmias, hypotension, and bleeding, potentially life-threatening symptoms (Choice D). The nurse would also perform neurologic assessments to monitor for stroke, but this assessment is not as important as vital sign monitoring (Choice B). Pain and fluid and electrolyte imbalance are not usually a problem after this procedure but would be part of a head-to-toe assessment for all clients (Choices A and C).

## Chapter 28
**Answer Key**
*Chapter Review*
**Pathophysiology Review**

#1

1. B
2. G
3. F
4. I
5. C
6. F
7. J
8. A
9. D
10. H

#2

1. T
2. T
3. F
4. T
5. T
6. T
7. F
8. T

## Activities

### Activity #1
Any four of these risk factors for the development of AF:

- Older age
- Hypertension
- Previous ischemic stroke
- Transient ischemic attack (TIA) or other thromboembolic event
- Coronary heart disease
- Diabetes mellitus
- Heart failure
- Obesity
- Hyperthyroidism
- Chronic kidney disease
- Excessive alcohol use
- Mitral valve disease

### Activity #2
1. T
2. T
3. T
4. F
5. T
6. T
7. T
8. T
9. T
10. F
11. T

### Activity #3
1. asystole
2. pulmonary embolism (or stroke)
3. Defibrillation
4. MAZE
5. Telemetry
6. andexanet alfa
7. heart failure
8. bradycardia (or decreased pulse)

### Activity #4
1. B
2. C
3. D
4. D
5. A
6. E
7. C
8. A

**Learning Assessments**

**NCLEX Examination Challenge #1**
Answer: A, B, C, E, F
Rationale: All of these nursing actions are appropriate for a client who had an electrical cardioversion except for Choice D. This procedure is not surgery or invasive, and, therefore, there is no incision to monitor.

**NCLEX Examination Challenge #2**
Answer: C
Rationale: Verapamil is a calcium channel blocker that can cause orthostatic hypotension, which can cause dizziness and result in a fall, especially for older adults. Therefore, the nurse would remind the client to move slowly when changing positions. The other statements are not related to verapamil (Choices A, B, and D).

**NCLEX Examination Challenge #3**
Answer: A
Rationale: Propranolol is a beta blocking agent that has beta$_2$ blocking effects on the lungs that can cause bronchospasm, resulting in shortness of breath and wheezing. The client has asthma that, when triggered, can result in bronchospasm, shortness of breath, and wheezing. Therefore, the drug is contraindicated in this client (Choice A). The other drugs are not beta blockers and would not have the same adverse effect on the client (Choices B, C, and D).

**NCLEX Examination Challenge #4**
Answer: D
Rationale: The client's ECG strip shows VF, a terminal rhythm. The nurse knows that the tracing is not artifact because the client is nonresponsive. Therefore, defibrillation is the appropriate action (Choice D). CPR would be initiated if the client had asystole (Choice A). A beta blocker decreases the heart rate, and this client has no effective heartbeat. Therefore, Choice B is not appropriate. Oxygen would not help restore normal sinus rhythm for the client (Choice C).

**NGN Challenge**
Answer:

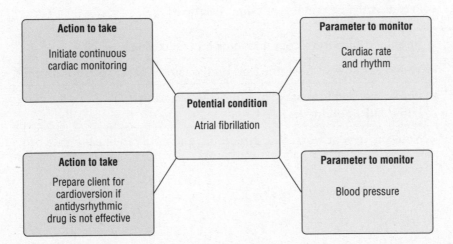

Rationale: The client has a rapid heart rate that was sustained for a time and caused palpitations, chest discomfort, and anxiety. The client was prescribed propranolol to lower the heart rate, indicating that the client most likely has AF or ventricular tachycardia. The client is able to communicate, so the dysrhythmia is not ventricular defibrillation. Premature ventricular contractions would cause an irregular heartbeat but not necessarily a rapid heart rate. The client's heart rate is irregular, and, therefore, the dysrhythmia is not a sinus dysrhythmia. When the client was admitted to the urgent care center, the client needed to begin continuous cardiac monitoring to diagnose which dysrhythmia was present. The client's SpO$_2$ was normal and there is no evidence of dyspnea. Therefore, oxygen therapy is not needed at this time. The nurse would prepare for cardioversion if antidysrhythmic medication did not lower the client's heart rate.

## Chapter 29
**Answer Key**
*Chapter Review*
**Pathophysiology Review**

#1
1. E
2. K
3. H
4. B
5. G
6. D
7. L
8. I
9. F
10. A
11. J
12. C

#2
1. F
2. T
3. T
4. T
5. T
6. T
7. F
8. T
9. T
10. T
11. T
12. T

**Activities**

**Activity #1**

| Component | Health Teaching Associated with Component (Any One of These Choices per Component) |
|---|---|
| Medications | • Take medications as prescribed and do not run out.<br>• Know the purpose and side effects of each drug.<br>• Avoid NSAIDs to prevent sodium and fluid retention. |
| Activity | • Stay as active as possible but don't overdo it.<br>• Know your limits.<br>• Be able to carry on a conversation while exercising. |
| Weight | • Weigh each day at the same time on the same scale to monitor for fluid retention. |
| Diet | • Limit daily sodium intake to 2 to 3 g as prescribed.<br>• Limit daily fluid intake to 2 L. |
| Symptoms | • Note any new or worsening symptoms, and notify the health care provider immediately. |

**Activity #2**
1. T
2. T
3. F
4. T
5. T
6. T
7. T
8. T
9. F
10. T

**Activity #3**
1. C
2. H
3. F
4. B
5. J
6. I
7. D
8. G
9. A
10. E

## Activity #4

1. C
2. F
3. D
4. G
5. A
6. E
7. B

## Activity #5

Any four of these symptoms that patients with a history of HF should report to the primary health care provider because they could indicate worsening or recurrent heart failure:

- Rapid weight gain (5 lb in a week or 2 to 3 lb in 24-hour period)
- Decrease in exercise tolerance lasting 2 to 3 days
- Cold symptoms (cough) lasting more than 3 to 5 days
- Excessive awakening at night to urinate
- Development of dyspnea or angina at rest or worsening angina
- Increased swelling in the feet, ankles, or hands

## Learning Assessments

### NCLEX Examination Challenge #1
Answer: D
Rationale: Weight is the most reliable indicator of fluid retention or loss (Choice D). Intake and output, edema, and pulse quality are not as reliable to determine fluid status (Choices A, B, and C).

### NCLEX Examination Challenge #2
Answer: B, C, D, E
Rationale: All of these actions are appropriate for the client experiencing dyspnea except that oxygen therapy should maintain the SpO$_2$ at 90% or above (Choice A).

### NCLEX Examination Challenge #3
Answer: C
Rationale: When the client's systolic BP falls below 90 mm Hg, the nurse would lie the client flat to increase blood flow to the brain and elevate the legs to promote venous return (Choice C). It would not be appropriate to wait 30 minutes to retake the client's BP because the systolic may continue to fall and shock could occur (Choice A). Continuous cardiac monitoring may be initiated later but not as the priority (Choice B). If the client's condition worsens, the client may be transferred to critical care, but that is not indicated at this time (Choice D).

### NCLEX Examination Challenge #4
Answer: B
Rationale: The client who develops hypokalemia while taking digoxin is at high risk for digoxin toxicity, including potentially life-threatening dysrhythmias (Choice B). It is not known if the client has a fluid imbalance (Choice A). Because the client is older, hyponatremia may cause confusion and weakness that could cause a fall (Choices C and D). However, this is likely not as potentially life-threatening as severe bradycardia or other cardiac dysrhythmia.

**NGN Challenge #1**
<u>Answer</u>:

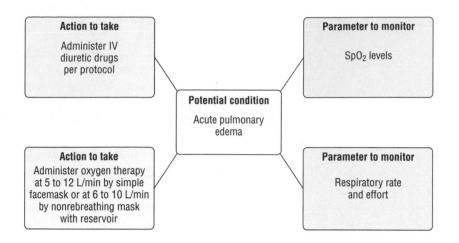

<u>Rationale</u>: Acute pulmonary edema is a life-threatening event that can result from HF (with fluid overload), acute myocardial infarction (MI), mitral valve disease, and possibly dysrhythmias. In pulmonary edema, the left ventricle fails to eject sufficient blood, and pressure increases in the lungs as a result. The increased pressure causes fluid to leak across the pulmonary capillaries and into the lung airways and tissues. Early symptoms of pulmonary edema include crackles in the lung bases, dyspnea at rest, disorientation, and confusion, especially in older clients. This client has these symptoms and a history of heart failure. Cor pulmonale is right-sided heart failure as a result of COPD, which this client does not have. The client has symptoms that are not associated with PE or MI. The primary desired outcome for the client is to reduce fluid overload and improve breathing. Giving an IV diuretic reduces fluid in the body, and a high concentration of oxygen helps to meet that outcome. The client's BP is not severely elevated such that IV antihypertensive drug therapy would be needed, and there is no indication that the client needs mechanical ventilation. Cardiac monitoring may be appropriate but is not a priority action for pulmonary edema at this time.

NGN Challenge #2
Answer:

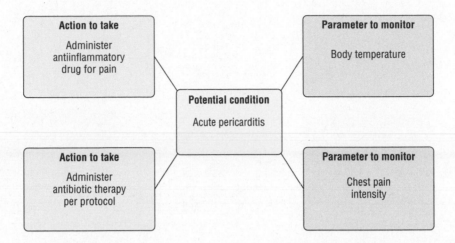

Rationale: Acute pericarditis is an inflammation or alteration of the pericardium (the membranous sac that encloses the heart). Assessment findings for patients with acute pericarditis include substernal precordial pain that radiates to the left side of the neck, the shoulder, or the back. The pain is classically grating and oppressive and is aggravated by breathing (mainly on inspiration), coughing, and swallowing. The pain is worse when the patient is in the supine position and may be relieved by sitting up and leaning forward. A pericardial friction rub may be heard with the diaphragm of the stethoscope positioned at the left lower sternal border. This client's report of pain meets this description, and the client has a pericardial friction rub. In addition, the client has a new ST elevation on ECG, a common finding for clients with acute pericarditis. Fever and tachycardia are also common. The nature of the client's pain is not consistent with any of the other cardiac conditions. Acute pericarditis is usually caused by bacteria, which explains the client's fever; therefore, antibiotic therapy to manage the infection and antiinflammatory drugs to manage pain are required. To evaluate the effectiveness of these medications, the nurse would monitor the client's temperature and pain level. Anticoagulants would not be given because of a risk of cardiac tamponade, a life-threatening complication. There are no data that indicate the need for oxygen therapy and antihypertensive medication.

## Chapter 30
### Answer Key
#### *Chapter Review*
#### Pathophysiology Review

#1
1. F
2. M
3. J
4. B
5. Q
6. H
7. N
8. D
9. O
10. R
11. G
12. A
13. K
14. E
15. L
16. C
17. P
18. I

#2
1. F
2. T
3. T
4. T
5. T
6. T
7. T
8. F
9. T
10. T

### Activities

#### Activity #1
Any four of these risk factors associated with the development of primary hypertension:
- Family history of hypertension
- Hyperlipidemia
- Black race
- Smoking
- Older than age 60 years or postmenopausal
- Excessive sodium intake
- Overweight/obesity
- Physical inactivity
- Excessive alcohol intake
- Excessive and continuous stress

#### Activity #2
1. T
2. T
3. F
4. T
5. T
6. T
7. F
8. T
9. T
10. T
11. T
12. T

## Activity #3

1. E
2. C
3. G
4. I
5. A
6. H
7. D
8. F
9. B
10. J

## Activity #4

1. F
2. B
3. D
4. G
5. E
6. A
7. C

## Activity #5

Any four of these areas of health teaching that the nurse would provide to help clients who have hypertension manage their care:

- Take medication(s) as prescribed with continual renewals.
- Report unpleasant drug side effects such as nagging cough.
- Obtain an ambulatory BP monitoring (ΛBPM) device for use at home so the pressure can be checked as recommended by the provider.
- If weight reduction is part of the treatment plan, be sure to have a scale for weight monitoring at home.
- Avoid foods high in sodium.
- Restrict alcohol use to the recommended maximum amount (one drink a day for women and two drinks a day for men).
- Engage in regular exercise.
- Manage stress as indicated.
- If needed, seek a smoking cessation program.

## Learning Assessments

### NCLEX Examination Challenge #1

Answer: B

Rationale: Clients who have a percutaneous vascular procedure have a catheter inserted most often in the femoral artery. The client returns from the procedure with an arterial plug, which the nurse carefully observes for signs of bleeding. Bleeding from an artery can cause shock in a very short period of time (Choice B). If bleeding occurs, the client's hematocrit would eventually decrease, but this is not a timely method to assess the client's condition (Choice C). The client's level of consciousness would also likely decrease if bleeding occurred because of hypoxemia from blood loss. Again, this is not a timely way to assess the client's condition. Femoral pulses would not be assessed, especially on the affected extremity that is patched with an arterial plug, and should not be disturbed (Choice D).

### NCLEX Examination Challenge #2

Answer: A, C, D, E

Rationale: All of these choices should be included in the nurse's health teaching about thiazide diuretics except for Choice B. HCTZ can cause hypokalemia, a loss of potassium, not hyperkalemia.

### NCLEX Examination Challenge #3

Answer: C

Rationale: The priority action after a femorotibial bypass is to ensure that any graft occlusion is caught early before damage to the extremity occurs. Therefore, the nurse would assess circulation in the affected extremity every 15 minutes for the first hour and then hourly (Choice C). Neurologic status and pain intensity would be assessed, but these assessments are not the priority when compared with extremity perfusion (Choices A and B). This surgery involves arteries and does not require a venous puncture. Therefore, Choice D is an incorrect response.

## NGN Challenge #1
Answer:

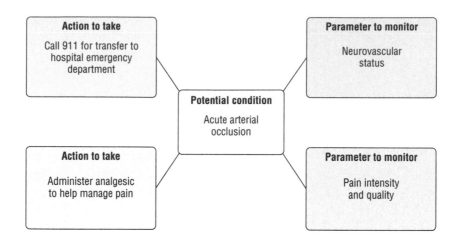

Rationale: The onset of acute arterial occlusion is sudden and dramatic, similar to what this client experienced. An embolus is the most common cause of peripheral occlusions, although a local thrombus may be the cause. Occlusion may affect the upper extremities, but it is more common in the lower extremities. Clients with an acute arterial occlusion describe severe pain below the level of the occlusion that occurs even at rest. The affected extremity is cool or cold, pulseless, and mottled. Peripheral arterial and venous disease have an insidious onset over time. Symptoms of deep vein thrombosis are due to inflammation and include warmth, swelling, redness, and pain. The level of care in an assisted living facility does not support care of this client. Therefore, the client needs to be admitted to an acute care hospital to have a procedure that will remove or bypass the arterial occlusion and restore adequate perfusion to the client's left leg and foot. Therefore, the nurse would call 911 because this problem is an emergency that, if not treated in a timely manner, can result in necrosis and gangrene with possible amputation. The nurse could provide oral analgesia to help with pain management; however, until the occlusion is removed, the client will likely continue to experience pain. The nurse would evaluate how well the analgesia helped to reduce pain and continue monitoring the client's left leg for neurovascular status.

**NGN Challenge #2**

<u>Answer</u>:

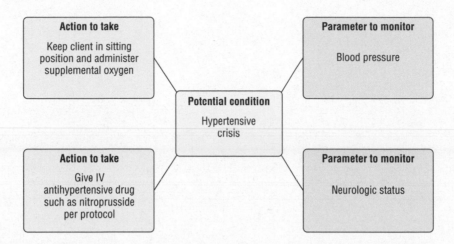

<u>Rationale</u>: Hypertensive crisis is a severe type of elevated BP that rapidly progresses with readings of 180/120 mm Hg or greater and is considered a hypertensive emergency. A person with this health condition may be asymptomatic or may have symptoms such as morning headaches, blurred vision, anxiety, nosebleeds, and dyspnea. This client meets this description and is experiencing most of these symptoms. This very high blood pressure can cause a hemorrhagic stroke rather than an acute ischemic stroke if hypertension is not treated quickly. The nurse would monitor the client's neurologic status frequently for signs and symptoms of stroke. There is no chest pain or other pulmonary symptoms that might indicate pulmonary hypertension or embolus. The client would receive an antihypertensive drug that works rapidly and is given IV, such as nitroprusside. To help reduce blood pressure, the client needs to be in a sitting position rather than lying down. The client's blood pressure needs to be monitored every 5 to 15 minutes until it lowers closer to the client's normal range. Every-4-hour BP monitoring is not adequate. Supplemental oxygen would also be useful to help reduce dyspnea. Morphine sulfate or fibrinolytic therapy is not necessary because there is no indication for either drug. Peripheral pulses and respiratory rate and effort are not the most essential parameters to monitor. Lab tests, such as aPTT and anti-factor Xa, would not need to be monitored because the client should not receive unfractionated heparin.

## Chapter 31
**Answer Key**
*Chapter Review*
**Pathophysiology Review**

#1

1. C
2. G
3. B
4. E
5. H
6. A
7. F
8. D

#2

1. T
2. T
3. F
4. T
5. T
6. T
7. T
8. F
9. T
10. T
11. T
12. F
13. T
14. F
15. T

## Activities

### Activity #1

Any three of these risk factors associated with the development of shock:

- Dehydration
- Trauma
- Infection
- Invasive procedures
- GI bleeding
- Surgery
- Anticoagulant therapy
- Antiplatelet therapy
- Impaired immunity (from illness or age)

### Activity #2

1. T
2. T
3. F
4. T
5. T
6. T
7. T
8. T
9. T
10. F

### Activity #3

1. A & B
2. A & B
3. A & B
4. A
5. A & B
6. A

**Activity #4**

| Body System | Physiologic Change(s) |
|---|---|
| Cardiovascular | • Increased diastolic blood pressure<br>• Increased heart rate<br>• Decreased peripheral pulse quality<br>• Decreased pulse pressure<br>• Decreased oxygen saturation<br>• Decreased capillary refill |
| Respiratory | • Increased respiratory rate |
| Kidney/urinary | • Decreased urinary output |
| Skin | • Cool, moist skin<br>• Dry mucous membranes<br>• Pallor or cyanosis |
| Central nervous system | • Thirst<br>• Acute confusion<br>• Decreased level of consciousness |

## Learning Assessments

### NCLEX Examination Challenge #1
Answer: A, B, D
Rationale: In the early stage of shock, vital signs begin to change. The heart and respiratory rates increase to compensate for decreasing tissue perfusion (Choices A and B). Diastolic blood pressure increases, but there is no significant change in the systolic pressure (Choices C and D). Therefore, pulse pressure is decreased. The oxygen saturation level does not increase but begins to decrease (Choice E) as tissue perfusion diminishes.

### NCLEX Examination Challenge #2
Answer: D
Rationale: A client experiencing sepsis and septic shock is critically ill. Client care is very complex, which requires the knowledge and experience of a registered nurse (RN) to make appropriate clinical judgments. The most appropriate nursing activity to delegate to an LPN/LVN is to monitor the peripheral oxygen saturation level using pulse oximetry (Choice D). Vital signs and CVP readings need to be measured and then interpreted by the RN (Choices A and B). Dopamine is a high-alert drug that needs to be monitored and titrated depending on the client's blood pressure and other assessments that would need to be performed by the RN (Choice C).

**NGN Challenge #1**
Answer:

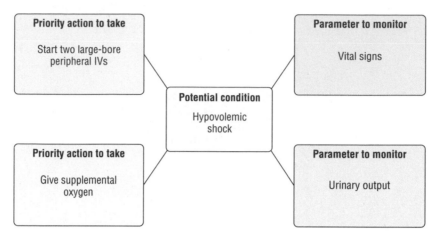

Rationale: The client has been vomiting has a headache, low blood pressure, low-grade fever, decreased voiding, and tachycardia. These findings are consistent with dehydration resulting from a lack of fluids in the body. In addition, the client has GI bleeding, which can deplete fluid volume in the vascular space, making the client at risk for hypovolemic shock. The client does not appear to have an infection and therefore septic and distributive shock are not potential conditions for this client. The notes do not indicate that the client has a heart condition, and therefore cardiogenic shock is not likely. For hypovolemic shock, the nurse and health care team would want to replace fluid volume, which would be accomplished by providing IV fluids and possibly a blood transfusion. Therefore, the nurse would start two large-bore IVs. With less blood volume to perfuse major body organs and peripheral tissues, the client would need supplemental oxygen. Lying the client flat would possibly cause aspiration in case of further vomiting. An NG tube may be needed if the GI bleeding and vomiting does not subside, but more evaluation is needed to determine this need. An ECG may be needed if the client has cardiac symptoms. The nurse would continue to monitor vital signs as fluids are restored and the SpO$_2$ as oxygen therapy continues. Lactate is a sensitive marker for septic shock for which this client is not at high risk. Neurovascular assessment is capillary refill assessment is not indicated at this time.

**NGN Challenge #2**
Answer: The nurse analyzes the assessment findings and determines that the client is at high risk for **septic shock** as evidenced by a(n) **increased lactate**, **tachycardia**, and **fever**.
Rationale: The client has an infected pressure injury and cellulitis. Cellulitis indicates that the infection has invaded surrounding body tissues, meaning that the infection has spread. The client's fever and tachycardia show evidence of systemic infection for which the client should be cultured. Clients who are at risk for sepsis and septic shock have an elevated serum lactate of greater than 18 mg/dL (2 mmol/L) in addition to these symptoms. The client is not hypotensive, and the WBC count is within normal limits. The oxygen saturation and capillary refill are not increased. An increased RR can occur with any type of shock or for other reasons.

# Chapter 32
## Answer Key
### *Pathophysiology Review*

#1.
1. G
2. I
3. C
4. H
5. D
6. F
7. A
8. J
9. E
10. B

#2.
1. T
2. T
3. T
4. F
5. F
6. T
7. T
8. T
9. T
10. T

## Activities

### Activity #1
Any four of these activities or lifestyle habits the nurse would include in health teaching about how to prevent coronary artery disease:
- If you smoke, vape, or use tobacco, quit.
- If you don't smoke, vape, or use tobacco, don't start.
- Consume sufficient calories for your body to include:
    o 5% to 6% from saturated fats
    o Avoiding *trans* fatty acids
- Limit your cholesterol intake to less than 200 mg/day.
- Limit your sodium intake as specified by your health care provider or under 1500 mg/day, if possible.
- Have your lipid levels checked regularly.
- If your cholesterol and LDL-C levels are elevated, follow your health care provider's advice, including taking statin medications as indicated.
- If you are middle-age or older or have a history of medical problems, check with your health care provider before starting an exercise program.
- Exercise periods should be at least 40 minutes long with 10-minute warm-up and 5-minute cool-down periods.
- If you cannot exercise moderately three to four times each week, walk daily for 30 minutes at a comfortable pace.
- If you cannot walk 30 minutes daily, walk any distance you can (e.g., park farther away from a site than necessary; use the stairs, not the elevator, to go one floor up or two floors down).
- Have your blood pressure checked regularly.
- If your blood pressure is elevated, follow your health care provider's advice.
- Continue to monitor your blood pressure at regular intervals.
- Restrict intake of saturated fats, sweets, sweetened beverages, and cholesterol-rich foods.

### Activity #2
1. T
2. T
3. T
4. T
5. F
6. T
7. T
8. F
9. T
10. T

### Activity #3
1. E
2. B
3. E
4. D
5. A
6. F
7. C

**Activity #4**
List three signs and symptoms associated with inadequate organ perfusion resulting from decreased cardiac output after a myocardial infarction.
- A change in orientation or mental status
- Urine output less than 0.5 to 1 mL/kg/h
- Cool, clammy extremities with decreased or absent pulses
- Unusual fatigue
- Recurrent chest pain

## Learning Assessment

### NCLEX Examination Challenge #1
Answer: A, D, E
Rationale: Clients who have experienced an MI may require dual antiplatelet therapy with aspirin and a P2Y12 inhibitor, a beta blocker, a statin drug, and, if the ejection fraction is below 40%, an ACEI and/or an ARB. Carvedilol CR is a long-acting, controlled release (CR) beta blocker. This group of drugs can cause heart failure and pulmonary symptoms, including wheezing, shortness of breath, and edema (Choice E). Beta blockers can cause bradycardia and hypotension. Therefore, the nurse would remind the client to not take the drug if the pulse rate is below 50 beats /min (Choice A). Although a beta blocker can be taken at any time with or without meals, most providers suggest taking the drug in the evening to minimize experiencing the side effects (Choice D). Beta blockers do not cause bleeding; bleeding can occur when taking antiplatelet and anticoagulant drugs (Choice B). A dry hacking cough is most common when taking an ACI inhibitor, not a beta blocker (Choice C).

### NCLEX Examination Challenge #2
Answer: B, D, E
Rationale: The three most common potential complications of PCI include hypotension (not hypertension in Choice A), hypokalemia, and dysrhythmias (Choices B and D). The nurse would monitor the catheter insertion site for any bleeding that can also occur (Choice E). Hypernatremia is not a complication of this invasive procedure (Choice C).

**NGN Challenge**
*Item #1*
Answer:

| Vital Signs | Nurses Notes | Orders | Laboratory Results |
|---|---|---|---|

**1010:** 911 to ED with report of severe substernal chest pain, nausea, and dyspnea. Alert and oriented × 4. Breath sounds clear in all lung fields. No wheezes or crackles. ECG shows irregular tachycardia with ST- and T-wave changes. Elevated cardiac troponins T and I. Current VS: T 100.4°F (37.4°C); HR 104 beats/min and irregular; RR 20 breaths/min; BP 152/84 mm Hg; $SpO_2$ 97% on $O_2$ 3 L/min via NC. History of heart failure (hospitalized × 2), high cholesterol, hypertension, and failed back syndrome (8 lumbar back surgeries over 30 years). Lives alone but family is local.

Rationale: Relevant client findings are those that are of immediate concern to the nurse. Chest pain can result from GI distress, musculoskeletal injury, or cardiac involvement. Therefore, any report of chest pain is a priority concern because the pain can result from lack of blood supply (perfusion) to the myocardium. If the myocardium is damaged, the client's cardiac output could decrease, resulting in poor perfusion to major organs, a potentially life-threatening condition. Nausea may be a sympathetic response to chest pain. Dyspnea could be due to anxiety from pain or as a result of myocardial ischemia or necrosis. Troponins T and I are sensitive and specific markers for myocardial ischemia or necrosis and would be of immediate concern. These data combined with ECG changes and tachycardia suggest that the chest pain is likely of cardiac origin. A low-grade fever is suggestive of inflammation or infection and would be concerning to the nurse. The client's blood pressure is elevated that, when combined with other client findings, it requires follow-up by the nurse at this time.

*Item #2*
Answer: The nurse analyzes the relevant assessment findings to determine that the client most likely has **NSTEMI** as evidenced by **elevated troponins** and **ECG ST- and T-wave changes**.
Rationale: A non–ST-elevation myocardial infarction (NSTEMI) is an MI in which the patient typically has ST- and T-wave changes on a 12-lead ECG; this indicates myocardial ischemia. This client has these changes plus elevated troponins. By contrast, a ST-elevation myocardial infarction (STEMI) is a myocardial infarction in which the patient typically has ST elevation in two contiguous leads on a 12-lead ECG; this indicates MI (necrosis). It is important to differentiate these two major types of MI to determine the severity and thus the need for emergency interventions. Troponins are not typically elevated in clients who have unstable angina. Dysrhythmias, fever, and dyspnea could occur from a number of conditions that are not specific for a cardiac problem.

*Item #3*
Answer: The *priority* for the client at this time is to increase **blood flow** to the myocardium to ensure adequate cardiac output.
Rationale: The client's symptoms are the result of myocardial ischemia, which is defined as a blockage of blood flow through a blood vessel, resulting in a lack of oxygen. To restore oxygenation to the myocardial tissue, the priority for the client's care is to increase blood flow by removing (if possible) the blockage or obstruction in one or more coronary arteries. These arteries supply the myocardium with oxygen and nutrients.

*Item #4*
Answer: A, B, C, E, F
Rationale: All of these interventions are appropriate (Choices A, B, C, E, and F) except that the client would not likely receive a heparin drip at this time because heparin does not remove a clot or plaque in the coronary arteries (Choice D).

*Item #5*

Answer: A, B, D, E, F

Rationale: All of these nursing actions are appropriate for a client after a PCI except for body position (Choices A, B, D, E, and F). Choice C is incorrect because most protocols require clients who have a PCI to be either in a flat supine or no more than a 30-degree elevation for several hours immediately after the procedure. Sitting upright could put stress on the insertion site.

*Item #6*

Answer:

| Client Findings on Hospital Admission (Before PCI) | Client Findings Today's Visit | Effective | Not Effective |
|---|---|---|---|
| Severe substernal chest pain | No chest pain since discharge | X | |
| Dyspnea | No dyspnea since discharge | X | |
| ECG ST- and T-wave changes | ECG: Normal sinus rhythm | X | |
| HR 104 beats/min and irregular | HR 88 beats/min and regular | X | |
| BP 152/84 mm Hg | BP 148/90 mm Hg | | X |

Rationale: Compared with assessment findings when the client was admitted to the hospital, the client's current findings have all improved with the exception of the blood pressure, which remains elevated. The cardiologist would likely re-evaluate the client's drug therapy and recommend other interventions that may help reduce blood pressure.

## Chapter 33
**Answer Key**
*Chapter Review*
**Anatomy & Physiology Review**
#1.

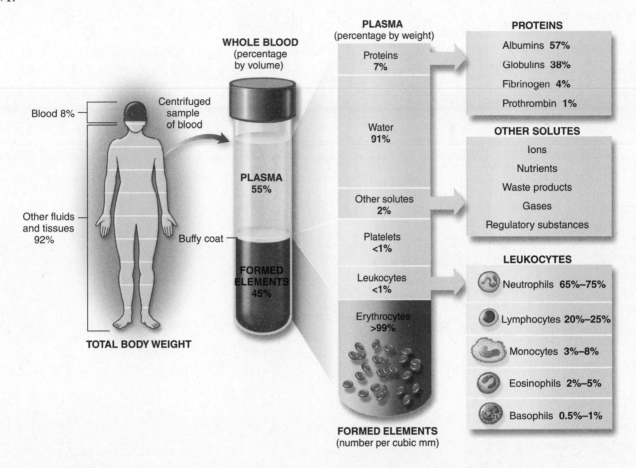

#2. Every laboratory has its own range for normal values. However, they should be very similar to the answers here.

1. RBC count (male)                $4.7–6.1 \times 10^6$/mcL
2. RBC count (female)              $4.2–5.4 \times 10^6$/mcL
3. Hemoglobin (male)               14–18 g/dL
4. Hemoglobin (female)             12–16 g/dL
5. Hematocrit (male)               42%–52%
6. Hematocrit (female)             37%–47%
7. WBC count                       5000–10,000/mm$^3$
8. Platelet count                  150,000–400,000/mm$^3$
9. D-dimer                         <0.4 mcg/mL
10. INR                            0.8–1.1
11. PT                             11–12.5 seconds

**Reference:**

Pagana, K., & Pagana, T. (2022). *Mosby's manual of diagnostic and laboratory tests* (7th ed.). St. Louis: Elsevier.

## Activities

### Activity #1
Answers may include five of these drugs that are associated with bone marrow suppression:
- Allopurinol
- Azathioprine
- Chemotherapeutic agents (almost all)
- Ciprofloxacin
- Colchicine
- Etanercept
- Hydroxychloroquine sulfate
- Interferon alfa
- Methotrexate
- Sulfamethoxazole/trimethoprim
- Zidovudine

### Activity #2
1. normal
2. 20%–40%
3. Allergies
4. O negative
5. O
6. Rh negative
7. Bone marrow suppression
8. Iron
9. Edema
10. Globulin

### Activity #3
1. T
2. T
3. F
4. F
5. F
6. T
7. F
8. T
9. F
10. T

### Activity #4
1. A+
2. A−
3. B+
4. B−
5. AB+
6. AB−
7. O+
8. O−

## Learning Assessments

**NCLEX Examination Challenge #1**
Answer: D
Rationale: ESAs are a synthetic form of erythropoietin, which is a growth factor for specific RBCs (erythrocytes). Its purpose is to raise a client's RBC count to normal or near-normal levels (4.2–6.1 $\times 10^6$/µL [4.2–6.1 $\times 10^{12}$/L]), so the nurse will use this value to determine efficacy (Choice D). The INR value (Choice A), platelet count (Choice B), and WBC count (Choice C) will not provide evidence of whether the RBC count has raised.

**NCLEX Examination Challenge #2**
Answer: A
Rationale: Clients with AB+ blood (called the universal recipient) can receive packed RBCs from any donor. The nurse will begin the infusion (Choice A). There is no need to return the unit to the blood bank (Choice B), complete an incident report (Choice C), or call the health care provider (Choice D).

**NCLEX Examination Challenge #3**
Answer: D
Rationale: A recipient client whose blood type is O negative can only receive blood from a donor whose blood type is O negative (Choice D). A positive (Choice A), B negative (Choice B), AB positive (Choice C), and AB negative (Choice E) blood is incompatible with a client who has O negative blood.

## Chapter 34
### Answer Key
*Pathophysiology Review*
#1.

1. E
2. A
3. C
4. D
5. F
6. B

#2. Precepitating factors should mirror the answers below.

| Potential Transfusion Reaction | Precipitating Factor(s) |
|---|---|
| Acute hemolytic transfusion reaction | Incompatibility of ABO blood type or Rh factor that usually occurs in the first 15 minutes after transfusion |
| Acute pain transfusion reaction | Some degree of hemolysis occurs during or shortly after transfusion but is not widespread |
| Allergic transfusion reaction (mucocutaneous) | Plasma protein sensitivity |
| Allergic transfusion reaction (anaphylactic transfusion reaction) | Plasma protein sensitivity |
| Febrile reaction (nonhemolytic) | Occurs most often in patients with anti-WBC antibodies |
| Transfusion-associated circulatory overload (TACO) | Pulmonary reaction that may be difficult at first to differentiate from transfusion-related acute lung injury (TRALI) can occur when a blood product is infused too quickly, especially in an older adult |
| Transfusion-associated graft-versus-host disease | Occurs most often in immunocompromised patients when donor T-cell lymphocytes attack host tissues |
| Transfusion-related acute lung injury (TRALI) | Occurs most often when donor blood contains antibodies against the recipient's neutrophil antigens, HLA, or both |

## Activities

### Activity #1

1. T
2. T
3. F
4. T
5. T
6. F
7. T
8. T
9. F
10. T

### Activity #2

| Patient (Recipient) Blood Group | Blood Donor Groups |
|---|---|
| O negative | O negative |
| O positive | O negative, O positive |
| B negative | O negative, B negative |
| B positive | O negative, O positive, B negative, B positive |
| A negative | O negative, A negative |
| A positive | O negative, O positive, A negative, A positive |
| AB negative | O negative, A negative, B negative, AB negative |
| AB positive | O negative, O positive, A negative, A positive, B negative, B positive, AB negative, AB positive |

### Activity #3

Things the nurse will teach a patient about preventing sickle cell crisis include:

- Drink at least 3 to 4 L of liquids every day.
- Avoid consuming alcoholic beverages and illicit substances.
- Avoid smoking cigarettes or using tobacco or nicotine in any form.
- Practice deep breathing to facilitate gas exchange.
- Avoid strenuous physical exercise.
- Avoid exposure to hot and cold temperature extremes.
- Avoid getting overheated and overexposure to the sun.
- Wear socks, hats, gloves, and a coat when going outside on cold days to avoid getting too cold.
- Avoid airplanes with unpressurized passenger cabins.
- Avoid traveling to areas of high altitudes.
- When you are not in crisis, engage in mild, low-impact exercise three times a week.
- See your primary health care provider for regular checkups.
- Be sure to get an influenza immunization and COVID-19 immunization every year.
- Ask your primary health care provider about receiving the pneumonia vaccine.
- Contact your primary health care provider at the first sign of illness or infection.
- Be sure all your health care providers know that you have sickle cell disease, especially the anesthesia provider and radiologist.

## Activity #4

Descriptions should resemble the information.

| Phase | Description |
|---|---|
| **Phase 1** <br> Conditioning | Chemotherapy and/or radiation is given. |
| **Phase 2** <br> Transplant day to engraftment | Stem cells are given. |
| **Phase 3** <br> Engraftment to day of discharge | RBC, WBC, and platelet counts begin to recover <br> Healing process begins. |
| **Phase 4** <br> Early convalescence | RBC, WBC, and platelet counts continue to recover; risk for infection is still high, as the immune system is not fully functioning yet. <br> Prophylactic antibiotics are given. |
| **Phase 5** <br> Late convalescence | The immune system is fully recovered. <br> Vaccination begins. |

## Activity #5

1. Assess the patient's **circulation, kidney function,** and **fluid** status before transfusion.
2. Use a needle no larger than **20** gauge.
3. Use blood that is less than **1 week** old.
4. Vital signs must be collected every **15** minutes during the transfusion.
5. Each unit of whole blood, packed red blood cells, or plasma is infused between **2 and 4** hours.
6. Do not transfuse whole blood, packed red blood cells, or plasma for more than **4** hours.
7. When possible, allow **2** hours between infusions of units.
8. Change blood tubing after every **2** units transfused.

## Learning Assessments

### NCLEX Examination Challenge #1

Answer: D

Rationale: The nurse will immediately report the WBC count of 20,000/mm³ because this indicates the presence of an acute infection (Choice D). The hematocrit value (Choice A), hemoglobin value (Choice B), and platelet count (Choice C) are within expected ranges and do not require provider notification.

### NCLEX Examination Challenge #2

Answer: A

Rationale: Older adults are at risk for developing fluid overload during transfusion therapy, especially when receiving multiple units of packed RBCs. Packed RBCs have a high osmotic pressure that draws interstitial fluid into the vascular space. The nurse will slow the infusion rate to as low as possible (Choice A), even before the client's circulatory status is assessed (Choice B), to prevent worsening of the problem. After those actions, the nurse can discontinue the infusion if necessary (Choice C) and document the occurrence (Choice D).

## NCLEX Examination Challenge #3
Answer: A, B, E
Rationale: In acute leukemia, there is an overproduction of immature WBCs. Other blood counts are also low, inducing fatigue (Choice A). The rapid production of WBCs in the marrow contributes to bone pain (Choice B). Low platelet counts cause bleeding and excessive bruising (Choice E). Facial pallor, not flushing, is usually present (Choice C). Finger clubbing is not expected (Choice D).

## NGN Challenge #1
Answer: C, F
Rationale: Based on the declining trend in the RBC count, hemoglobin, hematocrit, MCV, MCH, and ferritin, the client likely has iron deficiency anemia. This correlates with her symptoms of unexplained fatigue despite eating well and exercising regularly. The nurse will notify the primary health care provider (Choice C), who will likely prescribe iron supplementation; the nurse will teach the client how to take iron and explain that it can be taken with Vitamin C to increase absorption (Choice F). Monoclonal antibody therapy is not indicated (Choice A). Red meat should be encouraged–not discouraged–for clients with iron- deficiency anemia, because red meat contains valuable amounts of iron (Choice B). There is no need for an appointment with the diabetic educator (Choice D), as the client's glycohemoglobin A1C values are consistently within normal limits. The client's platelet count has been consistently normal so there is no need to educate about potential easy bruising (Choice E). Hydroxyurea is a treatment used for clients with SCD, not iron deficiency anemia (Choice G).

## NGN Challenge #2
Answer: B, C, F
Rationale: Chemotherapy decreases the platelet count. The client is at risk for bleeding once the platelet count falls below $50,000/mm^3$ ($50 \times 10^9$/L), and spontaneous bleeding may occur when the count is lower than $20,000/mm^3$ ($20 \times 10^9$/L). The nurse will teach the client about the risk for bleeding because their platelet count is declining (Choice B), explain the need to assess the stool at home for blood (Choice C), and encourage the client to increase the intake of dark green vegetables such as spinach, asparagus, and broccoli, which can serve to increase the platelet count (Choice F). Foods high in Vitamin D are not necessary (Choice A). The client will not be injecting Vitamin $B_{12}$; that is a treatment for Vitamin $B_{12}$ deficiency, not a low platelet count (Choice D). Fluid restriction is not necessary (Choice E). A low platelet count does not indicate that a client has SCD (Choice G). The Raynaud-like response occurs in cold antibody anemia, a type of immunohemolytic anemia (Choice H).

## Chapter 35

**Answer Key**
*Chapter Review*
**Anatomy & Physiology Review**
#1.
1. C
2. D
3. E
4. F
5. A
6. B

#2.

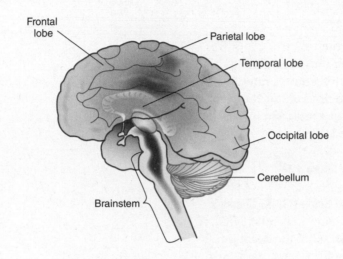

**Activities**

**Activity #1**
1. Any four of these physiologic changes of aging:
   - Slower cognitive processing time
   - Recent memory loss
   - Decreased sensory perception of touch
   - Possible change in perception of pain
   - Change in sleep patterns
   - Altered balance and/or decreased coordination
   - Increased risk for infection

**Activity #2**
1. physical disability
2. trigeminal neuralgia
3. Glasgow Coma Scale
4. pain, weakness, numbness, cognitive impairment (any two of these answers)
5. comatose
6. muscle strength
7. constrict
8. Nystagmus
9. IX, X
10. depression

**Activity #3**
1. T
2. F
3. T
4. F
5. F
6. T

**Activity #4**
1. D
2. A
3. C
4. E
5. B

## Learning Assessments

### NCLEX Examination Challenge #1
Answer: B

Rationale: A lumbar puncture is performed by inserting a spinal needle between the third and fourth lumbar vertebrae to obtain a cerebrospinal fluid (CSF) sample for analysis. The nurse's priority after the procedure is to monitor the client carefully for CSF leakage at the insertion site (Choice B). The nurse would also monitor the client's neurologic status frequently, including movement, to ensure that nerve damage did not occur during the procedure (Choice D). However, in a fetal side-lying position, the spinal nerves move and the vertebral space opens; spinal nerve injury rarely occurs. It is not necessary to assess vital signs every 2 hours after this procedure (Choice C). Infection is rare after the procedure; the nurse would monitor the client's temperature and other signs of infection before the WBC count would increase (Choice A).

### NCLEX Examination Challenge #2
Answer: C

Rationale: A Glasgow Coma Scale (GCS) helps to determine a client's level of consciousness (LOC). A maximum score of 15 denotes that the client is fully awake, alert, and aware (Choice C). As the client's condition deteriorates and LOC declines (lethargy, stupor, coma), the GCS score decreases (Choices A, B, and D).

### NCLEX Examination Challenge #3
Answer: D

Rationale: The frontal lobe contains the motor (movement) and speech centers. Therefore, a client who has speech difficulty and muscle weakness most likely has damage to the frontal lobe (Choice D). The other lobes of the cerebrum have other functions and are not affected by the client's brain cancer (Choices A, B, and C).

## Chapter 36

### Answer Key
#### *Pathophysiology Review*

#1
1. C
2. D
3. A
4. E
5. B

#2
1. D
2. C
3. B
4. E
5. A

## Activities
### Activity #1
1. T
2. F
3. T
4. T
5. F
6. T
7. T
8. T

### Activity #2
Any three of these tips for communicating with patients who have AD:
- Ask simple, direct questions that require only a "yes" or "no" answer if the patient can communicate.
- Provide instructions with pictures in a place that the patient will see if he or she can read them.
- Use simple, short sentences and one-step instructions.
- Use gestures to help the patient understand what is being said.
- Validate the patient's feelings as needed.
- Limit choices; too many choices cause frustration and increased confusion.
- Never assume that the patient is totally confused and cannot understand what is being communicated.
- Try to anticipate the patient's needs, and interpret nonverbal communication.

### Activity #3
Any four of these typical client assessment findings associated with PD:
- Hand and arm resting tremors
- Bilateral limb involvement
- Masklike face
- Slow, shuffling gait
- Postural instability
- Increased gait disturbances
- Akinesia
- Muscle rigidity

### Activity #4
1. B
2. C
3. A
4. C
5. B
6. B
7. A

### Activity #5
Any three of these health teaching points related to triptans:
- Do not take these drugs if you have a history of heart disease or Prinzmetal angina.
- After taking a triptan, contact the primary health care provider if you experience chest pain.
- Expect common side effects that include flushing, tingling, and a hot sensation.
- Triptan drugs should not be taken with selective serotonin reuptake inhibitor (SSRI) antidepressants or St. John's wort.
- Use contraception (birth control) while taking the drugs because they may not be safe for women who are pregnant.

### Activity #6
Any three of these complications for which the nurse monitors when caring for a patient who has bacterial meningitis:
- Decreased level of consciousness
- Seizures
- Fluid and electrolyte imbalances
- Vascular dysfunction (thrombus/embolus)
- Gangrene/potential amputation
- Shock

**Learning Assessments**

**NCLEX Examination Challenge #1**
Answer: A, D, E
Rationale: The client who has continuous seizure activity for more than 5 minutes is experiencing status epilepticus, which can be a life-threatening condition. Establishing an airway is the most important intervention (Choice A). To prevent aspiration and help maintain a patent airway, the nurse would turn the client on the side to rather than placing the client in a sitting position (Choice B). The nurse needs IV access to administer one or more antiepileptic drugs (Choices D and E). Vital signs should be taken after seizure activity is resolved rather than every 15 minutes or while the client is having a seizure (Choice C).

**NCLEX Examination Challenge #2**
Answer: A, C, D
Rationale: As a result of long-term levodopa-carbidopa therapy, the client with PD often develops one or more adverse drug events. The most common are orthostatic hypotension, dyskinesia (inability to perform voluntary movement), and psychosis, including hallucinations and delusions. Clients who are not taking this drug combination may also experience one or more of these symptoms.

**NCLEX Examination Challenge #3**
Answer: A, B, C, D, E, F
Rationale: As delineated in Box 36.1 in Chapter 36, the client who has moderate-stage AD may have all of these clinical manifestations, which continue into the late-stage of the disease or worsen.

**NGN Challenge #1**
<u>Answer:</u>

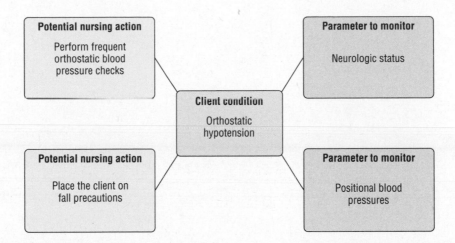

<u>Rationale:</u> The client has a history of PD with a recent episode of dizziness and lightheadedness that likely caused the fall this morning. The current blood pressure is low at 98/56 mm Hg and was likely taken while the client was in a recumbent position. Blood pressure tends to decrease when one moves from a recumbent position to a sitting or standing position. A low systolic blood pressure causes decreased perfusion to the brain resulting in dizziness, lightheadedness, or fainting. Orthostatic hypotension is common in clients who have PD because of sympathetic nervous system involvement. Additionally, orthostatic hypotension is an adverse drug effect of levodopa/carbidopa. The client is alert but oriented to person only. Cognitive impairment can occur in clients who have PD, but there is no other evidence that the client is delirious, has dementia, or had a seizure. The client is taking pimavanserin for hallucinations and should continue taking it to prevent this psychotic behavior. Given that the client likely has orthostatic hypotension, the nurse would perform orthostatic checks and place the client on fall precautions. Reorientation would be appropriate for the client but not for the client's current condition of orthostatic hypotension. Physical therapy may help with muscle strengthening and balance but would not be appropriate for managing hypotension. As a result of appropriate actions, the nurse would continue to monitor positional blood pressures during orthostatic checks and monitor the client's neurologic statis each shift. The client would not likely experience hallucinations if the prescribed medication is effective. Monitoring the client's gait and right arm injury are not appropriate parameters to monitor for the client's immediate problem of orthostatic hypotension.

**NGN Challenge #2**
<u>Answer:</u>

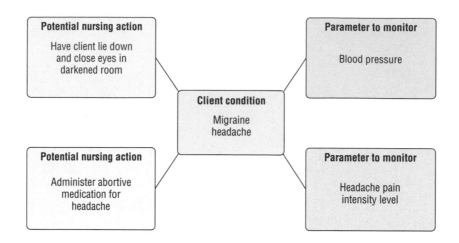

<u>Rationale:</u> The client's sequence of symptoms is suggestive of the phases of a migraine with aura, also called the classic migraine headache. The neurologic changes that occurred initially yesterday are common in the prodromal phase; in the migraine phase, the client has a severe headache with nausea and photophobia. Migraines are often accompanied by associated symptoms such as nausea or sensitivity to light, sound, or head movement and can last 4 to 72 hours. Vasodilation in the brain allows prostaglandins and other intravascular molecules to leak, contributing to widespread tissue swelling and the sensation of throbbing head ***pain.*** Although the neurologic changes the day before seeking medical attention can occur in clients who have transient ischemic attacks, the client experienced additional symptoms of severe headache, nausea, and photophobia, which are consistent with migraines. The client's neurologic changes resolved, which would rule out having a stroke. The presence of a cerebral aneurysm may or may not result in symptoms. If the aneurysm ruptures, the client would likely have longer lasting neurologic symptoms. The priority for care of the patient having migraines is pain management. Abortive drug therapy is aimed at alleviating pain during the aura phase or soon after the headache has started. The nurse would monitor the effectiveness of the drug to reduce pain by monitoring headache pain intensity. At the beginning of a migraine attack, the client may be able to reduce pain by lying down and darkening the room. The client may want both eyes covered and a cool cloth on the forehead to be undisturbed for a time. Oxygen therapy is not indicated and the client does not need admission to an acute care setting. A head CT scan is performed most often to rule out a stroke and is not necessary. The client's acute pain may have caused the client's increased blood pressure and, therefore, would be monitored by the nurse.

## Chapter 37
### Answer Key
*Pathophysiology Review*

#1
1. A
2. A
3. B
4. A
5. B
6. B
7. A

#2
1. remissions and exacerbations
2. demyelination, plaque
3. primary progressive MS
4. vision, mobility, sensory perception
5. respiratory musclc paralysis

## Activities

### Activity #1
1. F
2. E
3. D
4. J
5. A
6. I
7. G
8. H
9. B
10. C

### Activity #2
1. T
2. F
3. T
4. F
5. T
6. T
7. T
8. T
9. T
10. T

### Activity #3
Any three of these complications for which the nurse would monitor:
- Cerebrospinal leakage
- Dehydration
- Urinary retention
- Paralytic ileus
- Fat embolism syndrome
- Persistent or progressive lumbar radiculopathy
- Infection

### Activity #4
1. C
2. E
3. D
4. A
5. B

### Activity #5
Any four of these health promotion activities that can help prevent low back injury:
- Use safe manual handling practices, with specific attention to bending, lifting, and sitting.
- Assess the need for assistance with your household chores or other activities.
- Participate in a regular exercise program, especially one that promotes back strengthening, such as swimming and walking.
- Do not wear high-heeled shoes.
- Use good posture when sitting, standing, and walking.
- Avoid prolonged sitting or standing. Use a footstool and ergonomic chairs and tables to lessen back strain. Be sure that equipment in the workplace is ergonomically designed to prevent injury.
- Keep weight within 10% of ideal body weight.
- Ensure adequate calcium intake. Consider Vitamin D supplementation if serum levels are low.
- Stop smoking. If you are not able to stop, cut down on the number of cigarettes or decrease the use of other forms of tobacco.

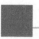

## Learning Assessments

### NCLEX Examination Challenge #1
Answer: B
Rationale: A halo ring around the dressing's edge indicates a likely CSF leak, which can cause severe headache or more severe life-threatening complications. Therefore, the nurse would **first** immediately lie the client flat to prevent the effect of gravity on the leaking CSF (Choice B). Then the surgeon or RRT would be contacted (Choices A and C). The dressing could be reinforced depending on how wet the surgical dressing is (Choice D), but this is not the nurse's first concern.

### NCLEX Examination Challenge #2
Answer: C
Rationale: All of the medications used to help create a remission for MS, including fingolimod, are immunomodulating drugs. When the immune system is suppressed, the client is at increased risk for infection and therefore should avoid crowds and individuals who are infected (Choice C). Choice A is an incorrect response because fingolimod is an oral drug and not given by injection. This drug does not cause liver damage, and therefore laboratory values to assess liver function are not necessary (Choice B). Fingolimod can be taken with or without food and therefore does not need to be taken with meals (Choice D).

### NCLEX Examination Challenge #3
Answer: A, C, D, E, F
Rationale: A complete C5-C6 SCI causes quadriplegia, which means that the client's mobility is markedly compromised. To help prevent complications of impaired mobility, the client is placed on a number of medications for 4 to 6 weeks or longer, depending on the client. Pantoprazole or a similar proton pump inhibitor is given to prevent stress ulcers following this traumatic event (Choice A). High SCIs lead to muscle spasticity, which can interfere with rehabilitation; therefore, baclofen is often given to decreases muscle spasms (Choice C). Calcium supplements or a bisphosphonate may be given to help prevent heterotopic ossification and osteoporosis (Choice D). Apixaban is an anticoagulant that helps to prevent venous thromboembolism complications (Choice E). Docusate sodium is a stool softener that facilitates bowel elimination, an important part of bowel retraining (Choice E). The client would not be taking an opioid such as morphine sulfate for the rehabilitation phase (Choice B).

### NGN Challenge #1
Answer: The nurse analyzes the data and determines that the client is most likely experiencing **neurogenic shock,** as evidenced by **bradycardia** and **hypotension**.
Rationale: The client's findings over a 12-hour period show a progressive decrease in BP until the systolic BP is below 90 mm Hg (hypotension). Initially, the client's heart rate increased to compensate for the decreasing BP but then decreased (bradycardia) because of hypoperfusion of the spinal cord. Additional evidence of neurogenic shock is the client's decreased LOC from alert and oriented ×4 to drowsy and oriented ×2. The client's urinary output also decreased to less than the minimum of 30 mL/h, indicating kidney dysfunction. These changes are also due to decreased perfusion to major organs of the body. The client does not have spinal shock, which is a temporary loss of motor, sensory perception, reflex, and autonomic function because this problem would not affect LOC or kidney function. Autonomic dysreflexia causes very high BP rather than hypotension.

### NGN Challenge #2
Answer: A, B, C, D, E
Rationale: The client has neurogenic shock, which indicates decreased perfusion to the spinal cord and vital organs of the body. Therefore, the client would receive increased IV fluids (Choice B). Dextran to expand blood plasma (fluid volume) would also be appropriate for this client to improve perfusion (Choice C). Atropine is the first-line drug for clients who have bradycardia to increase heart rate (Choice D). Dopamine or a similar drug helps to increase BP to maintain MAP to adequately perfuse vital organs (Choice E). Placing a client in a sitting position would lower blood pressure, which is contraindicated for this client (Choice F). Instead, the nurse would lie the client flat in a supine position.

# Chapter 38
## Answer Key
### *Chapter Review*
**Pathophysiology Review**

**#1**
1. C
2. A
3. B
4. A
5. B

**#2**
1. B
2. A
3. B
4. A
5. A
6. B
7. B

## Activities

### Activity #1
1. G
2. D
3. J
4. E
5. H
6. B
7. A
8. F
9. I
10. C

### Activity #2
Any three symptoms of increasing ICP for which the nurse monitors in patients who have strokes, TBIs, or other brain lesions:
- Severe headache
- Restlessness
- Irritability
- Decreased level of consciousness
- Pupil changes
- Increased BP
- Widened pulse pressure
- Bradycardia
- Nausea and vomiting (often projectile)

### Activity #3
1. F
2. T
3. T
4. T
5. T
6. T
7. F
8. T
9. T
10. T

### Activity #4
Any four of these essential interventions for providing patient-centered care for patients who have physical disability (from Chapter 38, Box 38.1):
- Ask patients what their goals are for care, and assist them in meeting those goals.
- Assess patient preferences, values, and beliefs, and incorporate them into care.
- Recognize that patients are experts in their disability.
- Communicate effectively with the patient and family, including keeping them informed at all times.
- Maintain mobility, if possible, by providing assistance while ensuring patient safety.
- Ensure that patients have access to devices and aids to assist with mobility and ADL performance.
- Collaborate with physical and occupational therapy as needed to ensure that the patient's disability needs are met.

### Activity #5
Any four of these six core principles of trauma-informed care that nurses need to incorporate into their practice:
- *Safety*: Provide a safe space, including the environment, for the patient without judgment regarding age, sexual orientation, gender identify, socioeconomic status, or social determinants of health. Be sure to ask patients how they want to be addressed.
- *Trustworthiness and transparency*: Transparency in communication helps to foster trust, which increases patient participation in their care. Use clear, plain terminology using knowledge of

the patient's health literacy, preferences, and values.

- *Peer support:* Peer support for patients who survive trauma and their families usually includes other individuals who are trauma survivors. Assist patients and families to locate community resources for effective peer support to help them understand their experience and reaction to it.
- *Collaboration and mutual support:* Patients should be active partners in their care, including being supported about their health care decisions. Nurses need to be aware of the patient's goals and recognize that patients are experts on their lived trauma experience.
- *Empowerment:* This core principle is integral to all other principles in that patients should have a voice to make informed decisions about their

care. Nurses and other health care staff should respect and support patients, even if they don't agree with those decisions.

- *Culture and historical sensitivity:* Patients bring their life experiences, including a history of traumatic events, when they seek health care. Many patients who experienced one or more traumatic events have resulting emotional and mental health problems, including anxiety, depression, and insomnia. They may also use harmful or unhealthy strategies, such as smoking, excess alcohol use, and overeating, to help cope with their stress. Be sure not to judge patients regarding their habits, but help them develop more healthy behaviors by referring them to appropriate resources.

**Activity #6**

| Potential Complication | Nursing Assessments and/or Actions (Any 2 for Each Complication) |
|---|---|
| Cardiac dysrhythmias | 1. Continuous cardiac monitoring<br>2. Frequent vital signs |
| Syndrome of SIADH | 1. Fluid restriction<br>2. Strict intake and output |
| Venous thromboembolism | 1. Early ambulation<br>2. Intermittent sequential pneumatic devices<br>3. Leg exercises |
| Hypernatremia/DI | 1. Monitor for seizure activity<br>2. Strict intake and output<br>3. Monitor laboratory values |

**Learning Assessments**

**NCLEX Examination Challenge #1**

Answer: D

Rationale: Supratentorial tumors are located within the cerebral hemispheres above the tentorium (dural fold). After surgery to remove a tumor in this location, the client needs to be in a semisitting position at about 30 degrees to facilitate venous drainage and prevent cerebral edema that would increase intracranial pressure (Choice D). Choices A and B are not sitting positions and would not allow gravity to help with venous drainage. The position in Choice C may cause the client's BP to become too low and may be uncomfortable for the client.

**NCLEX Examination Challenge #2**

Answer: A, B, C

Rationale: Choices A, B, and C have been shown through research to be high risk factors for clients to have a stroke if they have had a TIA. For general health, alcohol consumption should be no more than a moderate level, which is usually defined as no more than 7 drinks a week for a woman and no more than 14 drinks a week for men. Three drinks a week is acceptable and is not considered a risk factor for strokes (Choice D). Age is a major risk factor for predicting who is most likely to have a stroke, but the risk is greater for individuals older than 60 years of age rather than 75 (Choice E).

## NCLEX Examination Challenge #3
Answer: C

Rationale: The nurse caring for a client who is receiving alteplase, a "clot busting" drug, would discontinue the infusion if the client experiences bleeding, has a severe headache (which could indicate a hemorrhagic stroke), or has nausea and vomiting, which may be indicative of increasing intracranial pressure (Choice C). Neurologic assessments should be performed every 15 to 30 minutes, not every 2 hours (Choice A). The client's BP should be maintained below 185/110 mm Hg rather than 130/80 mm Hg (Choice B). IV heparin or any other anticoagulant drug that can cause bleeding would not be given with alteplase, which is a fibrinolytic drug that can cause bleeding (Choice D).

## NGN Challenge #1
Answer:

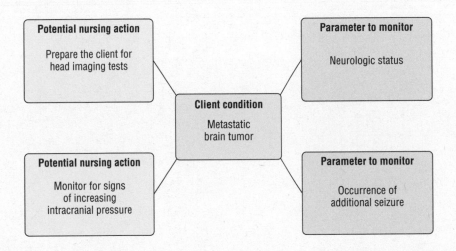

Rationale: The client has a history of lung cancer that was apparently successfully treated 2 years ago. However, he has new onset of neurologic symptoms over the past several months, including a seizure today at home. These symptoms have been episodic and suggest brain pathology that is worsening. Stroke symptoms would not occur and resolve. Although symptoms of a TIA usually resolve, they do so in 24 hours. This client's symptoms have not followed that pattern. One seizure is not indicative of a seizure disorder such as epilepsy. Therefore, given the client's history of lung cancer and the pattern of symptoms, the client most likely has a metastatic brain tumor. Brain metastasis is common in clients who have lung cancer. After evaluation in the ED, the client would be sent for a CT scan to rule out stroke or another acute neurologic event. The client is oriented ×2 and does not require frequent reorientation. Seizure precautions would be indicated if the client had a history of seizures, but at this point, the client only had one seizure reported by family. The client may need a physical therapy consult later, but the client needs a confirmation of the medical diagnosis. However, given the neurologic changes the client has experienced and the concern that the client may have a space-occupying brain tumor, the nurse would monitor the client for any signs of increased intracranial pressure as an action. The client's neurologic status would be monitored to determine any further changes, including the occurrence of another seizure. The client is not reporting pain at this time, so a pain assessment is not the best parameter for the nurse to monitor. The GCS is used if a stroke is suspected; carotid bruits would not be monitored because there is no indication that the client has this pathophysiologic change.

**NGN Challenge #2**

Answer: The nurse analyzes the assessment data and determines that the client is most likely experiencing a **decreased level of consciousness** as evidenced by **increased drowsiness** and **restlessness**.

Rationale: Based on the data provided, there is no evidence that the client has had an embolic stroke of TIA. However, the data support a decreasing LOC, especially the client's increased drowsiness and restlessness. The client is not bradycardic because the heart rate is between 76 and 80 beats/min. The client's respiratory rate is between 18 and 22 breaths/min. Although 22 breaths/min is above normal, tachypnea is not a symptom of decreased LOC. The $SpO_2$ is normal at 95% on RA. The client's BP is increasing, but it does not provide evidence of a decreased LOC.

## Chapter 39

### Answer Key
#### *Chapter Review*
**Pathophysiology Review**

#1
1. H
2. A
3. G
4. D
5. B
6. I
7. C
8. E
9. F

#2
1. F
2. T
3. T
4. T
5. F
6. F
7. F
8. T
9. T
10. F

## Activities

### Activity #1

Changes that occur to these eye structures as a result of the aging process should resemble these answers.

| Structure/Function | Change |
|---|---|
| Appearance | Eyes appear "sunken." |
| | Arcus senilis forms. |
| | Sclera yellows or appears blue. |
| Cornea | Cornea flattens, which blurs vision and can cause or worsen astigmatism. |
| Ocular muscles | Muscle strength is reduced, making it more difficult to maintain an upward gaze or a focus on a single image. |
| Lens | Elasticity is lost, increasing the near point of vision (making the near point of best vision farther away). |
| | Lens hardens, compacts, and forms a cataract. |
| Iris and pupil | Decrease in ability to dilate results in small pupil size and poor adaptation to darkness. |

## Activity #2

1. Once in the 30s unless there are eye or vision problems
2. Annually
3. Now, and every 2 to 4 years thereafter (unless eye or vision problems arise)
4. In 2 more years; then every 3 to 5 years (unless eye or vision problems arise)
5. Now, and every 2 to 4 years thereafter (unless eye or vision problems arise)
6. As frequently as recommended by the eye care provider
7. Every 1 to 2 years (unless eye or vision problems arise)
8. As frequently as recommended by the eye care provider
9. Once in the 20s unless there are eye or vision problems
10. Every 1 to 2 years (unless eye or vision problems arise)

## Activity #3

1. B
2. A
3. F
4. H
5. G
6. E
7. D
8. C

## Activity #4

Activities or actions the nurse will teach to patients who have increased intraocular pressure to avoid should resemble these examples. This is not an exhaustive list.

- Bending from the waist
- Lifting objects weighing more than 10 lb
- Sneezing, coughing
- Blowing the nose
- Straining to have a bowel movement
- Vomiting
- Having sexual intercourse
- Keeping the head in a dependent position
- Wearing tight shirt collars or ties

## Activity #5

Descriptions and signs/symptoms of each condition should reflect the information below.

1. Cataract
   a. Description–a lens opacity that distorts vision
   b. Signs/symptoms–slightly blurred vision and decreased color perception

2. Open-angle glaucoma
   a. Description–condition in which intraocular pressure (IOP) is increased
   b. Signs/symptoms–may be asymptomatic in the early stages; initially, a gradual loss of visual fields occurs without affect to central vision. Late signs and symptoms occur after irreversible damage to optic nerve function and include seeing halos around lights, losing peripheral vision, and having decreased visual sensory perception that does not improve with eyeglasses.

3. Corneal abrasion
   a. Description–scrape or scratch injury of the cornea; can be caused by a small foreign body, trauma, contact lens use, malnutrition, dry eye syndromes, and certain cancer therapies. Organisms entering the eye can lead to corneal infection or corneal ulceration.
   b. Signs/symptoms–pain, reduced vision, photophobia, and eye secretions often occur; cloudy or purulent fluid may be present on the eyelids or lashes.

4. Age-related macular degeneration (dry)
   a. Description–deterioration of the macula; leading cause of blindness in the United States.
   b. Signs/symptoms–mild blurring and visual distortion occurs in the early stages; then central and night vision decline, and reading ability is impaired. Eventually, all central vision is lost.

5. Retinal hole
   a. Description–break in the retina caused by trauma (or can occur with aging)
   b. Signs/symptoms–sudden bright flashes of light (sometimes with "floaters"); may feel like a curtain is being pulled over part of the visual field.

6. Myopia
   a. Description–nearsightedness
   b. Signs/symptoms–difficulty in seeing images clearly that are further away.

7. Hyperopia
   a. Description–life-long condition of having farsightedness
   b. Signs/symptoms–difficulty in seeing images clearly that are close to the eyes

8. Presbyopia
   a. Description–age-related problem in which lens elasticity is lost
   b. Signs/symptoms–difficulty seeing images clearly at a reading distance

9. Astigmatism
   a. Description–uneven corneal curve
   b. Signs/symptoms–blurry or distorted images seen at all distances

## Learning Assessments

### NCLEX Examination Challenge #1

Answer: A

Rationale: Myopia (nearsightedness) occurs when the eye overbends the light and images converge in front of the retina (Choice A). Near vision is normal, but distance vision is poor. Myopia is corrected with a concave lens in eyeglasses or contact lenses. In hyperopia (farsightedness), the client has poor near vision (Choice B); emmetropia is the perfect refraction of the eye in which light rays from a distant source are focused into a sharp image on the retina (Choice C); and astigmatism is caused by unevenly curved surfaces on or in the eye, especially the cornea (Choice D). These uneven surfaces distort vision.

### NCLEX Examination Challenge #2

Answer: B

Rationale: OAG, the most common form of primary glaucoma, usually affects both eyes and has no signs or symptoms in the early stages. It develops slowly, with gradual loss of visual fields (Choice B) that may go unnoticed because central vision at first is unaffected. Flashes of light accompanied by floaters often occur with a retinal hole, tear, or detachment (Choice A). Sudden severe pain is associated with hemorrhagic detachment (Choice C). The sensation of a curtain closing over vision is associated with a retinal detachment (Choice D).

### NCLEX Examination Challenge #3

Answer: A, B, D, E

Rationale: The client who has undergone keratoplasty must be taught to avoid activities that increase IOP, such as bending at the waist (Choice A). Jogging, running, dancing, and any other activity that promotes rapid or jerky head motions should be avoided for several weeks after surgery (Choice B). Purulent drainage may be an indication of infection, so this needs to be reported immediately to the surgeon (Choice E). The eye should be examined daily for signs of infection or graft rejection (Choice D). An ongoing leak of clear fluid from the graft site (not tears) and light sensitivity need to be reported to the surgeon right away because these may be signs of complications (Choice C).

## NGN Challenge #1
Answer:

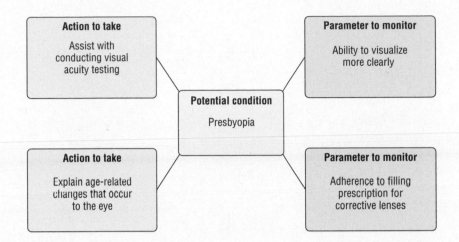

**Rationale:** The 49-year-old client with a recent onset of visual disturbances that include difficulty reading and no other concerning symptoms most likely has presbyopia. Presbyopia is the age-related problem in which the lens loses its elasticity and is less able to change shape to focus the eye for close work. As a result, images fall behind the retina. This problem usually begins in adults in their 40s. The nurse will assist with conducting visual acuity testing because this can demonstrate a difference from baseline and can explain age-related changes that occur to the eye, especially presbyopia. Parameters to monitor include determining the client's ability to visualize more clearly once corrective lenses are obtained.

Glaucoma is unlikely at this age; it also often has a silent onset without symptoms. Macular degeneration is unlikely at this age. There are no symptoms such as a decline in central vision. Without the symptoms of a sudden onset of bright lights in the visual field, retinal detachment is unlikely.

Emergency eye surgery is not necessary to treat presbyopia. Corneal staining, done by placing fluorescein or other topical dye into the conjunctival sac and followed by viewing of the eye through a filter, is done to detect corneal abrasions. The client has no symptoms of corneal abrasion. Gonioscopy is a test performed when a high IOP is found and determines whether open-angle or closed-angle glaucoma is present. There are no symptoms indicating that IOP is high or that glaucoma is present. Therefore, IOP does not need to be monitored because surgery will not be necessary. Monitoring for a reduction in light flashes in the visual field is not necessary. Eye drops will not be used to treat presbyopia.

**NGN Challenge #2**
<u>Answer</u>:

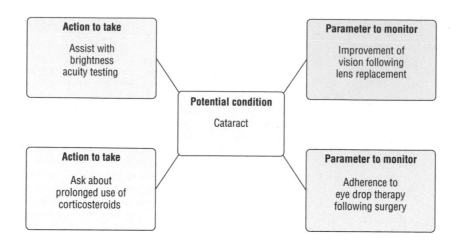

<u>Rationale</u>: The incidence of cataract formation increases with age. By age 75 years, more than half of all Americans have had a cataract. Although both eyes may develop cataracts, the rate of progression is usually different in each eye. Early signs and symptoms include a slight blurring of vision in the affected eye. Later, double vision can occur, and driving at night becomes challenging. The nurse will conduct a full assessment that includes asking about factors that can predispose the development of cataracts, including whether there has been a prolonged use of corticosteroids. A brightness acuity test will be performed as part of an evaluation for cataracts; the nurse can assist with this process. A lens replacement will be conducted because the cataract is removed so the nurse will monitor for adherence to postsurgical eye drop therapy (e.g., antibiotic and corticosteroid eye drops) and for improvement of vision thereafter.

Myopia is nearsightedness. Astigmatism is an uneven corneal curvature. Macular degeneration is characterized by a loss of central vision. None of these conditions is characterized by the symptoms the client reported. Cataracts do not require antiviral eye drops. Increased intake of lutein is recommended for people at risk for dry age-related macular degeneration (AMD). This type of condition is not expected to resolve spontaneously. Vascular endothelial growth factor is used in the treatment of wet AMD. IOP is monitored for patients with glaucoma, not cataracts. This condition is not infectious in nature.

Chapter 40
**Answer Key**
*Chapter Review*
**Pathophysiology Review**

#1

1. F
2. I
3. A
4. D
5. B
6. H
7. J
8. C
9. E
10. G

#2

1. T
2. F
3. T
4. T
5. T
6. F
7. T
8. F
9. T
10. F

**Activities**

**Activity #1**

Changes that occur to the ear structures and findings as a result of the aging process should resemble these answers.

| Ear or Hearing Change |
|---|
| ***Pinna*** becomes elongated because of loss of subcutaneous tissues and decreased elasticity. |
| ***Hair in the canal*** becomes coarser and longer, especially in men. |
| ***Cerumen*** is drier and becomes impacted more easily, reducing hearing function. |
| ***Tympanic membrane*** loses elasticity and may appear dull and retracted. |
| ***Hearing acuity*** decreases (in some people). |
| ***Ability to hear high-frequency sounds*** is lost first. Older adults may have particular problems hearing the *f*, *s*, *sh*, and *pa* sounds. |

**Activity #2**

Nursing adaptations and actions that can be undertaken to address each ear or hearing change that can occur in older adults should resemble these.

| Ear or Hearing Change | Nursing Adaptations and Actions |
|---|---|
| Pinna | • Reassure the patient that this is normal.<br>• When positioning a patient on the side, do not "fold" the ear under the head. |
| Ear canal hair | • Reassure the patient that this is normal.<br>• Provide frequent ear irrigations (if needed) to prevent cerumen attaching to hairs. |
| Cerumen presence | • Request the health care provider perform an assessment and recommend if the patient should self-irrigate the ears.<br>• If recommended by the provider, teach the patient (and caregiver, as necessary) to irrigate the ear canal as often as ordered. |

| Ear or Hearing Change | Nursing Adaptations and Actions |
|---|---|
| Tympanic membrane | • Although this can indicate otitis media, do not use this as the only sign of this condition in older adults. |
| Hearing acuity | • Tell the patient you will speak three words softly, and then ask them to repeat them. You may have to repeat this test once or twice.<br>• If a deficit is assessed, refer the patient to a specialist to further assess hearing loss and recommend appropriate intervention.<br>• Do not assume that all older adults have hearing loss! |
| Ability to hear high-frequency sounds | • Provide a quiet environment when speaking (close the door to the hallway) and face the patient.<br>• Avoid standing or sitting in front of bright lights or windows, which may interfere with the patient's ability to see your lips move.<br>• If the patient wears glasses, be sure that they are using them to enhance speech understanding when reading lips.<br>• Speak slowly, clearly, and in a deeper voice while emphasizing beginning word sounds. |

## Activity #3
1. E—average business office
2. F—conversational speech
3. C—city traffic (from inside a car)
4. A—motorcycle
5. D—nightclub
6. B—sirens

## Activity #4
Ways the nurse will explain the difference between conductive hearing loss and sensorineural hearing loss to a patient should resemble these causes and assessment findings.

| Conductive Hearing Loss | Sensorineural Hearing Loss |
|---|---|
| *Causes* | *Causes* |
| Allergies<br>Cerumen<br>Eustachian tube dysfunction<br>External otitis<br>Fluid presence<br>Foreign body<br>Otitis media<br>Perforation of the tympanic membrane | Aging<br>Auditory tumors<br>Genetic hearing problems<br>Head injury<br>Health disorders (e.g., diabetes, Ménière disease, meningitis, stroke)<br>Ototoxic drugs<br>Prolonged noise exposure |

| Conductive Hearing Loss | Sensorineural Hearing Loss |
|---|---|
| *Assessment Findings* | *Assessment Findings* |
| Cerumen | Difficulty following conversations |
| Hears better out of one ear | Dizziness |
| Narrowing of ear canal | Ear structures appear normal |
| Obstruction with a foreign body | Hearing poorly in a loud environment |
| Otosclerosis | Reports that speech of others is mumbled |
| Otitis externa | Tinnitus |
| Pain in the ear | |
| Report that one's own voice sounds strange | |
| Rupture of tympanic membrane | |
| Rinne test: bone conduction greater than air conduction in affected ear (will not hear fork at ear), and air conduction greater than bone conduction in unaffected ear | Rinne test: air conduction greater than bone conduction in most patients; some with severe loss may report bone conduction greater than air conduction if one ear functions better than the other |
| Weber test: lateralization to affected ear | Weber test: lateralization to unaffected or better-hearing ear |

**Activity #5**

Information about diagnostic studies, as they would be explained to a patient by the nurse, should resemble this information.

| Diagnostic Study | Description |
|---|---|
| Audiometry | *Pure tone audiometry* is done to determine a patient's ability to hear sounds.<br>*Speech audiometry* is used to assess how loud speech must be before the patient can hear it well, and how clearly the patient can understand and distinguish words they hear. |
| BAER (also known as *auditory brainstorm response,* or ABR) | Used to measure brain wave activity that happens when sounds are heard<br>Can be used to help with the diagnoses of hearing loss and acoustic tumors |
| AEP | Used to detect and estimate a patient's hearing level or degree of impairment<br>Can be used to help with diagnosis of auditory disorders, multiple sclerosis, and neurologic disorders that affect balance |
| CDP, also called *balance board testing,* or *equilibrium platform testing* | Used to measure whether a patient can maintain steady balance as the platform they are standing on is manipulated<br>Can be used to identify problematic vestibular symptoms |
| ENG | Used to assess for central and peripheral disease of the vestibular system in the ear by detecting and recording nystagmus<br>Can be used to detect peripheral vestibular system disorders, or to determine the site of a known lesion |
| Tympanometry | Used to assess eardrum mobility, stiffness, or presence of puncture by changing air pressure in the external air canal |

## Learning Assessments

### NCLEX Examination Challenge #1

Answer: A, B, C, D, E

Rationale: The nurse will ask a variety of questions to determine if there may be a problem with a client's auditory sensory perception. It is appropriate to ask if the client has had ear trauma or surgery (Choice A), noticed a change in hearing (Choice B), has had problems with excessive wax (Choice C), has had recent pain or itching (Choice D), and whether they have been exposed to loud noises at work (Choice E). Any of these answered with "yes" by the client might indicate a problem with auditory sensory perception.

### NCLEX Examination Challenge #2

Answer: A, B, C, E

Rationale: To enhance communication with a client who has a hearing impairment, the nurse will sit in adequate lighting (Choice A), facing the client when speaking (Choice C). These actions allow the client to see the nurse's lips move. It is appropriate to use short, simple language that can be better understood (Choice B) as opposed to long sentences that may cause confusion. Talking in a quiet room with minimal distractions is optimum (Choice E). It is not appropriate to primarily address the client's caregiver (Choice D). The client has a hearing impairment, yet this does not mean that they cannot actively make choices about their own health.

### NCLEX Examination Challenge #3

Answer: C

Rationale: An acoustic neuroma is a benign tumor of the vestibulocochlear nerve (cranial nerve VIII). Depending on the size and exact location of the tumor, damage to hearing, facial movements, and sensation can occur. The client who expresses that the tumor is benign but acknowledges the potential implications including neurologic damage has demonstrated understanding (Choice C). Radiation may be part of the treatment, but chemotherapy is not (Choice A). An acoustic neuroma can cause many neurologic signs and symptoms as the tumor enlarges in the brain (Choice B). It can damage other structures as it grows (Choice D); hearing loss may not be the only thing that is affected.

**NGN Challenge #1**
<u>Answer:</u>

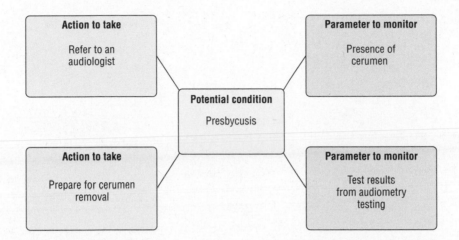

<u>Rationale:</u> This client likely has presbycusis and cerumen build-up. The client does not perceive the hearing degree to be significant other than needing to turn up the television, so further assessment needs to be done to determine if hearing loss is truly present. This testing is likely to be done by an audiologist after having cerumen removed. The nurse will monitor for more cerumen build-up in the future, as well as watch for audiometry test results to learn more about the client's diagnosed condition.

There is no evidence of infection, so the client is not likely to have mastoiditis. There is no vertigo nor tinnitus, so Ménière disease is unlikely.

Hearing aids will not be ordered until cerumen is removed and audiology testing is complete. There is no need for the spouse to drive the client home. CDP testing is done to determine if a client can maintain steady balance while the platform they are standing on is manipulated. Because the client does not report vertigo, this test is unnecessary.

Because vertigo is denied, this does not need to be monitored. Hearing aids are not ordered until testing confirms the need for such. There is no ear infection, so drops for this purpose will not be used.

NGN Challenge #2
Answer:

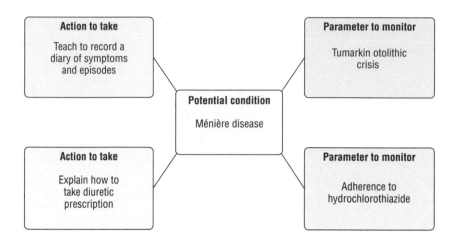

Rationale: Ménière disease is a condition that includes a classic trio of symptoms—episodic vertigo, tinnitus, and hearing loss, which this client reports. Initial treatment for this disorder includes diuretic therapy and symptomatic management. Although there is no discernable pattern yet, the nurse will teach the client to keep a diary of symptoms to determine if a pattern develops or triggers can be identified. The nurse will teach the client about and monitor for the onset of Tumarkin otolithic crisis, known as *sudden drop attacks* in where the client falls to the ground with no warning. It will also be important to monitor the client's adherence to hydrochlorothiazide, which is a diuretic, to see if symptoms decrease.

Because of vertigo, cerumen accumulation and conductive hearing loss are unlikely. Nystagmus is the involuntary movement of the eyes.

Acoustic neuroma is a benign tumor of the vestibulocochlear nerve. Intratympanic gentamicin and labyrinthectomy are treatments that may be considered later if diuretics and symptomatic management fails. This is not an infectious process so antibiotics will not be prescribed, and monitoring for recurrence of infection is unnecessary. There will be no tumor removal–that is an intervention for acoustic neuroma.

# Chapter 41
**Answer Key**
*Chapter Review*
**Anatomy & Physiology Review**
#1.

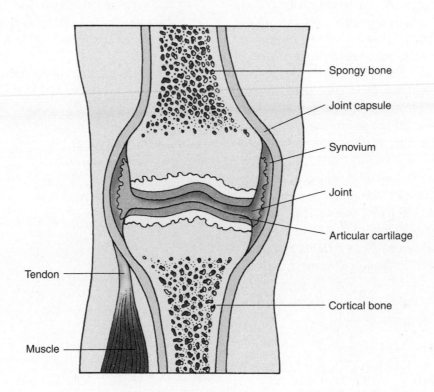

#2.
1. osteoblasts
2. calcium, phosphorus
3. joint
4. Synovial (or Diarthrodial)
5. osteomalacia
6. fascia
7. Muscle atrophy

## Activities

| Activity #1 | Activity #2 |
| --- | --- |

**Activity #1**

1. Any four of these physiologic changes of aging:
   - Decreased bone density
   - Bony prominence
   - Kyphosis
   - Widened gait
   - Joint cartilage degeneration
   - Muscle atrophy
   - Decreased range of motion
   - Slowed movement

**Activity #2**

1. D
2. F
3. H
4. G
5. A
6. E
7. C
8. B

**Activity #3**

Any three of these activities that help promote bone health:

- Teach the client to engage in weight-bearing activities, such as walking and strengthening exercises, to reduce risk factors for osteoporosis and maintain muscle strength.
- Ensure adequate intake of nutrients such as calcium and vitamin D to help prevent bone loss.
- Remind young adults, especially men, that they are at the greatest risk for traumatic injury related to motor vehicle or scooter crashes and should use these devices safely and avoid substance use.
- Teach older adults and their families or caregivers to prevent falls by implementing evidence-based strategies (see Chapter 4).
- Avoid excessive alcohol intake because it can decrease vitamins and nutrients that individuals need for bone and muscle tissue growth.
- Avoid or stop smoking because nicotine can slow bone healing and growth.

**Activity #4**

Any three of these nursing actions would be included in the client's immediate postoperative care, including discharge teaching:

- Perform frequent neurovascular assessments of the surgical extremity.
- Elevate affected extremity to reduce swelling.
- Apply ice to the surgical area to reduce swelling.
- Encourage clients to perform postoperative exercises as instructed, if able.
- Manage surgical pain appropriately, depending on intensity and quality.
- Monitor and teach the patient to observe for:
  o Swelling
  o Severe joint or limb *pain*
  o Thrombophlebitis
  o Infection

**Learning Assessments**

**NCLEX Examination Challenge #1**

Answer: B

Rationale: A painful and inflamed wrist may interfere with the client's ability to perform ADLs or other activity. Therefore, the nurse would observe how well the client can move the wrist as the priority (Choice B). The nurse would also assess the client's left wrist to determine if the client's condition affects other similar joints; however, this assessment would be done later (Choice A). A painful joint should not be palpated (Choice C). Documentation of the client findings would be done after the assessment is completed (Choice D).

**NCLEX Examination Challenge #2**

Answer: B, C, E

Rationale: As the name implies, muscular dystrophy affects muscles in the body, particularly skeletal muscle. When skeletal muscle is inflamed or affected by disease, enzymes in the muscle are produced, released in the bloodstream, and measured through laboratory testing. The muscle enzyme levels are elevated, and include aldolase, creatine kinase (CK-MM subtype), and lactate dehydrogenase (LDH) (Choices B, C, and E). Calcium and alkaline phosphatase are produced or stored in bone rather than in muscles (Choices A and D).

**NCLEX Examination Challenge #3**

Answer: D

Rationale: The nurse would perform neurovascular assessments to monitor for adequate perfusion of the surgical extremity. The radial pulse of 2+ is a normal finding and would not be reported to the surgeon (Choice A). Shoulder pain and the inability to move the affected shoulder would be expected as a result of surgery (Choices B and C). However, the client should not experience any numbness or tingling in the affected arm because this finding may indicate beginning hypoperfusion to the hands. Therefore, this finding would be reported to the surgeon immediately (Choice D).

## Chapter 42

**Answer Key**
*Chapter Review*
**Pathophysiology Review**

#1

1. E
2. H
3. B
4. J
5. D
6. A
7. I
8. G
9. C
10. F

#2

1. T
2. T
3. F
4. T
5. T
6. T
7. T
8. F

## Activities

### Activity #1

Any five of these risk factors that contribute to the development of primary osteoporosis:

- Older age (aged more than 50 years)
- Menopause or history of total hysterectomy, including removal of ovaries
- Parental history of osteoporosis, especially mother
- White or Pacific-Island/Asian ethnicity
- Eating disorders, such as anorexia nervosa
- Rheumatoid arthritis
- History of any fracture after age 50 years
- Low body weight, thin build
- Chronic low calcium and/or vitamin D intake
- Estrogen or androgen deficiency
- Current smoking (active or passive)
- High alcohol intake (two or more drinks a day)
- Drug therapy, such as chronic steroid therapy
- Poor nutrition
- Lack of physical exercise or prolonged decreased mobility

### Activity #2

Any three important teaching points that the nurse would include for a client starting alendronate:

- Teach patients to have an oral assessment and preventive dentistry before beginning any bisphosphonate therapy.
- Patients with poor renal function, hypocalcemia, or GERD should not take bisphosphonates.
- Teach patients to take bisphosphonates early in the morning with 8 ounces of water and wait 30 to 60 minutes in an upright position before eating.
- To promote safety, instruct them to inform any dentist who is planning invasive treatment, such as a tooth extraction or implant, that they are taking a bisphosphonate drug.

**Activity #3**
1. T
2. T
3. T
4. F
5. T
6. T
7. F
8. T

**Activity #4**
1. C
2. E
3. A
4. D
5. B

**Learning Assessments**

**NCLEX Examination Challenge #1**
Answer: A, C, D, E
Rationale: The client with a T-score below −1.5 has osteopenia and likely needs to be managed with drug therapy, such as bisphosphonates, to prevent further bone loss (Choice A). Calcium and vitamin D$_3$ may also be needed depending on the client's nutritional habits (Choice C). Older adults should ensure that interventions are taken to prevent falls, including removing environmental hazards (Choice D). The nurse would also assess the client for other risk factors that likely contributed to osteopenia so they could be prevented or avoided (Choice E). Female clients should avoid having more than one alcoholic drink per day, not two drinks a day. Therefore, Choice B is not correct. Weight-bearing exercises such as walking are better than swimming or other water exercise to help prevent bone loss. Therefore, Choice F is also incorrect.

**NCLEX Examination Challenge #2**
Answer: A
Rationale: The nurse would recognize that the client with advanced metastatic bone cancer typically has severe pain that is difficult to manage at the EOL. Therefore, the nurse would refer the client and family to hospice that specializes in EOL and palliative care, including pain management (Choice A). The nurse should not participate in passive or active euthanasia because this action is an ethical breach of professional conduct and may be illegal, depending on the geographic location (Choice B). Spiritual leaders or clergy may be requested, but the nurse should not assume the client and family want or need spiritual support (Choice D). The client should already be receiving opioids but not necessarily via the IV route at EOL. Many opioids are available as patches, suppositories, and/or sublingual tablets, depending on the presence of nausea and/or vomiting (Choice C).

**NGN Challenge #1**
Answer: The nurse analyzes the data and determines that the client is most likely experiencing **osteomyelitis, draining wound with cellulitis, and fever.**
Rationale: The client is an older client who has diabetes mellitus and a draining nonhealing ankle ulcer with cellulitis. In this case, cellulitis occurred when the wound infection entered the surrounding tissues, causing swelling, redness, heat, and pain. Additionally, this client has throbbing deep localized ankle pain when the foot is moved and has an increasing temperature to over 101°F (38.3°C). These classic symptoms indicate that the client most likely has osteomyelitis. The client may also have *chronic* peripheral vascular disease, which commonly occurs in clients who are diabetic. However, this is not the client's *acute* condition at this time. The client's blood glucose is elevated but not to the level that would cause a hyperglycemic complication. Given that the client most likely has osteomyelitis, the evidence for this condition is a draining wound with cellulitis and a fever of higher than 101°F (38.3°C). The other options are associated with other health conditions.

**NGN Challenge #2**
Answer: A, B, D, E
Rationale: The client has a fever and severe pain and therefore requires close monitoring of vital signs (Choice A) and pain medication around the clock on a regular basis. Bone pain can be very intense

and unrelenting (Choice B). A long course of IV antibiotic therapy is the main treatment for acute osteomyelitis. These drugs need to be administered in a timely manner to ensure a continuous and consistent serum drug concentration (Choice D). The client's blood glucose levels also need frequent monitoring before meals and at bedtime for the sliding scale insulin regimen (Choice E). The wound is infected and does not require the use of sterile technique when changing the dressing. Clean technique is required instead (Choice C).

Oxygen therapy is not needed because the $SpO_2$ is only slightly below normal, which is typical for older adults (Choice F). If the client has difficulty breathing or if the $SpO_2$ continues to decrease, the nurse would begin supplemental oxygen. The client's ankle should not be elevated on two pillows because the client has a nonpalpable pedal pulse indicating the presence of peripheral arterial disease. Elevation of the ankle would decrease perfusion to the distal foot, which is already compromised (Choice G).

## Chapter 43

**Answer Key**
*Chapter Review*
**Pathophysiology Review**

#1
1. G
2. E
3. H
4. D
5. B
6. I
7. A
8. C
9. F

#2
1. F
2. F
3. T
4. T
5. T

## Activities

### Activity #1
Any three lifestyle habits or activities that promote joint health and help prevent development of osteo-arthritis:
- Maintain proper nutrition to prevent obesity or participate in an evidence-based weight reduction program if needed.
- Take care to avoid injuries, especially those that can occur from professional or amateur sports.
- Avoid participating in risky behaviors that could cause trauma and subsequent arthritis.
- Take adequate work breaks to rest joints in jobs where repetitive motion or joint stress is common.
- Stay active and maintain a healthy lifestyle, including regular physical activity and exercise, if possible.

### Activity #2
Any four of these preoperative instructions the nurse would provide to help prevent infection in the client who has a total hip or knee arthroplasty:
- Expect to receive an IV antibiotic before surgery and possibly up to 24 hours after surgery.
- It is important to be screened for nares (nose) colonization of *Staphylococcus aureus* 2 to 4 weeks before surgery.
- Use nasal mupirocin ointment twice a day for 1 week (or longer depending on the nasal culture) before surgery.
- Bathe with chlorhexidine gluconate (CHG) solution or wipes for at least the night before and the morning of surgery (a longer time may be needed depending on agency or surgeon protocol).
- Sleep on clean linens and do not use lotions or powders after the CHG baths; avoid sleeping with pets in the bed.

## Activity #3

1. T
2. T
3. T
4. F
5. F
6. T
7. T
8. T
9. T
10. F

## Activity #4

1. D
2. C
3. H
4. B
5. I
6. E
7. A
8. G
9. F

## Activity #5

Any three of these ways to protect joints of patients with arthritis:

- Use large joints instead of small ones; for example, place your purse strap over your shoulder instead of grasping the purse with your hand.
- Do not turn a doorknob clockwise. Turn it counterclockwise to avoid twisting your arm and promoting ulnar deviation (especially for patients who also have rheumatoid arthritis).
- Use two hands instead of one to hold objects.
- Sit in a chair that has a high, straight back.
- When getting out of bed, do not push off with your fingers; use the entire palm of both hands.
- Do not bend at your waist; instead, bend your knees while keeping your back straight.
- Use long-handled devices, such as a hairbrush with an extended handle.
- Use assistive/adaptive devices, such as Velcro closures and built-up utensil handles to protect your joints.
- Do not use pillows in bed except a small one under your head.
- Avoid twisting or wringing your hands; use a device or rubber grip to open jars or bottles.

## Activity #6

Any two of these actions for each complication:

| Potential Complication | Nursing/Collaborative Actions |
|---|---|
| Venous thromboembolism | 1. Get patient out of bed on surgical day.<br>2. Administer anticoagulant as prescribed.<br>3. Apply sequential compression devices to lower extremities while in bed.<br>4. Ambulate patient as soon as possible.<br>5. Encourage fluid intake. |
| Skin breakdown | 1. Keep the patient's heels off the bed.<br>2. Get patient out of bed several times a day and change position every 1 to 2 hours while in bed.<br>3. Encourage increased protein and Vitamin C foods for skin health. |
| Infection | 1. Monitor vital signs, especially temperature.<br>2. Monitor WBC count for changes.<br>3. Monitor surgical incision for signs and symptoms of infection. |
| Decreased mobility | 1. Get the patient out of bed on the surgical day.<br>2. Collaborate with PT and OT as needed.<br>3. Teach patient how to perform active range-of-motion exercises.<br>4. Manage pain using a multimodal approach. |

### Activity #7

Any three of these nursing interventions to address physical disability:

- Assess the patient's mobility, ADL, and IADL function, and incorporate those abilities into the plan of care.
- If needed, refer the patient to appropriate rehabilitation therapists (PT and/or OT) for evaluation of mobility and/or ADL function.
- If the patient is able to ambulate with or without a walker or other gait aid, continue to ambulate the patient daily if in any inpatient setting, if possible.
- Assess the patient's coping skills in living with a physical disability; refer the patient to appropriate inpatient or community resources as needed to improve coping and quality of life.
- Determine if the patient is aware of or has obtained preventive health screenings and practices healthy lifestyle habits if the patient's living situation supports those activities.
- Assess any social determinants of health that impact the ability of the patient to have access to health care; incorporate these factors into the patient's plan of care, including providing community resources and referrals.

## Learning Assessments

### NCLEX Examination Challenge #1

Answer: D

Rationale: Osteoarthritis is caused by deterioration and degeneration of joint cartilage and is not a primary inflammatory condition. It is characterized by bony nodules, especially on the finger joints, which is consistent with Choice D. Choice A describes an inflammatory arthritis. Spongy joints indicate inflamed synovium (Choice B); subcutaneous nodules are common in clients who have late-stage rheumatoid arthritis (Choice C).

### NCLEX Examination Challenge #2

Answer: B

Rationale: Clients who have an anterior surgical approach for a traditional total hip arthroplasty do not commonly dislocate their new hip and, therefore, abduction with a pillow or splint is not needed (Choices A and D). The postoperative client should not be placed flat to aid in lung expansion (Choice C). The head of the bed should be raised slightly to between a 15- and 30- degree elevation and the legs kept in a neutral position to prevent hip rotation (Choice B).

### NCLEX Examination Challenge #3

Answer: C

Rationale: The client likely is having an acute gout attack, which requires either colchicine or an NSAID such as indomethacin or ibuprofen to get pain under control (Choice C). Methotrexate is used to treat rheumatoid arthritis (Choice A). Allopurinol is given to manage chronic gout and is not effective for acute gout (Choice B). Acetaminophen is an analgesic but has no antiinflammatory properties, which this client needs at this time (Choice D).

**NGN Challenge**
*Item #1*
Answer:

| Health History | Nurses Notes | Orders | Laboratory Results |
|---|---|---|---|

**1405:** Client returned from PT at 1320 reporting feeling "very tired." 6/10 right hip pain; pain medication administered. Assisted to bed by UAP.

**1650:** UAP reported that client fell while going to the bathroom without assistance. Client did not use call light to seek assistance after fall and tried to ambulate back to bed using a walker. Could not bear weight and yelled for help. States right hip pain currently 9/10. New pain in posterior left calf. Left leg calf has 3-in (7.6-cm) reddened, tender, and warm intact area. Right (surgical) leg slightly shorter than left and internally rotated. Client crying and asking for family. VS: T 98.2°F (36.8°C); HR 88 beats per minute; RR 20 breaths per minute; BP 135/74 mm Hg; $SpO_2$ 94%.

Rationale: The nurse would be concerned that the client fell, which resulted in increased right hip pain (9/10), an inability to bear weight, and a shorter, rotated right leg, suggesting injury from the fall. In addition, the client has a left calf area that is reddened, tender, and warm. This finding is a new finding that would be of immediate concern to the nurse because it suggests a possible postoperative complication. The client's VS are within normal limits with the exception of the BP and oxygen saturation. The BP elevation is likely from the client's acute pain as a sympathetic response causing vasoconstriction. The client's BP is not at a life-threatening level and would not need follow up at this time. When the client's pain is reduced, the BP will likely also decrease. The client's $SpO_2$ is only slightly lower than the adult normal of more than or equal to 95%, but the client has no respiratory changes. Older adults often have slightly lower peripheral oxygen saturation levels without any respiratory distress.

*Item #2*
Answer: Based on the <u>assessment</u> findings, the nurse determines that the client most likely has **right hip dislocation** and **left deep vein thrombosis**.
Rationale: The client dislocated the surgical hip prosthesis as evidenced by intense right hip pain, affected leg shortening and rotation, and inability to bear any weight on the hip. The client also has evidence of left calf DVT, which is manifested by redness, swelling, warmth, and pain. DVT is a common postoperative complication for clients who have a total hip or knee arthroplasty. Although the client may have hypertension, the elevated BP could be the result of the typical sympathetic response when one has severe acute pain. The client is not oriented ×4 as expected, but this problem could be due to the client experiencing severe pain and a fall. There is no other indication that the client has dementia. Stage 1 pressure injuries often appear as reddened areas with warmth and possible <u>tenderness</u>, but they are not usually swollen. Additionally, pressure injuries rarely occur on a client's calf. Instead, they tend to occur over bony prominences such as the sacrum and heels.

*Item #3*
Answer: Based on the client's condition, the nurse determines that the *priority* for care is most likely managing the client's **deep vein thrombosis** because this condition can lead to **pulmonary embolism**.
Rationale: Of the two current client conditions, the most potentially life-threatening condition is the client's DVT because a piece of the clot can dislodge and travel to the lungs, causing pulmonary embolism, or to another major organ. Because this condition is potentially life-threatening, it is the *priority* for the client's care. Managing the hip dislocation is also important but it not life-threatening, although very painful. It is not known if the client has hypertension, and the current BP level is not extremely high such that it could cause life-threatening complications such as a stroke.

## Item #4
Answer:
Which of the <u>following</u> orders would the nurse anticipate to be included? **Select all that apply.**

- **X** Establish peripheral IV access.
- **X** Prepare for administration of moderate sedation.
- o Administer supplemental oxygen 2 L/min via nasal cannula.
- **X** Initiate continuous pulse oximetry.
- o Maintain continuous cardiac monitoring via telemetry.
- o Give IV antibiotic therapy to begin after wound culture is obtained.
- **X** Begin drug therapy with a DOAC per protocol.

<u>Rationale:</u> The nurse would ensure that the client is treated for the DVT as the priority for care by starting the client on a higher dose of apixaban or administering a different DOAC, depending on the surgeon's preference or agency protocol. The affected leg would be elevated to decrease swelling. IV access would be needed for moderate sedation and any emergency drugs that may be required later. Moderate sedation is needed for reduction of the hip dislocation. Oxygen <u>saturation</u> monitoring would be appropriate during this procedure to ensure adequate oxygenation. Oxygen therapy and cardiac monitoring are not indicated at this time because the $SpO_2$ is currently close to normal range. The client does not require antibiotic therapy because there is no evidence that the hip incision is infected.

## Item #5
Answer:
Select **two** interventions that the nurse would implement based on these client findings.

- o Administer supplemental oxygen at 2 L/min via nasal cannula.
- **X** Rub the client's sternum several times until respirations increase.
- **X** Speak in a loud voice to remind the client to keep breathing.
- o Place the client in a flat supine position.
- o Stop the procedure and reschedule for another day.

<u>Rationale:</u> The client's findings during the hip dislocation reduction procedure indicate that the client was experiencing respiratory depression: the $SpO_2$ decreased from 94% to 88%, the client's RR decreased to 10 breaths/min, and the end-<u>tidal</u> carbon dioxide level dropped to 26 mm Hg (normal range is 30–45 mm Hg). The nurse would first rub the client's sternum and tell the client to breathe to provide stimulate respirations. For many clients, these interventions are effective. If not effective, the client may need oxygen supplementation but not at this point. The client would not be placed supine but likely would have the head slightly elevated to promote lung expansion. If possible, the procedure would be completed as quickly as possible.

## Item #6
Answer:

| Previous Client Findings | Current Client Findings (Today) | Improving | Not Improving/ Declining |
|---|---|---|---|
| 9/10 right hip pain | 4/10 right hip pain | X | |
| Left swollen calf that is reddened, warm, and tender | Slight redness and tenderness; no swelling | X | |
| Alert and oriented ×1 | Alert and oriented ×1 | | X |
| Able to ambulate with walker until fall | Not able to ambulate with walker | | X |
| BP 135/74 | BP 120/70 | X | |
| $SpO_2$ 94% on RA | $SpO_2$ 96% on RA | X | |

<u>Rationale:</u> As a result of nursing and collaborative interventions, the client's right hip pain decreased because the hip was relocated into the correct anatomical position. The left DVT improved because the calf is less red and tender, and there is now no swelling. The client's BP and $SpO_2$ are now within normal range for an adult. However, the client is not able to ambulate yet and is still disoriented. The client would likely return to rehabilitation to resume PT and OT.

## Chapter 44

### Answer Key
#### *Chapter Review*
**Pathophysiology Review**

#1

1. D
2. H
3. B
4. E
5. G
6. A
7. F
8. C

#2

1. T
2. T
3. T
4. T
5. F
6. T
7. T
8. F

### Activities

#### Activity #1
Any five of these areas would be included by the nurse in a neurovascular assessment:
- Capillary refill
- Skin temperature
- Skin color
- Presence of edema
- Pain level
- Distal pulses
- Ability to move

#### Activity #2
The six Ps include **p**ain, **p**ressure, **p**aralysis, **p**aresthesia, **p**allor, and **p**ulselessness.

#### Activity #3
1. T
2. T
3. T
4. F
5. T
6. T
7. F
8. T
9. T
10. T

#### Activity #4
Any three of these health teaching statements the nurse would provide to help adults promote health to prevent an elective or traumatic amputation:
- Maintain a healthy weight.
- Engage in regular exercise.
- Avoid smoking.
- Take safety precautions at work or home.
- Avoid speeding.
- Avoid driving while drinking alcohol.

#### Activity #5
**R:** Rest
**I:** Ice
**C:** Compression
**E:** Elevation

## Learning Assessments

### NCLEX Examination Challenge #1
Answer: D

Rationale: By lying prone several times a day, the client would be keeping the affected hip joint in a neutral position to counteract the natural tendency of the hip flexor muscles to create a contracture (Choice D). A firm mattress would also help, but by itself is not the most effective method to help prevent a hip contracture (Choice A). The nurse would teach the client to perform active ROM exercises but not perform passive exercises (Choice B). The surgical leg should not be highly elevated on two firm pillows because this position would promote hip contracture (Choice C).

### NCLEX Examination Challenge #2
Answer: B

Rationale: Phantom limb pain is real to the client and needs to be promptly managed by the nurse by giving medication (Choice B). Choice C is a response that allows the nurse to collect more data about the pain, but it is not addressing the client's immediate need. Choices A and D are nontherapeutic responses because they do not acknowledge the client's pain as real.

### NCLEX Examination Challenge #3
Answer: B, C, D, E

Rationale: All of the symptoms are consistent with complex regional pain syndrome (CRPS) except for Choice A, which is a decreased pedal pulse. CRPS is a poorly understood dysfunction of the central and peripheral nervous systems that leads to severe, persistent pain and other symptoms. It does not affect perfusion to distal extremities.

### NGN Challenge
*Item #1*
Answer:

| Health History | Nurses Notes | Orders | Laboratory Results |
|---|---|---|---|

**0755:** Client reports severe throbbing pain in left lower leg that radiates into the foot. Rates pain at 7/10. Left leg immobilized via splint and bulky gauze wrap after closed fracture reduction. Analgesic administered an hour ago. Left lower leg significantly swollen when compared with right. Right pedal pulse 2+; left pedal pulse 1+. Left leg less pigmented when compared to right. Cap refill >3 seconds in left leg; <3 seconds in right leg. Client alert and oriented × 4. Lung sounds clear in all fields. $S_1$ and $S_2$ present. Bowel sounds present × 4. VS: T 98.2°F (36.8°C); HR 92 beats/min; RR 20 breaths/min; BP 125/66 mm Hg; SpO$_2$ 97% on RA.

Rationale: The nurse would be concerned that analgesia an hour ago did not significantly reduce the client's pain because it is reported as 7 on a 1 to 10 pain intensity scale (7/10). Additionally, the nurse would be concerned because the pain radiates, and the affected leg is swollen and less pigmented than the unaffected leg. Pedal pulses are unequal with a normal pulse in the right foot and a diminished pulse in the left foot. Capillary refill is also unequal in that it is normal in the right foot but not normal in the affected left foot. All of these findings are unexpected and abnormal. The other physical assessment data are within normal range except for the systolic BP, which is slightly elevated. This client finding is most likely the result of a sympathetic response because the client is experiencing acute pain.

*Item #2*
Answer: Based on the assessment findings, the nurse determines that the client is at high risk for **acute compartment syndrome,** which causes **hypoperfusion**.

Rationale: The client has a number of findings that suggest that the affected leg is not receiving adequate perfusion to supply oxygen to distal tissues, including decreased pedal pulse, pallor, and prolonged capillary refill. If this neurovascular compromise worsens, the client is at high risk for acute compartment syndrome (ACS). Cellulitis and necrotizing fasciitis are infections that would be consistent with reddened rather than less pigmented or pale skin. The client would also likely have a fever. Although peripheral vascular disease (PVD) can also cause the pedal pulse to be diminished, it is usually bilateral and both pulses would likely be diminished. Additionally, the pain of PVD is usually not as severe as the acute intense pain associated with ACS.

### Item #3
Answer: Based on the client's condition, the nurse determines that the **_priority_** for care is to prevent **tissue necrosis**.

Rationale: When body tissue has prolonged hypoperfusion, the lack of oxygen and glucose results in cellular death, or tissue necrosis. If this condition occurs, the client can develop gangrene and may need an amputation. Therefore, preventing tissue necrosis by increasing perfusion is the client's **_priority_** for care. Necrosed tissue can become infected and, if not treated effectively, can cause sepsis. However, this process occurs after tissue necrosis occurs and is not the priority. There is no indication that the client has hypovolemia, and, therefore, the client is presently not at risk for hypovolemic shock. Complex regional pain syndrome (CRPS) is a chronic condition that usually occurs weeks after the traumatic event. It does not affect distal pulses.

### Item #4
Answer: A, B, F

Rationale: The surgeon would likely prescribe additional pain medication while ensuring that the nurse would perform more frequent neurovascular assessments (Choices A and B). Currently, the pedal pulse for the affected foot is diminished at 1+, but the client's foot is still being perfused. However, if the pulse becomes nonpalpable, the surgeon would want to be notified because this change indicates that hypoperfusion is worsening (Choice F). The nurse would not elevate the affected leg because this position would slow arterial blood flow to the affected leg and foot (Choice C). Although the bulky dressing of a splint may be loosened by the surgeon, nurses would not remove the splint because the reduced fracture is not yet healed (Choice D). The client's heels should be kept off the bed to prevent heel pressure injury; however, this action is not associated with the client's current acute issue of neurovascular compromise (Choice E).

### Item #5
Answer: A, B, C, D, E

Rationale: All of these actions are needed in preparation for the client's surgery. The client needs to be informed and understand what is involved with the surgical procedure and postoperative care and sign the informed consent to have the procedure performed (Choices C and D). The nurse would notify the family or ensure that the client contacted the family, depending on how the client feels (Choice B). The nurse would also continue to perform frequent neurovascular assessments and keep the client on NPO status (Choices A and E).

### Item #6
Answer:

| Previous Client Findings | Current Client Findings (Today) | Improving | Not Improving |
|---|---|---|---|
| Severe pain reported at 10/10 | Pain reported at 2/10 | X | |
| Left leg capillary refill >3 seconds | Left leg capillary refill <3 seconds | X | |
| Left nonpalpable pedal pulse | Left pedal pulse 1+ | X | |
| Left lower leg and ankle edema | Left lower leg and ankle edema | | X |

Rationale: The client had an open fasciotomy to relieve the pressure in the lower left leg and increase perfusion to the distal tissues of the foot and ankle. The current findings of 2/10 pain, left capillary refill <3 seconds, and a left pedal pulse of 1+ indicate that perfusion to the affected foot is increased to prevent tissue necrosis. However, the client continues to have edema, which demonstrates that assessment finding has not improved.

## Chapter 45
**Answer Key**
*Chapter Review*
**Anatomy & Physiology Review**
#1.

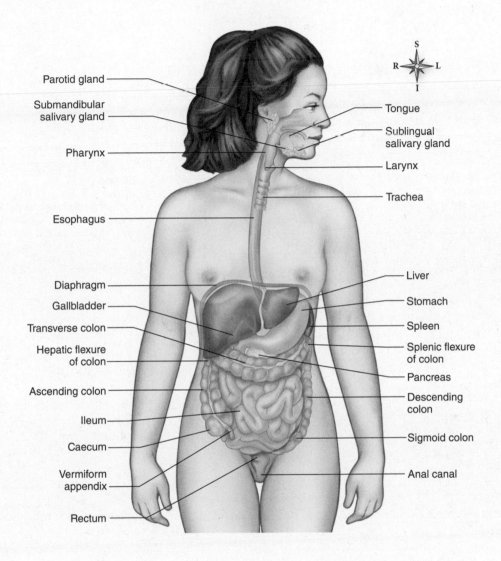

Parotid gland

Submandibular
salivary gland

Pharynx

Esophagus

Diaphragm

Gallbladder

Transverse colon

Hepatic flexure
of colon

Ascending colon

Ileum

Caecum

Vermiform
appendix

Rectum

Tongue

Sublingual
salivary gland

Larynx

Trachea

Liver

Stomach

Spleen

Splenic flexure
of colon

Pancreas

Descending
colon

Sigmoid colon

Anal canal

#2. Labels include:

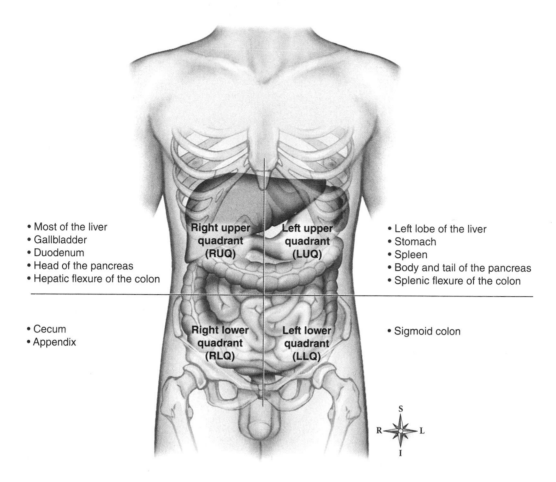

- Most of the liver
- Gallbladder
- Duodenum
- Head of the pancreas
- Hepatic flexure of the colon

**Right upper quadrant (RUQ)**

**Left upper quadrant (LUQ)**

- Left lobe of the liver
- Stomach
- Spleen
- Body and tail of the pancreas
- Splenic flexure of the colon

- Cecum
- Appendix

**Right lower quadrant (RLQ)**

**Left lower quadrant (LLQ)**

- Sigmoid colon

## Activities

### Activity #1

Answers should resemble changes in the gastrointestinal system that are associated with aging, and their associated implications.

| Physiologic Change | Implications |
|---|---|
| Atrophy of the gastric mucosa leads to decreased hydrochloric acid levels (hypochlorhydria). | Decreased absorption of iron and Vitamin $B_{12}$ and proliferation of bacteria. Atrophic gastritis occurs as a consequence of bacterial overgrowth. |
| Peristalsis decreases and nerve impulses are dulled. | Decreased sensation to defecate can result in postponement of bowel movements, which leads to constipation and impaction. |
| Distention and dilation of pancreatic ducts change. Calcification of pancreatic vessels occurs with a decrease in lipase production. | Decreased lipase level results in decreased fat absorption and digestion. Steatorrhea (fatty stool) occurs because of decreased fat digestion. |

| Physiologic Change | Implications |
|---|---|
| A decrease in the number and size of hepatic cells leads to decreased liver weight and mass. This change and an increase in fibrous tissue lead to decreased protein synthesis and changes in liver enzymes. Enzyme activity and cholesterol synthesis are diminished. | Decreased enzyme activity depresses drug metabolism, which leads to accumulation of drugs—possibly to toxic levels. |
| Intestinal microbiota abnormalities occur during the aging process. | Dysfunctional microbial activity contributes to anorexia and subsequent undernutrition. |

## Activity #2

Examples of drugs or substances that irritate the gastrointestinal system include, but are not limited to:

1. NSAIDs
2. Aspirin
3. Alcohol
4. Caffeine

## Activity #3

1. Borborygmus
2. Flatulence
3. Bruit
4. NPO
5. Steatorrhea

## Activity #4

1. T
2. F
3. T
4. T
5. F
6. T
7. F
8. T
9. F
10. T

## Activity #5

1. Virtual colonoscopy
2. Sigmoidoscopy
3. Guaiac-based fecal occult blood test
4. Esophagogastroduodenoscopy
5. Enteroscopy
6. Endoscopy
7. Endoscopic retrograde cholangiopancreatography
8. Colonoscopy

## Learning Assessments

### NCLEX Examination Challenge #1

Answer: B

Rationale: Midazolam is commonly used for sedation with procedures such as an esophagogastroduodenoscopy or a colonoscopy. Drugs such as this can depress the rate and depth of respirations. Thus the nurse's priority assessment is checking the client's rate and depth of respirations (Choice B). If the client's respiratory rate is below 10 breaths/min or the exhaled carbon dioxide level falls below 20%, the nurse uses a stimulus such as a sternal rub to encourage deeper and faster respirations. After the nurse has assessed the client's respiratory status, the level of consciousness (Choice A), heart rate and rhythm (Choice C), and bowel sounds (Choice D) can be assessed.

### NCLEX Examination Challenge #2

Answer: A, B, C, D, E

Rationale: All of these options must be included in the care provided to the client immediately after colonoscopy. Vital signs must be monitored (Choice A), and assessment for abdominal pain and guarding must be done (Choice B); these could indicate early signs of a complication. To prevent aspiration, the client must be maintained on NPO status (Choice C). The top rails of the bed should be kept up until the client regains consciousness (Choice D) because they are at risk for falls until the anesthesia wears off. Left lateral position facilitates the passing of flatus (Choice E).

**NCLEX Examination Challenge #3**
Answer: C
Rationale: Gastrointestinal causes of decreased potassium include vomiting, gastric suctioning (Choice C), diarrhea, and drainage from intestinal fistulas. Liver disease (Choice A), malabsorption (Choice B), and acute pancreatitis (Choice D) are not associated directly with hypokalemia.

## Chapter 46
### Answer Key
### *Chapter Review*
**Pathophysiology Review**

#1
1. H
2. D
3. B
4. J
5. C
6. F
7. E
8. I
9. A
10. G

#2 Any of these factors can contribute to decreased lower esophageal sphincter pressure.
- Caffeinated beverages
- Coffee, tea, and cola
- Chocolate
- Nitrates
- Citrus fruits
- Tomatoes and tomato products
- Alcohol
- Peppermint, spearmint
- Smoking and other tobacco products
- Calcium channel blockers
- Anticholinergic drugs
- High levels of estrogen and progesterone
- Nasogastric tube placement

## Activities

**Activity #1**
1. T
2. F
3. T
4. T
5. T
6. F
7. F
8. F
9. T
10. F

**Activity #2**
Actions the nurse will take when caring for a patient with an oral cavity include, but are not limited to:
- Remove dentures if the patient has severe stomatitis or oral pain.
- Encourage the patient who is able to do so to perform oral hygiene twice daily, after meals, and as often as needed. Ensure mouth care is provided if the client is unable.
- Increase oral care frequency to every 2 hours or more if stomatitis is not controlled.
- Teach patient to use a soft toothbrush or gauze, to use toothpaste free of sodium lauryl sulfate (SLS), and to avoid commercial mouthwashes and lemon-glycerin swabs, which can irritate mucosa.

- Encourage frequent rinsing of the mouth with warm saline, sodium bicarbonate (baking soda) solution, or a combination of these solutions.
- Help the patient select soft, bland, and nonacidic foods.
- Apply topical analgesics or anesthetics as prescribed by the primary health care provider, and document effectiveness.

**Activity #4**
1. F
2. E
3. C
4. A
5. D
6. B

### Activity #3
Actions that are contained within the PASS acronym for dysphagia include:
- Assess if it is **P**robable that the patient will have swallowing difficulty.
- **A**ccount for previous swallowing problems.
- **S**creen for signs and symptoms.
- Obtain a **S**peech-language pathologist (SLP) referral.

## Learning Assessments

### NCLEX Examination Challenge #1
Answer: D
Rationale: Chemical injury is usually a result of the accidental or intentional ingestion of caustic substances (Choice D). The damage to the mouth and esophagus is rapid and severe. Acid burns tend to affect the superficial mucosal lining, whereas alkaline substances cause deeper penetrating injuries. Strong alkalis can cause full perforation of the esophagus within 1 minute. Additional complications may include aspiration pneumonia and hemorrhage. Esophageal strictures may develop as scar tissue forms. Nasogastric tube placement (Choice A), esophageal ulcers (Choice B), and impact from a foreign object (Choice C) are not associated with intentional causes for esophageal trauma.

### NCLEX Examination Challenge #2
Answer: A, B, C, D
Rationale: The client with GERD can benefit from restricting or avoiding caffeinated or carbonated beverages (Choice A), which can irritate tissues. Eating slowly and chewing food thoroughly can assist with digestion (Choice B), as can consuming small meals daily instead of large meals that can induce reflux (Choice C). Avoidance of eating for at least 3 hours before bed can minimize the incidence of GERD (Choice D). The client must be taught to sleep propped up to promote gas exchange and prevent regurgitation rather than laying on the side (Choice E). This can be done by placing blocks under the head of the bed or by using a large, wedge-style pillow instead of a standard pillow.

### NCLEX Examination Challenge #3
Answer: A
Rationale: Tobacco use increases the chance of development of leukoplakia. The nurse will ask the client about any current or historical tobacco use as the priority (Choice A). Asking about alcohol use (Choice B), fast food meals (Choice C), and dental checkups (Choice D) can all be done after learning whether the client uses tobacco products.

**NGN Challenge**
**Item #1**
Answer:

| Health History | Nurses Notes | Vital Signs | Laboratory Results | |
|---|---|---|---|---|

**1202:** Client moved here from another state; wishes to establish care with this primary health care provider. All health records from previous provider are accessible in the electronic health record. Client reports no preexisting medical history other than removal of tonsils as a child. Family history of type 2 diabetes. Lives at home with spouse and 2-year-old child. States, "I feel pretty good overall but lately I've been burping a lot after meals, and I have some burning in my chest." Indicates a preference for fast food because of traveling extensively for work. Drinks 1 to 2 glasses of water daily and about 3 to 4 cans of soda. Denies change in usual dietary habits and bowel or bladder patterns. Denies abdominal pain.

Rationale: Information that requires the nurse to assess further includes burping after meals, having chest burning, eating fast food regularly, drinking only 1 to 2 glasses of water daily, and consuming 3 to 4 cans of soda daily. Burping after meals with a burning in the chest is indicative of reflux. Eating fast food regularly could be a contributor to these symptoms because fast food often is fried or contains spices, both of which aggravate reflux. Drinking only 1 to 2 glasses of water daily is much less than the recommended 6 to 8 glasses; drinking 3 to 4 sodas instead can increase lower esophageal sphincter pressure and further contribute to reflux. This much soda is also nutritionally unhealthy, requiring the nurse to further assess.

**Item #2**
Answer: The client is at high risk for **reflux** as evidenced by **burning in the chest.**
Rationale: Burping excessively with chest burning are characteristic signs of reflux. There are no symptoms that indicate the presence of esophageal tumor or stomatitis. Gas bloat syndrome occurs when clients have difficulty belching to relieve distention. The client's heart rate and oral cavity assessments are within normal parameters. Although the client's blood pressure is elevated, it is not the option that predisposes the client to reflux.

**Item #3**
Answer: The *priority* for the client at this time is to manage **reflux** to prevent **Barrett esophagus**.
Rationale: Nighttime reflux causes prolonged exposure of the esophagus to acid when the client is in the supine position. Secretions do not drain back down with gravity. This causes erosion to the esophageal tissues. As the tissues heal, the body may substitute Barrett epithelium (columnar epithelium) for the normal squamous cell epithelium of the lower esophagus; this becomes known as Barrett esophagus. Although this new tissue is more resistant to acid and supports esophageal healing, it is premalignant and is associated with an increased risk for cancer in patients with prolonged GERD.

Therefore, the nurse will prioritize management of reflux to prevent development of Barrett esophagus.

**Item #4**
Answer: A, F, G
Rationale: Carbonated, spicy, fried, fatty, and acidic foods and beverages can aggravate reflux. The nurse will teach the client to avoid these kinds of foods and beverages, which include soda (carbonated), orange juice (acidic), and fried chicken (fried and fatty). Yogurt, applesauce, baked fish, cooked rice, mashed potatoes, and grilled hamburgers are foods that the client can enjoy that usually do not contribute to reflux.

**Item #5**
Answer: A, C, D, E, F, G, I
Rationale: The nurse will teach the client ways to manage gastroesophageal reflux disease following diagnosis. Bending at the abdomen increases lower esophageal sphincter (LES) pressure, so the nurse will teach the client to avoid doing this. The nurse will also encourage keeping a food diary because this can help the client to trend intake and identify foods that cause symptoms. Spicy foods and foods containing things like mint should be avoided because these can contribute to reflux. Weight loss can lower LES pressure. Propping up on a pillow

when lying down helps to facilitate digestion because food does not travel backward through the esophagus. A registered dietitian nutritionist can work with the client to plan meals that do not aggravate reflux. The nurse will teach the client to avoid eating 3 hours before bed, not 1 hour. This does not allow enough time for the food to begin digestion. Acidic foods and beverages such as grapefruit juice can increase the incidence of reflux and create substernal burning. The client will be taught to eat 4 to 6 small meals daily to facilitate digestion rather than eating 2 to 3 large meals.

*Item #6*
<u>Answer:</u>

| Previous Client Finding | Current Client Finding | Effective | Not Effective |
|---|---|---|---|
| Burping after meals | Reports incidence of burping has decreased | X | |
| Feels burning in chest | Says burning in chest occurs less often than it did previously | X | |
| Eats at fast food locations often | Eats at fast food locations often | | X |
| Drinks 1 to 2 glasses of water daily | Drinks 3 glasses of water daily | X | |
| Consumes 3 to 4 cans of soda daily | Drinks 2 cans of soda daily | X | |

<u>Rationale:</u> Reports of a decreasing incidence of burping and less frequent episodes of burning in the chest help to verify that earlier nursing interventions were effective. It is favorable that the client is drinking more water and less soda; these changes also indicate intervention efficacy. The client's eating habits at fast food locations has not changed, indicating that earlier nursing interventions for this behavior were not effective.

## Chapter 47
### Answer Key
*Chapter Review*
**Pathophysiology Review**
#1
1. E
2. C
3. G
4. A
5. D
6. F
7. B

#2
1. F
2. T
3. T
4. F
5. T
6. T
7. T
8. T
9. F

## Activities

### Activity #1

Any four lifestyle habits that the nurse would include in health teaching to help individuals prevent gastritis:

- Eat a well-balanced diet and exercise regularly, if possible.
- Avoid drinking excessive amounts of alcoholic beverages.
- Avoid long-term use of aspirin, other NSAIDs (e.g., ibuprofen), or corticosteroids.
- Avoid excessive intake of coffee (even decaffeinated).
- Be sure that foods and water are safe and free from contamination.
- Manage stress levels using complementary and integrative therapies such as relaxation and meditation techniques.
- Stop smoking and/or using other forms of tobacco.
- Protect yourself against exposure to toxic substances in the workplace such as lead and nickel.
- Seek medical treatment if you are experiencing symptoms of gastroesophageal reflux disease (GERD).

### Activity #2

1. C
2. E
3. B
4. A
5. D
6. A

### Activity #3

1. T
2. T
3. T
4. T
5. T
6. F
7. F
8. T
9. T
10. T

### Activity #4

Any three actions that the patient should implement to prevent dumping syndrome:

- Eat small, frequent meals.
- Avoid drinking liquids with meals.
- Avoid foods that cause discomfort.
- Eliminate caffeine and alcohol consumption.
- Begin a smoking-cessation program, if needed.
- Receive $B_{12}$ injections, as prescribed.
- Lie flat for a short time after eating.

## Learning Assessments

### NCLEX Examination Challenge #1
Answer: A

Rationale: Melena is dark, "tarry" (sticky) stool, indicating occult blood caused by digestion of blood within the small intestine. This blood is likely from the client's peptic ulcer disease (PUD) causing upper GI bleeding and is a medical emergency. Therefore, the nurse would immediately report the presence of melena to the primary health care provider (Choice A). Epigastric pain and dyspepsia are expected for clients with PUD (Choices B and D) and are not life-threatening. Intolerance to certain foods can occur, particularly in clients who have gastric ulcers with gastritis. However, this finding is not potentially life-threatening or an emergent situation (Choice C).

### NCLEX Examination Challenge #2
Answer: C

Rationale: All of the statements except C are correct. Clients who have acute gastritis need to avoid any food or other substance that causes stimulation of gastric acid. They also need to reduce stress and use effective coping strategies. Smoking is not an effective coping method and can stimulate gastric acid production. Therefore, the client needs further education about managing this client condition.

### NGN Challenge #1
Answer:

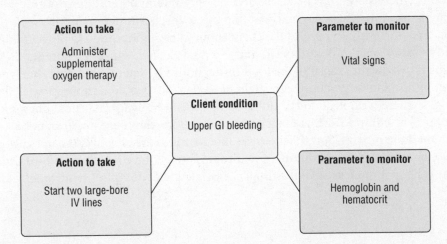

Rationale: The client has a history of PUD treated with a PPI. Today, the client has hematemesis and dizziness, most likely from low blood pressure in which the systolic blood pressure is below 100 mm Hg. The client's HR is 96 to compensate for hypotension. These symptoms indicate the client most likely has upper GI bleeding. It is also possible that the client has mild gastroenteritis given that the client experienced occasional diarrhea after eating fast-food seafood. However, this condition is not the priority for the client's care. The client's $SpO_2$ is low (below 95%) and requires the nurse to administer supplemental oxygen, especially in the presence of a high HR and low BP. The client may develop dyspnea if lowered in a flat supine position, so the nurse would likely elevate the head of the bed or stretcher. Two IV lines with large-bore catheters are needed in case the client requires a blood transfusion. Intake and output documentation is not needed at this time but may be needed later if the client's condition worsens. The nurse would not need to insert a urinary catheter at this time due to the risk of catheter-associated urinary tract infection (CAUTI). To ensure that the client is responding to nursing and collaborative interventions, the nurse would monitor the client's vital signs, especially HR and BP, and hemoglobin and hematocrit. Body weight is not related to the client's condition at this time. Pain is expected for clients who have PUD and does not help monitor the status of the client's upper GI bleeding. Although urinary output may need monitoring if the client's condition worsens, the nurse would not measure intake and output at this time.

**NGN Challenge #2**
<u>Answer:</u>

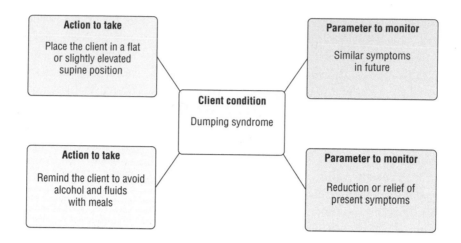

**Action to take**

Place the client in a flat or slightly elevated supine position

**Parameter to monitor**

Similar symptoms in future

**Client condition**

Dumping syndrome

**Action to take**

Remind the client to avoid alcohol and fluids with meals

**Parameter to monitor**

Reduction or relief of present symptoms

<u>Rationale:</u> The client had a gastrectomy for gastric cancer and reported eating a large holiday meal with alcohol. These factors caused dumping syndrome, as evidenced by the client's dizziness, sweating, weakness, and heart palpitations. These sensations occur because a large amount of food moves from the esophagus directly into the small intestine. There are no client findings that support hyponatremia, pyloric obstruction, or pernicious anemia. The nurse would remind the client about interventions to help prevent dumping syndrome, including the need to avoid any fluids with meals and avoiding alcohol, which is a stimulant. After eating, the client should lie down to slow the transit of the food through the GI system. Therefore, having the client in a flat supine position or in a supine position with slight head elevation would be appropriate. The client has no nausea or vomiting, so there is no need for IV fluids or an antiemetic drug. The client does not have respiratory distress, and their SpO$_2$ is within a normal range at 95%. Therefore, the client does not need supplemental oxygen. To determine if the nursing and collaborative interventions are effective, the nurse would observe the client for reduction of symptoms of dumping syndrome and tell the client to monitor for these symptoms going forward. The other parameters are not strongly associated with dumping syndrome.

**Chapter 48**

**Answer Key**
*Chapter Review*
**Pathophysiology Review**

#1

1. E
2. I
3. K
4. B
5. G
6. L
7. D
8. J
9. A
10. H
11. C
12. F

#2

1. T
2. T
3. T
4. T
5. F
6. T
7. T
8. T

## Activities

### Activity #1

Any three of these actions that the nurse would include in health teaching to help individuals promote bowel health:

- Consume adequate fluids.
- Get regular exercise at least 3 days a week.
- Consume a high-fiber diet and, if needed, a stool softener.
- Avoid excessive fat, refined carbohydrates, red meat, and low-fiber foods.
- Have regular colon screenings, especially a colonoscopy as recommended.
- Avoid smoking and excessive alcohol.

### Activity #2

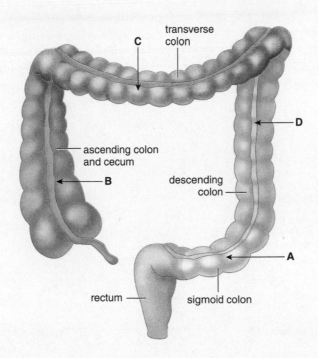

### Activity #3

1. F
2. T
3. T
4. T
5. T
6. T
7. T
8. F
9. F
10. T

### Activity #4

1. F
2. D
3. B
4. B
5. E
6. C
7. A
8. G

**Learning Assessments**

**NCLEX Examination Challenge #1**

Answer: D

Rationale: All of the choices are correct and would be included in teaching about FOBT except for D. This test is usually done for 3 consecutive days rather than 5 days. Following the other three instructions (Choices A, B, and C) helps to prevent false-positive FOBT results.

**NCLEX Examination Challenge #2**

Answer: A and D

Rationale: The procedure performed for an abdominoperineal (AP) resection requires cutting of multiple nerves that control urinary and sexual function. Therefore, Choices A and D are the correct responses. There is no ostomy involved in an AP resection; therefore, there is no stoma (Choice C). Although the client needs to take actions to help prevent constipation, obstipation is not usually a complication of this surgery (Choice E). Wound infection can also occur, but antibiotics and meticulous wound care are given to help prevent this complication (Choice B).

**NCLEX Examination Challenge #3**

Answer: C

Rationale: All of the statements are appropriate for discharge teaching for a client who had a hernioplasty. However, the most important statement is to avoid excessive coughing because coughing increases intra-abdominal pressure, which could damage the surgical area (Choice C).

**NGN Challenge #1**

Answer:

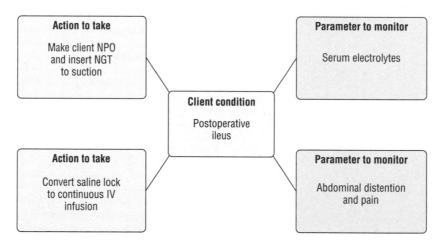

Rationale: The client had surgery 2 days ago and is having significant GI symptoms, including nausea and vomiting, anorexia, 9/10 pain, abdominal distention, and lack of flatus and bowel sounds, all of which indicate decreased or lack of peristalsis. Postoperative ileus (POI), or nonmechanical intestinal obstruction, is a fairly common complication of abdominal surgery, which the client had 2 days earlier. The loss of GI fluids, especially gastric contents, resulted in a loss of electrolytes as expected. The client's tachycardia may be due to acute pain or dehydration from fluid loss. The body temperature would be elevated if the client had a surgical wound infection, but it is within normal limits at this time. There is no evidence of abdominal hernia or mechanical intestinal obstruction. However, if the client's malignant tumor had not been surgically removed 2 days ago, the client could have developed a mechanical obstruction. The most effective management for POI is to make the client NPO, insert an NGT connect to low suction, and support with IV fluids and electrolytes. The nurse would monitor the client's electrolyte levels and continue assessing the abdomen and pain level for improvement. Urinary output and daily weight may help monitor fluid status, but the client is receiving IV therapy to replace both fluids and electrolytes. Vital signs may also help to assess fluid status but would not be as helpful for determining the effectiveness of POI management.

## NGN Challenge #2
<u>Answer:</u>

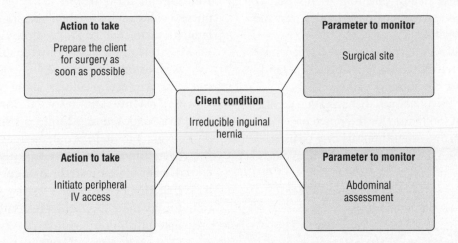

<u>Rationale:</u> The client's nonmovable bulging mass is probably an irreducible, or incarcerated, inguinal hernia. The client likely acquired the hernia at work given the lifting and other heavy work the client's occupation requires. Although umbilical hernias can occur, the client's hernia is located in the inguinal area rather than more centrally located at the umbilicus. There is no evidence that the client has either appendicitis (which would likely cause a fever) or intestinal obstruction. An irreducible hernia requires surgery as soon as possible to prevent strangulation in which blood supply to the intestines can be compromised. The nurse would make the client NPO and start IV fluids in preparation for surgery. There is no indication at this time that an NGT, urinary catheter, or antibiotic therapy would be needed. However, during surgical opening or immediately before surgery, the client would likely receive one dose of IV antibiotic to prevent infection. The nurse would observe the surgical site for intactness, swelling, and drainage and perform frequent abdominal assessments. Vital signs would be monitored, but body temperature was within normal limits before surgery. Oxygen saturation is also monitored but does not indicate if the client is making progress as a result of surgery.

## Chapter 49
### Answer Key
### *Chapter Review*
**Pathophysiology Review**

#1
1. E
2. H
3. K
4. C
5. G
6. A
7. I
8. L
9. D
10. J
11. B
12. F

#2
1. F
2. T
3. T
4. T
5. F
6. T
7. T
8. T
9. F
10. T

## Activities

### Activity #1

Any three of these health teaching points that the nurse would provide to help prevent the transmission of gastroenteritis:

- Wash hands well for at least 30 seconds with soap, especially after a bowel movement, and maintain good personal hygiene.
- Restrict the use of glasses, dishes, eating utensils, and tubes of toothpaste for their own use. In severe cases, disposable utensils may be used.
- Maintain clean bathroom facilities to avoid exposure to stool.
- Inform the primary health care provider if symptoms persist beyond 3 days.
- Do not prepare or handle food that will be consumed by others. If the patient is employed as a food handler, the public health department should be consulted for recommendations about the return to work.

### Activity #2

1. T
2. T
3. T
4. F
5. T
6. T
7. T
8. F
9. T
10. T

### Activity #3

Any three of these factors that help to explain the poor outcomes of care for non-White individuals who have chronic inflammatory bowel disease:
- Delay in disease diagnosis
- Lack of health insurance coverage
- Difficulty accessing an IBD specialist (gastroenterologist)
- Less likely to receive biologic modifying drugs

### Activity #4

1. E
2. A
3. B
4. D
5. C
6. A

### Activity #5

Any four of these health teaching points that the nurse would include when teaching a patient and family how to care for an ileostomy at home:

- Use a skin barrier to protect skin from contact with ostomy excretions.
- Use skin-care products, such as skin sealants and ostomy skin creams. If skin continues to be exposed to ostomy contents, select a product to fill in problem areas and provide an even skin surface.
- Watch skin around the ostomy for any irritation or redness.
- Empty the pouch when it is one-third to one-half full.
- Change the pouch during inactive times, such as before meals, before retiring at night, on waking in the morning, and 2 to 4 hours after eating.
- Change the entire pouch system every 3 to 7 days.
- Chew food thoroughly.
- Be cautious about high-fiber and high-cellulose foods. These foods may need to be eliminated from the diet if they cause severe problems (diarrhea, constipation, or blockage). Examples include coconut, popcorn, tough-fiber meats, rice, cabbage, and vegetables with skins (tomatoes, corn, and peas).
- Avoid taking enteric-coated and capsule medications.
- Inform any primary health care provider who is prescribing medications about the ostomy. Before having prescriptions filled, inform the pharmacist about the ostomy.
- Do not take any laxatives or enemas. Loose stools are normal, contact your primary health care provider if no stool has passed in 6 to 12 hours.
- Report any drastic increase or decrease in drainage to the primary health care provider.
- If stomal swelling, abdominal cramping, or distention occurs or if ileostomy contents stop draining:
  - Remove the pouch with faceplate.
  - Lie down, assuming a knee-chest position.
  - Begin abdominal massage.
  - Apply moist towels to the abdomen.
  - Drink hot tea.
- If none of these maneuvers is effective in resuming ileostomy flow or if abdominal pain is severe, call the primary health care provider right away.

## Learning Assessments

### NCLEX Examination Challenge #1
<u>Answer</u>: A, C, D

<u>Rationale</u>: The client who has any type of chronic inflammatory bowel disease, such as Crohn's disease, typically has elevations of inflammatory laboratory markers, including WBC count, erythrocyte sedimentation rate (ESR), and C-reactive protein (CRP) (Choices A, C, and D). Blood urea nitrogen (BUN) is often increased when a client is dehydrated, has increased protein intake or catabolism, or kidney disease (Choice B). Serum creatinine is a specific indicator of kidney function and increases when the kidneys are damaged (Choice E).

### NCLEX Examination Challenge #2
<u>Answer</u>: B

<u>Rationale</u>: Bleeding from any area of the body can cause decreased fluid volume in the intravascular compartment. If it is not managed or does not respond to treatment, hypovolemia can result in decreased perfusion to major organs and shock can occur (Choice B). Although the client who has GI bleeding may become anemic, pernicious anemia occurs from the lack of intrinsic factor in gastric juices and is not related to bleeding (Choice A). Pulmonary embolus is the presence of a life-threatening clot in a pulmonary blood vessel and is not a complication of GI bleeding (Choice C). Toxic megacolon is a massive dilation of the colon and subsequent colonic ileus that can lead to gangrene and peritonitis (Choice D).

### NCLEX Examination Challenge #3
<u>Answer</u>: A

The small intestinal effluent is rich in enzymes that can irritate and possibly excoriate the skin around the stoma. Meticulous and frequent skin care is essential and, therefore, would be included in the health teaching provided by the nurse (Choice A). A pouch for the continuous effluent will be needed at all times (Choice B), and dietary restrictions to avoid high-fiber foods are important (Choice C). Clients who have ileostomies should physically be able to have sexual intercourse (Choice D). The psychological impact of the bowel diversion may impact libido, however.

## NGN Challenge #1
<u>Answer:</u> The nurse analyzes the client data and determines that the client has a **<u>fistula</u>** that could lead to **<u>sepsis</u>**.
<u>Rationale:</u> The client has an exacerbation of Crohn's disease, a fever, an elevated WBC count, and a draining abdominal wound for which the client is hospitalized. In Crohn's disease, strictures and deep ulcerations (cobblestone appearance) occur, which put the client at risk for developing a bowel fistula (abnormal opening [tract] between two organs or structures). In this case, the client's fistula connects the small bowel and skin (enterocutaneous fistula). The client with multiple fistulas often has complications such as systemic infections (sepsis), skin problems (including abscesses and fissures), and malnutrition. Therefore, even though the client is losing weight, at this time there is no indication that the client is malnourished and could become cachexic. A fissure is a tear, crack, or split in skin and underlying tissue, usually in the anal area. A toxic megacolon is a massive dilation of the colon and subsequent colonic ileus that can lead to gangrene and peritonitis. There are no data to confirm that this client has this condition.

## NGN Challenge #2
<u>Answer:</u>

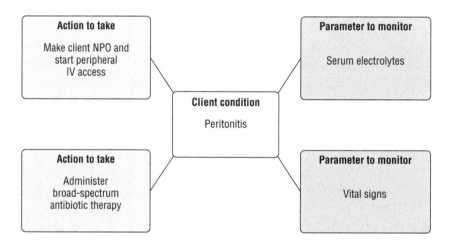

<u>Rationale:</u> The client has the classic sign of peritonitis—a rigid and distended abdomen. The x-ray showed air and fluid in the abdominal cavity indicating a bowel perforation caused leakage of contents into the abdomen and caused inflammation and infection of the peritoneum. There is no evidence of chronic pancreatitis (that would cause severe, boring pain), intestinal obstruction, or Crohn's disease. The client has a history of diverticulosis, which apparently became inflamed and perforated. Surgery will likely be needed but at this time the client needs broad-spectrum IV antibiotic therapy to treat the infection and fluid and electrolyte replacement. There is no indication that the client needs supplemental oxygen at this time and a urinary catheter would not be inserted unless absolutely needed to prevent CAUTI. The nurse would monitor the client's vital signs frequently, especially to track body temperature to determine the effectiveness of drug therapy and monitor for systemic infection or sepsis. RBC count should not be affected by the client's condition unless lower GI bleeding occurs. Urinary output would be carefully monitored if the client becomes septic. There is no indication for a need to monitor gastric pH unless the client has a nasogastric tube inserted, which may be part of the client's plan of care.

## Chapter 50
### Answer Key
### *Chapter Review*
**Pathophysiology Review**

| #1 | | | #2 | |
|----|----|---|----|---|
| 1. | E | | 1. | T |
| 2. | H | | 2. | T |
| 3. | B | | 3. | T |
| 4. | J | | 4. | T |
| 5. | F | | 5. | F |
| 6. | I | | 6. | T |
| 7. | A | | 7. | T |
| 8. | D | | 8. | T |
| 9. | G | | 9. | T |
| 10. | C | | 10. | F |

## Activities

### Activity #1
Any three of these health teaching points the nurse would provide to help prevent hepatitis A:
- Proper handwashing, especially after handling shellfish
- Avoiding contaminated food or water (including tap water in countries with high incidence)
- Receiving immunoglobulin within 14 days if exposed to the virus
- Receiving the HAV vaccine before traveling to areas where the disease is common (e.g., Mexico, Caribbean)
- Receiving the vaccine if living or working in enclosed areas with others, such as college dormitories, correctional institutions, day-care centers, and long-term care facilities

### Activity #2
1. T
2. F
3. T
4. T
5. T
6. T
7. T
8. T
9. F
10. T

### Activity #3
Any three of these populations should receive the hepatitis B vaccine:
- People who have sexual intercourse with more than one partner
- People with sexually transmitted infection (STI) or a history of STI
- Men having unprotected sex with men (MSM)
- People with any chronic liver disease (such as hepatitis C or cirrhosis)
- Patients with HIV infection
- People who are exposed to blood or body fluids in the workplace, including health care workers, firefighters, and police
- People in correctional facilities (prisoners)
- Patients needing immunosuppressant drugs
- Family members, household members, and sexual contacts of people with HBV infection

### Activity #4
1. C
2. D
3. F
4. G
5. B
6. E
7. A
8. A

Learning Assessments

| NCLEX Examination Challenge #1 | NCLEX Examination Challenge #2 |
|---|---|

**NCLEX Examination Challenge #1**

Answer: A, B, C, D, E, F

Rationale: All of the choices are common findings that occur in adults who have end-stage or advanced liver disease. Box 50.2 in the textbook chapter provides a complete list of signs and symptoms for end-stage cirrhosis.

**NCLEX Examination Challenge #2**

Answer: D

Rationale: The nurse would need to be alert to signs and symptoms of transplant rejection, including tachycardia, fever, jaundice, and elevated liver enzymes (Choice D). A temperature of 99°F (37.2°C) may be normal for the client and would not be considered a fever (Choice B). Abdominal discomfort is likely from the surgical procedure (Choice A); the cause of the client's nausea and vomiting would need to be determined, but it is possibly a side effect of analgesic medication (Choice C).

**NGN Challenge**

*Item #1*

Answer:

| Body System | Client Finding |
|---|---|
| Neurologic | o Alert<br>**X** Oriented ×1 (person) |
| Gastrointestinal | o Jaundice<br>**X** Increased abdominal girth<br>o Distal bowel sounds ×4 |
| Respiratory | **X** Shortness of breath<br>**X** RR 24 breaths/min<br>**X** SpO$_2$ 94% on RA |

Rationale: The client has advanced cirrhosis and would be expected to have jaundice, icterus, and ascites. Increasing ascitic fluid, as evidenced by an increased abdominal girth, could cause a number of other problems, including respiratory distress. The client demonstrates respiratory distress by new onset shortness of breath, RR of 24 breaths/min, and a low peripheral oxygen saturation level (normal is 95% or higher). The nurse would be concerned about the respiratory changes, especially in view of increased ascites. The client's neurologic status has also changed. Although the client is alert, the client is oriented to person only. This change could indicate another complication of cirrhosis.

## Item #2

Answer:

The nurse analyzes the relevant assessment findings to determine the client's current conditions. Select **four** conditions that the client likely has at this time.

- o   Upper GI bleeding
- X   Hepatic encephalopathy
- X   Respiratory distress
- o   Heart failure
- X   Hypertension
- X   Pruritis

Rationale: The client's neurologic status has changed, causing the client to be disoriented. Cognitive impairment for a client who has advanced cirrhosis likely indicates that the client has hepatic encephalopathy. The client's more immediate problem is respiratory distress as evidenced by increased RR and shortness of breath. The $SpO_2$ is slightly decreased at this time. The client also has elevated blood pressure, or hypertension, and reports dry, itchy skin, which is also called pruritis. There is no evidence that the client has active GI bleeding or heart failure, although both of these conditions can occur in clients with advanced or end-stage liver disease.

## Item #3

Answer: The nurse determines that the *priority* for care at this time is to manage the client's **respiratory distress** as evidenced by **shortness of breath** and **increased respiratory rate**.

Rationale: Of the four client conditions determined by the nurse's analysis, respiratory distress can be quickly life-threatening. Clients can die from complications of hypertension such as stroke, but there is no indication that the client has any of them. Over time, clients may die as a result of hepatic encephalopathy if they become comatose. This client's level of consciousness is drowsy.

## Item #4

Answer:

| Potential Nursing Actions | Indicated | Not Indicated |
|---|---|---|
| Initiate supplemental oxygen therapy. | X | |
| Place the client in a sitting or high-Fowler's position. | X | |
| Administer analgesic medication. | | X |
| Reorient the client frequently. | X | |
| Monitor respiratory rate and $SpO_2$ frequently. | X | |

Rationale: The client's respiratory distress requires oxygen therapy to ease the client's breathing effort, decrease the RR, and increase peripheral oxygen saturation. The nurse would monitor these indices frequently to determine client progress and the effectiveness of appropriate actions, including having the client remain upright in a sitting position. A sitting or high-Fowler's position allows for improved lung expansion as the diaphragm lowers from gravity. The nurse would also reorient the client frequently to ensure that the client does not get OOB without assistance and perhaps sustain a fall. Ascites can be uncomfortable because the client often expresses a feeling of fullness or heaviness. However, analgesic medications are usually metabolized by the liver. Advanced cirrhosis causes severe liver damage, preventing drugs to be adequately metabolized.

*Item #5*

Answer:

Which of the following orders would the nurse anticipate from the primary health care provider based on the latest client findings? **Select all that apply.**

- **X** Begin IV antibiotic therapy.
- **X** Prepare client for paracentesis.
- o Prepare client for transfer to the ICU.
- o Insert nasogastric tube for decompression.
- **X** Draw STAT ammonia level.
- o Type and crossmatch two units packed RBCs.

Rationale: The client's body temperature has increased, the client's HR is 100 beats/min (tachycardia), and the client is sweating. These changes indicate possible infection, such as spontaneous bacterial peritonitis. Starting the client on IV antibiotics may be appropriate, especially because the client has esophageal varices that can begin bleeding. The client would likely need a paracentesis because of increasing ascites that has caused respiratory distress. Changes in neurologic status may be due to increases in ammonia level, although increased ammonia does not always occur in clients who have hepatic encephalopathy. At this time, there is no need to move the client to critical care or prepare for a blood transfusion. There is also no indication that the client needs an NGT inserted.

*Item #6*

Answer:

| Current Client Findings | Improving | Not Improving |
|---|---|---|
| Alert and oriented ×4 | X | |
| Uses continuous ambulatory oxygen therapy | | X |
| T 98.4°F (36.9°C) | X | |
| RR 20 breaths/min | X | |
| SpO$_2$ 97% on O$_2$ at 2 L/min | X | |

Rationale: The client's condition is markedly improved as evidenced by being oriented ×4 rather than only to person and having a normal temperature, RR, and SpO$_2$. However, the client continues to need supplemental oxygen therapy, which was also needed when the client was hospitalized.

# Chapter 51

**Answer Key**
*Chapter Review*
**Pathophysiology Review**

#1

1. E
2. C
3. G
4. H
5. A
6. D
7. F
8. B

#2

1. T
2. T
3. F
4. T
5. F
6. T
7. T
8. T
9. T
10. T

## Activities

### Activity #1

Any three of these health teaching points the nurse would provide to help prevent biliary and pancreatic conditions:

- Practice lifestyle habits that help prevent obesity, including avoiding excessive high-fat/high-cholesterol foods and exercising regularly.
- For patients who are obese, lose weight slowly under the care of a qualified health care professional.
- Avoid excessive alcohol.
- Avoid smoking and other tobacco use.

### Activity #2

1. Acute pancreatitis
2. Ultrasonography
3. Pain
4. Pancreatitis
5. Amylase
6. Pleural effusion
7. Pancreatic enzyme replacement therapy
8. Diabetes mellitus
9. Whipple
10. Fistula

### Activity #3

1. B
2. B
3. A
4. B
5. A
6. B
7. A
8. B

### Activity #4

Any three of these factors that help to explain the poor outcomes of care for non-White individuals who have pancreatic conditions.

- Most non-White patients tend to have their surgery more often in low-volume hospitals, meaning that the surgical team is less specialized or experienced than those in a high-volume hospital.
- Some non-White patients may not have adequate insurance coverage.
- Some non-White patients may not have the same access to health care when compared with other patients.
- Non-White patients often have a lower income than White patients, resulting in more food insecurity and less ability to eat a healthy diet.

### NCLEX Examination Challenge #1
Answer: B

Rationale: Biliary colic is severe acute pain that can cause the client to go into shock with tachycardia, diaphoresis, and hypotension. Shock is a life-threatening condition for which the nurse monitors carefully. Therefore, Choice B is the priority for client care. The nurse would assess pain intensity, but this action is not the priority (Choice A). The client in severe pain would not want to lie flat because a sitting position would relax the abdominal muscles (Choice C). However, if the client develops shock, the nurse would lower the head of the bed and lie the client flat to help increase blood pressure. Ursodiol is a drug used for chronic gallstones and would not be useful in this client situation (Choice D).

### NCLEX Examination Challenge #2
Answer: C

Rationale: The primary problem for clients who have acute pancreatitis is severe, acute boring abdominal pain. Therefore, the nurse's priority for care is pain management (Choice C). Nutritional support and oxygen therapy are usually required more for clients who have chronic pancreatitis (Choices A and D). The nurse would monitor laboratory enzyme levels for any client who has acute pancreatitis, but this is not the priority for the client's care (Choice B).

### NGN Challenge #1
Answer:

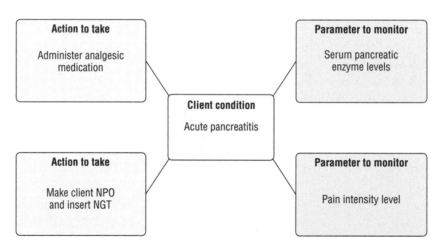

Rationale: The pain described by the client is consistent with acute pancreatitis. Clients who have chronic pancreatitis have a burning or gnawing pain. The client's history of cholelithiasis and elevated alanine transaminase (ALT) suggest that the client may be experiencing biliary obstruction. However, there is no indication that the client is experiencing biliary colic because the client is not tachycardic or having other symptoms associated with this condition. The client's elevated amylase and lipase further support the diagnosis of acute pancreatitis. The symptoms associated with pancreatic cancer are slow and vague rather than having an acute onset. The nurse's priority for care is to manage the client's pain by administering analgesic medication. Because the client likely has biliary obstruction that has caused the pancreatitis, the client should be NPO and have an NGT inserted and connected to low continuous suction for gastric decompression to rest the GI system. Surgery, antibiotic therapy, and oxygen are not indicated at this time but may be added later if the client has an abscess or cyst. The nurse would monitor the client's pain level, which should decrease as a result of drug therapy, NPO and an NGT for decompression. As the pancreas begins to heal and inflammation decreases, the client's serum pancreatic enzyme levels should also decrease. Therefore, the nurse needs to monitor labs carefully. The other assessments would apply if the client had an infection or other complication.

**NGN Challenge #2**
<u>Answer:</u>

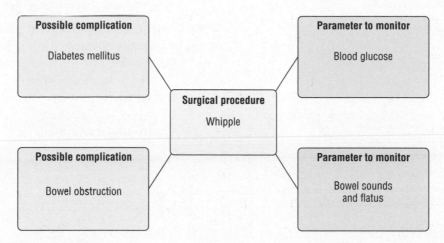

| Possible complication | | Parameter to monitor |
|---|---|---|
| Diabetes mellitus | | Blood glucose |
| | **Surgical procedure**<br>Whipple | |
| **Possible complication** | | **Parameter to monitor** |
| Bowel obstruction | | Bowel sounds<br>and flatus |

<u>Rationale:</u> A Whipple surgical procedure is commonly performed for pancreatic cancer. This radical procedure entails removal of the proximal head of the pancreas, the duodenum, a portion of the jejunum, the stomach (partial or total *gastrectomy)*, and the gallbladder, with anastomosis of the pancreatic duct *(pancreaticojejunostomy)*, the common bile duct *(choledochojejunostomy)*, and the stomach *(gastrojejunostomy)* to the jejunum. Most of the insulin-producing cells are beta cells located mostly in the tail of the pancreas. However, diabetes mellitus is a possible complication of a Whipple procedure. The nurse would monitor finger stick blood sugars frequently to detect this problem. The manipulation of the small bowel during the procedure can cause a nonmechanical bowel obstruction, or adynamic ileus. Therefore, the nurse needs to monitor bowel sounds and the passage of flatus. Diabetes insipidus occurs when there is damage to or dysfunction of the pituitary gland, which is within the cranium. Sepsis could only occur if the client acquired an infection. The client who has an infection usually experiences increased pain and fever. Clients receive at least one dose of IV antibiotics before surgery to help prevent infection. Acute kidney injury may occur in the presence of sepsis, but sepsis is very unlikely for this procedure, particularly if it is performed as a minimally invasive procedure. An increased serum creatinine level with changes in urinary output indicates decreased kidney functioning.

## Chapter 52

**Answer Key**
*Chapter Review*
**Pathophysiology Review**
#1

1.  G
2.  A
3.  N
4.  H
5.  E
6.  L
7.  K
8.  D
9.  I
10. B
11. M
12. J
13. C
14. F

#2 Common complications of obesity can include any of these:

**Cardiovascular**
- Coronary artery disease
- Hyperlipidemia
- Hypertension
- Peripheral artery disease (PAD)

**Endocrine**
- Insulin resistance
- Metabolic syndrome
- Type 2 diabetes

**Gastrointestinal**
- Cholelithiasis

**Genitourinary/reproductive**
- Erectile dysfunction in men
- Menstrual irregularities in women
- Urinary incontinence

**Integumentary**
- Delayed wound healing
- Susceptibility to infections

**Musculoskeletal**
- Chronic back and/or joint pain
- Early onset of osteoarthritis

**Neurologic**
- Stroke

**Psychiatric**
- Depression

**Respiratory**
- Obesity hypoventilation syndrome
- Obstructive sleep apnea

#3 Common complications of undernutrition can include any of these:

**Cardiovascular**
- Reduced cardiac output

**Endocrine**
- Cold intolerance

**Gastrointestinal**
- Anorexia
- Diarrhea
- Impaired protein synthesis
- Malabsorption
- Vomiting
- Weight loss

**Immunologic**
- Susceptibility to infectious disease

**Integumentary**
- Dry, flaky skin
- Various types of dermatitis
- Poor wound healing

**Musculoskeletal**
- Cachexia
- Decreased activity tolerance
- Decreased muscle mass
- Impaired functional ability

**Neurologic**
- Weakness

**Psychiatric**
- Substance misuse

**Respiratory**
- Reduced vital capacity

## Activities

### Activity #1
1. F
2. T
3. T
4. F
5. F
6. F
7. T
8. T
9. F
10. F

### Activity #2

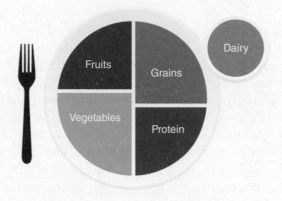

### Activity #3
Foods eaten and avoided by each type of vegetarian include:

1. **Lacto-vegetarian**—allows dairy[a]; avoids meat, poultry, seafood, eggs, and foods that contain those items
2. **Ovo-vegetarian**—allows eggs; avoids meat, poultry, seafood, and dairy[a]
3. **Lacto-ovo vegetarian**—allows eggs and dairy[a]; avoids meat, poultry, seafood
4. **Pescatarian**—allows fish; avoids meat, poultry, dairy,[a] eggs
5. **Vegan**—consumes a plant-based diet only; avoids meat, poultry, seafood, dairy,[a] and eggs, and foods that contain those items (note = some vegans also avoid honey)

[a]Dairy = milk, cheese, yogurt, butter, etc.

### Activity #4
1. G
2. A
3. E
4. H
5. D
6. I
7. C
8. J
9. F
10. B

## NCLEX Examination Challenge #1
Answer: A, B, C, D
Rationale: The nurse will monitor the client's oxygen saturation and airway as a priority following surgery (Choice A). The nurse will also apply an abdominal binder to prevent wound dehiscence (Choice B), place the patient in semi-Fowler's position to promote comfort (Choice C), and assess the skin folds for any type of breakdown that can occur following surgery (Choice D). The client will not be maintained on bedrest for 24 to 48 hours after surgery (Choice E); evidence shows that patients recover more successfully when they are ambulated soon after surgery.

## NCLEX Examination Challenge #2
Answer: A, B, E
Rationale: The nurse will teach techniques that encourage nutrition because clients are more likely to eat when they enjoy the experience and have some control over the process. Clients are encouraged to feed themselves whenever it is possible (Choice A) and to eat food that they like (Choice B). Wearing prescribed glasses and hearing aids increase sensory perception, which can help hold the client's interest in eating (Choice E). Clients are more likely to eat if they are not in pain (Choice C), so the nurse will teach that giving prescribed pain medication an hour to 30 minutes before meals can increase the comfort level. The family will be taught to let the client eat at their own pace (Choice D). Hurrying the client can result in an increased risk for aspiration, as well as make the experience less pleasant.

## NCLEX Examination Challenge #3
Answer: B
Rationale: Weight change is the most reliable indicator of fluid status (Choice B). A liter of water weighs 1 kg (2.2 lb). An actual weight gain or loss can account for a daily change of only about a half lb (~240 g). More than that indicates fluid increase, and less than that indicates fluid loss. Although intake and output (Choice A), changes in skin turgor (Choice C), and presence of dependent edema (Choice D) can be used as additional indicators of fluid status, weight change is the most reliable independent measure.

## NGN Challenge #1
Answer: B, C, F, G, H
Rationale: Information analyzed from the trended documentation demonstrates that the client is recovering as expected. The nurse will monitor for dumping syndrome (Choice B), which can occur even when the client who is postbariatric surgery consumes full liquids; assess the dressing and incision site (Choice C) to monitor for any infection; administer prophylactic anticoagulants (Choice F), which are prescribed following surgery to prevent venous thromboembolism; encourage use of incentive spirometer hourly (Choice G) to decrease the risk for pulmonary complications following surgery; and assist the client with walking the hallway (Choice H) because evidence demonstrates that clients who ambulate regularly soon after surgery recover more quickly. The nurse will not provide a tray with pureed foods (Choice A) because this type of food is not introduced until a week after bariatric surgery. There is no need for an antibiotic (Choice D) because the trended information does not demonstrate any type of finding that is consistent with an infection. The nurse will not decrease fluids (Choice E); rather, fluids will be encouraged to prevent dehydration.

## NGN Challenge #2
Answer: Based on this history and assessment, the client is at risk for developing **malnutrition** and **undernutrition**.
Rationale: Malnutrition is characterized by deficiencies, excesses, or imbalances in a person's intake of energy and/or nutrients. Because the client is barely eating, the risk for malnutrition is increased because there is a deficiency in the intake of sources of energy and/or nutrients. The client is also at risk for undernutrition, which is a state of being underweight. The client is 5 feet, 3 inches tall (63 cm); a female client of this height would normally weigh 107 to 135 pounds (48.5–61.2 kg), so she is already underweight with a continued downward trend noted over the past several days. Anorexia nervosa is an eating disorder in which someone engages in self-induced starvation. This client's lack of intake is related to radiation for cancer. Dumping syndrome is associated with bariatric surgery, not diminished intake. Kwashiorkor is a lack of protein quality despite having adequate caloric intake. Refeeding syndrome occurs when nutrition is restarted for a client who is in a starvation state.

# Chapter 53
**Answer Key**
***Chapter Review***
**Anatomy & Physiology Review**
#1.

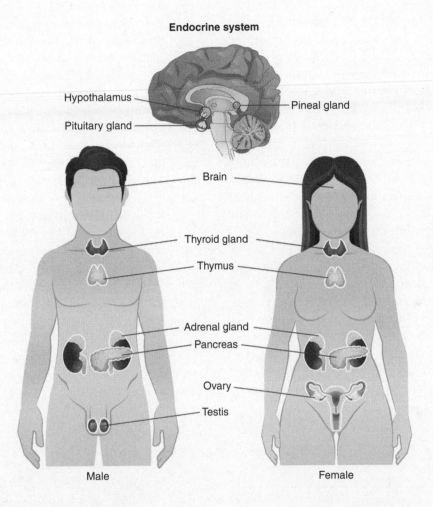

**Endocrine system**

Hypothalamus

Pineal gland

Pituitary gland

Brain

Thyroid gland

Thymus

Adrenal gland

Pancreas

Ovary

Testis

Male

Female

#2. A negative feedback mechanism signals an endocrine gland to secrete a hormone in response to a body change to *oppose* the action of the initial condition change and restore homeostasis.

## Activities

### Activity #1

Answers should resemble these functions:

1. Mineralocorticoids are produced and secreted by the adrenal cortex to help control fluid and electrolyte balance.
2. The adrenal medulla is a sympathetic nerve ganglion that has secretory cells. Stimulation of the sympathetic nervous system causes the release of adrenal medullary hormones, the catecholamines (epinephrine and norepinephrine [NE]). These hormones travel to all areas of the body through the blood and exert their effects on target cells.
3. The hypothalamus produces regulatory hormones. Some of these hormones are released into the blood and travel to the anterior pituitary, where they either stimulate or inhibit the release of anterior pituitary hormones.
4. In response to the releasing hormones of the hypothalamus, the anterior pituitary secretes some tropic (trophic) hormones that have as their target tissues other endocrine glands. Other pituitary hormones, such as prolactin, produce their effect directly on final target tissues. The hormones of the posterior pituitary—vasopressin (antidiuretic hormone [ADH]) and oxytocin—are produced in the hypothalamus and delivered to the posterior pituitary, where they are stored. These hormones are released from the posterior pituitary into the blood when needed.
5. The exocrine function of the pancreas involves the secretion of digestive enzymes through ducts that empty into the duodenum. The cells in the islets of Langerhans perform the pancreatic endocrine functions. The islets have three distinct cell types: alpha cells, which secrete glucagon; beta cells, which secrete insulin; and delta cells, which secrete somatostatin. Glucagon and insulin affect carbohydrate, protein, and fat metabolism.
6. The parathyroid glands consist of four small glands located close to or within the back surface of the thyroid gland that secrete parathyroid hormone (PTH). PTH regulates calcium and phosphorus metabolism by acting on bones, the kidneys, and the GI tract.
7. This gland secretes melatonin when it is dark, thereby helping to regulate circadian rhythm and the sleep-wake cycle.
8. Control of metabolism occurs through $T_3$ and $T_4$, which are produced by follicular cells of the thyroid gland.

### Activity #2

Answers should resemble these changes in the endocrine system that are associated with aging, and their associated implications.

| Change | Nursing Considerations |
|---|---|
| **Decreased antidiuretic hormone (ADH) production** | |
| Urine is more dilute and may not concentrate when fluid intake is low. | The patient is at greater risk for dehydration; assess frequently for this condition. If not contraindicated by another health condition, teach assistive personnel (AP) to offer fluids at least every 2 hours while the patient is awake. |

| Change | Nursing Considerations |
|---|---|
| **Decreased ovarian production of estrogen** | |
| Bone density decreases.<br>Skin is thinner, drier, and at greater risk for injury.<br>Perineal and vaginal tissues become drier, and the risk for cystitis increases. | Teach about the importance of regular exercise and weight-bearing activity to maintain bone density.<br>Encourage intake of healthy foods with adequate protein and to drink 2 L of fluid daily (if not contraindicated by another health condition).<br>Protect skin integrity as noted in Chapter 21.<br>Perform or assist the patient to perform perineal care at least twice daily.<br>Teach sexually active older women to urinate immediately after sexual intercourse and how vaginal lubricants can reduce discomfort and tissue damage during intimacy. |
| **Decreased glucose tolerance** | |
| Weight becomes greater than ideal, along with:<br>• Elevated fasting blood glucose level<br>• Elevated random blood glucose level<br>• Slow wound healing<br>• Frequent yeast infections<br>• Polydipsia<br>• Polyuria | Assess for family history for obesity and type 2 diabetes mellitus.<br>Teach about the importance of regular exercise and maintenance of a healthy weight.<br>Teach the signs and symptoms of diabetes that should be reported to the primary health care provider.<br>Suggest diabetes testing for any patient with:<br>• Persistent vaginal candidiasis<br>• Failure of a wound to heal in 2 weeks or less (especially of the leg or foot)<br>• Increased and persistent hunger and thirst<br>• Noticeable and persistent decrease in energy level |
| **Decreased general metabolism** | |
| Patient has less tolerance for cold.<br>Appetite is decreased.<br>Heart rate and blood pressure are decreased. | Teach patients to dress in layers so that they can be added or removed based upon temperature.<br>Assess for additional signs and symptoms of an endocrine disorder including for:<br>• lethargy<br>• constipation (as a change from usual bowel habits)<br>• decreased cognition<br>• slowed speech<br>• body temperature consistently below 97°F (36°C)<br>• heart rate consistently below 60 beats/min |

**Activity #3**

1. H
2. G
3. D
4. E
5. B
6. C
7. A
8. F
9. J
10. I

**Activity #4**

1. T
2. T
3. F
4. T
5. T
6. F
7. T
8. T
9. T
10. F

**Activity #5**

Any of these functions of thyroxine ($T_4$) and triiodo-thyronine ($T_3$) are correct.

• Regulate metabolic rate of all cells
• Regulate body heat production
• Serve as insulin antagonists
• Maintain growth hormone secretion and skeletal maturation
• Affect central nervous system development
• Influence muscle tone and vigor
• Maintain calcium mobilization
• Affect RBC production
• Maintain cardiac rate, force, and output
• Affect respiratory rate and oxygen utilization
• Maintain secretion of the GI tract
• Regulate protein, carbohydrate, and fat metabolism
• Stimulate lipid turnover, free fatty acid release, and cholesterol synthesis

**Learning Assessments**

**NCLEX Examination Challenge #1**

Answer: B

Rationale: Cortisol must be present for catecholamine (epinephrine, norepinephrine [NE]) action and maintaining the normal excitability of the heart muscle cells (Choice B). These are not the actions of insulin (Choice A), oxytocin (Choice C), or glucagon (Choice D).

**NCLEX Examination Challenge #2**

Answer: C

Rationale: An unintentional weight loss in excess of 5 lb is significant; this client has lost 15 lb, which requires further assessment for a potential endocrine problem (Choice C). It may indicate an increase in metabolic rate or a problem with excessive fluid loss, either of which could be associated with an endocrine disorder. Receiving a new eyeglasses prescription at the age of 45 years is most likely an age-related change (Choice A). The father's diagnosis of prostate cancer is irrelevant to this client's presentation (Choice B). Taking oral contraceptives without problems does not indicate a potential endocrine problem (Choice D).

**NCLEX Examination Challenge #3**

Answer: A, B, C, D, E

Rationale: Decreased estrogen levels increase bone density loss and make skin drier and thinner; using a skin moisturizer can decrease discomfort and flaking associated with dry skin (Choice A). Decreased estrogen levels also increase the risk for cystitis. Drinking at least 2 L of water daily and urinating immediately after intercourse help prevent cystitis (Choices B and E). Weight-bearing activity and increasing intake of calcium and vitamin D can help slow problems associated with bone density loss (Choices C and D).

Chapter 54
**Answer Key**
*Chapter Review*
**Pathophysiology Review**
#1
1. E
2. C
3. G
4. H
5. D
6. F
7. A
8. B

#2 Causes of primary adrenal insufficiency, and three causes of secondary adrenal insufficiency can contain any of these:

| Primary Causes | Secondary Causes |
|---|---|
| • Autoimmune disease[a] | • Pituitary tumors |
| • Tuberculosis | • Postpartum pituitary necrosis |
| • Metastatic cancer | • Hypophysectomy |
| • HIV-III (AIDS) | • High-dose pituitary or whole-brain radiation |
| • Hemorrhage | • Cessation of long-term corticosteroid drug therapy[a] |
| • Gram-negative sepsis | |
| • Adrenalectomy | |
| • Abdominal radiation therapy | |
| • Drugs (mitotane) and toxins | |

[a]Most common cause

#3 Laboratory test values in the presence of *hypofunction* or *hyperfunction* of the adrenal glands include:

| Test | Normal Range | Hypofunction | Hyperfunction |
|---|---|---|---|
| Sodium | 136–145 mEq/L (mmol/L) | Low | High |
| Potassium | 3.5–5.0 mEq/L (mmol/L) | High | Low |
| Glucose (fasting) | 70–110 mg/dL (4–6 mmol/L) | Normal to low | Normal to high |
| Calcium | Total: 9–10.5 mg/dL (2.25–2.75 mmol/L) Ionized: 4.5–5.6 mg/dL (1.05–1.30 mmol/L) | High | Low |
| Bicarbonate | 23–30 mEq/L (mmol/L) | High | Low |

| Test | Normal Range | Hypofunction | Hyperfunction |
|---|---|---|---|
| BUN | 10–20 mg/dL (3.6–7.1 mmol/L) | High | Normal |
| Cortisol (serum) | 6 a.m. to 8 a.m.: 5–23 mcg/dL (138–635 nmol/L)<br>4 p.m. to 6 p.m.: 3–13 mcg/dL (83–359 nmol/L) | Low | High |
| Cortisol (salivary) | 7 a.m. to 9 a.m.: 100–750 ng/dL<br>3 p.m. to 5 p.m.: <401 ng/dL | Low | High |

## Activities

### Activity #1

1. F
2. T
3. T
4. T
5. F
6. T
7. F
8. F
9. T
10. T

### Activity #2

Drug or drug classes that can cause syndrome of inappropriate antidiuretic hormone secretion (SIADH) includes hydrocodone, levofloxacin, vincristine, carbamazepine, amitriptyline, halothane, ciprofloxacin, methoxyflurane, and oxycodone.

### Activity #3

Expected findings in a patient with Cushing syndrome include any of the following:

#### General Appearance

- Moon face
- Buffalo hump
- Truncal obesity
- Weight gain

#### Cardiovascular Symptoms

- Hypertension
- Frequent dependent edema
- Bruising
- Petechiae

## Immune System Symptoms
- Increased risk for infection
- Reduced immunity
- Decreased inflammatory responses
- Signs and symptoms of infection and inflammation possibly masked

## Musculoskeletal Symptoms
- Muscle atrophy (most apparent in extremities)
- Osteoporosis with:
  - Fragile fractures
  - Decreased height and vertebral collapse
  - Aseptic necrosis of the femur head
  - Slow or poor healing of bone fractures

## Skin Symptoms
- Thinning skin
- Increased facial and body hair
- Striae and increased pigmentation

## Activity #4
Blanks should be completed as follows:
- Take your medication with <u>meals or snacks</u> to prevent stomach irritation.
- Weigh yourself <u>daily</u> and keep a record to show your primary health care provider.
- If you have persistent vomiting or severe diarrhea and cannot take your medication by mouth for <u>24</u> to <u>36</u> hours, call your primary health care provider.
- Always wear your <u>medical alert bracelet or necklace</u>.
- Learn how to self-administer an <u>intramuscular</u> injection of hydrocortisone in case you cannot take your oral drug.
- Avoid <u>crowds and/or others with infection</u> to minimize your chance of getting an infection.

## Learning Assessments

### NCLEX Examination Challenge #1
<u>Answer</u>: D
<u>Rationale</u>: The client has demonstrated understanding when they acknowledge that leg pain or swelling must be immediately reported to their primary health care provider (Choice D). The use of exogenous estrogen and progesterone increases the risk for thrombus and emboli formation. Persistent leg pain and swelling without trauma are an indication of deep vein thrombosis in the extremity. This risk is even greater for women who use nicotine in any form (even vaping), so vaping should be discouraged (Choice A). Exogenous estrogen and progesterone therapy are more likely to promote adequate skin oil production rather than dry skin (Choice B). Breast size increases are an expected side effect of this hormone replacement therapy (Choice C); a mammogram will not be needed unless there are other accompanying findings of concern.

### NCLEX Examination Challenge #2
<u>Answer</u>: C
<u>Rationale</u>: Clients with acute adrenal insufficiency are hypotensive and dehydrated with hypoglycemia, hyponatremia, and hyperkalemia. Their level of consciousness is altered to the point of lethargy and confusion, so finding the client alert and oriented indicates that treatment has been effective

(Choice C). Anorexia is present with adrenal insufficiency (Choice B), so this does not indicate effective therapy. Urine output can be excessive so an increase demonstrates ineffective therapy (Choice A). A blood glucose level of 60 mg/dL (3.3 mmol/L) is still low, demonstrating that treatment is not yet effective (Choice D).

**NCLEX Examination Challenge #3**
Answer: B
Rationale: Increased serum sodium due to fluid restriction indicates effective therapy (Choice B). Restricting fluid would result in increasing hematocrit levels as the fluid volume excess resolves, rather than decreased levels (Choice A). Plasma osmolality is decreased as a result of SIADH, so treatment would result in this level rising to near normal rather than remaining low (Choice C). Urine specific gravity is increased with SIADH and would decrease to near normal with treatment, rather than increasing (Choice D).

**NGN Challenge #1**
Answer:
Based on this history and assessment, the client is at risk for developing **syndrome of inappropriate antidiuretic hormone secretion (SIADH)** as evidenced by **a urine specific gravity of 1.040**.
Rationale: SIADH is a problem in which antidiuretic hormone (ADH, vasopressin) is secreted even when plasma osmolarity is low or normal, resulting in water retention and fluid overload. A decrease in plasma osmolarity normally inhibits ADH production and secretion. SIADH occurs with many conditions (e.g., cancer therapy, pulmonary infection or impairment) and with select antidepressants, antiseizures, antipsychotics, anticancer drugs, antidiabetic drugs, and vasopressin analogues, and when using illicit drugs such as opiates and methylenedioxymethylamphetamine (MDMA, or Ecstacy). This client has started opioid medication and takes an antidepressant and antidiabetic drug. The client's headache is most likely caused by the

decreasing serum sodium level. The elevated urine specific gravity value is characteristic of SIADH. This client has no symptoms of hyperpituitarism, Cushing syndrome, or acute adrenal insufficiency. The history of type 2 diabetes mellitus does not place her at risk for SIADH. The potassium value and urine WBC counts are both within normal parameters.

**NGN Challenge #2**
Answer: A, B, C, E, F, G, H
Rationale: The client is likely experiencing acute adrenal insufficiency. This condition often occurs in response to a stressful event (e.g., surgery, trauma, severe infection), especially when the adrenal hormone output is already reduced. Unless intervention is initiated promptly, sodium levels fall and potassium levels rise rapidly. For this reason, potassium should not be given (Choice D). Severe hypotension results from the blood volume depletion that occurs with the loss of aldosterone. The client's blood pressure continues to drop, she is tachycardic, and her level of consciousness is deteriorating. The nurse will contact the primary health care provider to see the client and to provide further orders (Choice F). The nurse will also apply a heart monitor (Choice A) and listen closely to the client's heart sounds (Choice C) because hyperkalemia can cause dysrhythmias with an irregular heart rate, which can result in cardiac arrest. For this reason, a request for a laboratory order for serum potassium is important (Choice H). The nurse will obtain a glucose reading (Choice B) because tachycardia and tremors can indicate the presence of hypoglycemia in a client with acute adrenal insufficiency. The nurse will anticipate administration of IV steroids (Choice E) because cortisol and aldosterone deficiencies are corrected with this type of therapy. It is important to monitor the level of consciousness for any further changes (Choice G).

**Chapter 55**
**Answer Key**
*Chapter Review*
**Pathophysiology Review**
#1

1. E
2. H
3. F
4. I
5. C
6. B
7. J
8. A
9. D
10. G
11. K

#2

| Test | Normal Range (Will Vary by Laboratory) | Hypothyroidism | Hyperthyroidism |
|------|----------------------------------------|----------------|-----------------|
| Serum $T_3$ | *Age >50 years old:* 40–180 ng/dL (0.6–2.8 nmol/L) | Decreased | Increased |
| | *Age 20–50 years old:* 70–205 ng/dL (1.2–3.4 nmol/L) | | |
| Serum $T_4$ (total) | *Males* 4–12 mcg/dL (59–135 nmol/L) | Decreased | Increased |
| | *Females* 5–12 mcg/dL (71–142 nmol/L) | | |
| | *Older adults >60 years old* 5–11 mcg/dL (64–142 nmol/L) | | |
| "Direct" free $T_4$ | 0.8–2.8 ng/dL (10–36 pmol/L) | Decreased | Increased |

#3

| Test | Normal Range | Hypoparathyroidism | Hyperparathyroidism |
|---|---|---|---|
| Serum calcium | Total: 9.0–10.5 mg/dL (2.25–2.62 mmol/L)* *Values may be slightly lower in older adults | Decreased | Increased (primary hyperparathyroidism) |
| Serum magnesium Critical levels <0.5 or >3 mEq/L mg/dL | 1.3–2.1 mEq/L (0.65–1.05 mmol/L) | Decreased | Increased |
| Serum parathyroid hormone | 10–65 pg/mL (10–65 ng/L) | Decreased | Increased |
| Serum phosphorus Critical level <1 mg/dL | 3–4.5 mg/dL | Increased | Decreased |
| | (0.97–1.45 mmol/L) | | |
| Vitamin D | *Natal sex males:* 18–64 pg/mL | Decreased | Variable |
| | *Natal sex females:* 17–78 pg/mL | | |

## Activities

### Activity #1
1. T
2. T
3. F
4. T
5. T
6. F
7. T
8. F
9. F
10. T

### Activity #2
Findings in each system that the nurse would expect to see in a client with hypothyroidism include:
1. Cardiovascular symptoms
   - Bradycardia
   - Decreased activity tolerance
   - Diastolic hypertension
   - Pericardial effusion
2. Respiratory symptoms
   - Dyspnea
   - Hypoventilation
   - Pleural effusion
3. Gastrointestinal symptoms
   - Abdominal distention/ascites
   - Constipation
   - Weight gain
4. Metabolic symptoms
   - Decreased basal metabolic rate
   - Decreased body temperature
   - Cold intolerance
5. Reproductive symptoms
   *Women*
   - Anovulation
   - Decreased libido
   - Menstrual changes (amenorrhea or prolonged periods)
   
   *Men*
   - Decreased libido
   - Impotence
6. Psychosocial symptoms
   - Apathy
   - Depression
7. Integumentary symptoms
   - Cool, pale, dry, coarse, scaly skin
   - Decreased hair growth, with loss of eyebrow hair

- Dry, coarse, brittle hair
- Poor wound healing
- Thick, brittle nails
8. Neuromuscular symptoms
    - Confusion
    - Decreased tendon reflexes
    - Hearing loss
    - Impaired memory
    - Inattentiveness
    - Lethargy or somnolence
    - Muscle aches and pain
    - Paresthesia of the extremities
    - Slowing of intellectual functions:
    - Slowness or slurring of speech

## Activity #3
Findings in each system that the nurse would expect to see in a client with hyperthyroidism include:
1. Cardiovascular
    - Chest pain
    - Dysrhythmias
    - Increased systolic blood pressure
    - Palpitations
    - Rapid, shallow respirations
    - Tachycardia
2. Gastrointestinal symptoms
    - Increased appetite
    - Increased stools
    - Weight loss
3. Metabolic symptoms
    - Fatigue
    - Heat intolerance
    - Increased basal metabolic rate
4. Reproductive symptoms
    *Women*
    - o Amenorrhea
    *Men*
    - o Erectile dysfunction
    - o Gynecomastia
5. Psychosocial symptoms
    - Anxiety
    - Hyperactivity
    - Restlessness
6. Integumentary symptoms
    - Diaphoresis
    - Fine, soft, silky body hair
    - Smooth, warm, moist skin
    - Thinning of scalp hair
7. Neuromuscular symptoms
    - Eyelid retraction, eyelid lag
    - Hyperactive deep tendon reflexes
    - Insomnia
    - Muscle weakness
    - Tremors

## Activity #4
Causes of hyperparathyroidism and hypoparathyroidism can include:

| Causes of Hyperparathyroidism | Causes of Hypoparathyroidism |
|---|---|
| • Calcium absorption difficulties (e.g., as present in celiac disease or those who have had bariatric surgery)<br>• Chronic kidney disease with hypocalcemia<br>• Congenital hyperplasia<br>• Drug therapy (e.g., diuretics, bisphosphonates)<br>• Inherited conditions (e.g., multiple endocrine neoplasia type 1 [MEN1])<br>• Neck trauma or radiation<br>• Parathyroid hormone–secreting carcinomas of the lung, kidney, or GI tract<br>• Parathyroid tumor or cancer<br>• Vitamin D deficiency | • Autoimmune conditions<br>• Congenital dysgenesis<br>• Parathyroidectomy<br>• Thyroid ablation (surgical or radiation-induced) |

## Learning Assessments

### NCLEX Examination Challenge #1

Answer: A

Rationale: In clients with hypothyroidism, the serum $T_3$ value is usually decreased. The normal range for clients older than 50 years of age is 40–180 ng/dL and 70–205 ng/dL for those between 20 and 50 years old. The serum $T_3$ of 30 ng/dL is low regardless of the client's age (Choice A). The serum calcium of 9.2 mg/dL is within normal limits. In a client with hypothyroidism, this value is expected to be decreased (Choice B). The "Direct" free $T_4$ of 1.4 ng/dL is within normal limits. In a client with hypothyroidism, this value is expected to be decreased (Choice C). The total serum $T_4$ of 6 mcg/dL is within normal limits. In a client with hypothyroidism, this value is expected to be decreased (Choice D).

### NCLEX Examination Challenge #2

Answer: B

Rationale: Urine darkening when taking propylthiouracil can be a sign of liver toxicity or failure; this must be reported to the health care provider (Choice B). Monitoring the pulse should occur; however, the nurse will teach the client to monitor for bradycardia, not tachycardia (Choice A). Taking the drug 1 hour after methimazole (Choice C) and diluting the drug in a glass of water or beverage (Choice D) are instructions the nurse would provide for a client who is prescribed iodine therapy.

### NCLEX Examination Challenge #3

Answer: C, D, E

Rationale: The pulse (Choice C) and blood pressure (Choice D) are in an acceptable range, which would indicate improvement during myxedema coma because both of these values would have been much lower before the start of therapy. An increasing core body temperature (Choice E) is a strong indication that the client's rate of metabolism is increasing in response to appropriate therapy; again, this value would have been lower pretherapy. The $SpO_2$ is well below normal and an indication of ongoing poor perfusion and gas exchange (Choice A). Cool dry skin is a characteristic of hypothyroidism, not an indication of improvement in myxedema coma (Choice B).

### NGN Challenge #1

Answer: D, F, G

Rationale: The client's laboratory values have consistently trended toward normal since the beginning of thyroid replacement therapy. This indicates to the nurse that treatment is successful. Because treatment is life-long, the nurse will emphasize the need to continue taking medication as directed (Choice F). It can be helpful to discuss the benefit of consistent mild to moderate exercise because this is often a very successful nonpharmacologic intervention to address fatigue (Choice D). Before providing this teaching, the nurse will assess to learn more information about the client's perception of fatigue, such as when it occurs and how bothersome it seems to be (Choice G). There is no need to moderate calcium in the diet (Choice A); calcium excess is a concern for clients with hyperparathyroidism. Pretibial edema is a concern related to myxedema coma, which can occur when hypothyroidism is undertreated or untreated (Choice B). There is no need for medication adjustment because the laboratory values confirm that medication therapy is successful (Choice C). Therapy is life-long, so the nurse will not recommend discontinuation (Choice E).

**NGN Examination Challenge #2**

Answer:

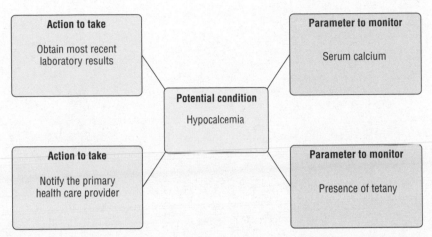

Rationale: The client's presentation is characteristic of hypocalcemia following removal of some or all of the parathyroid glands because of hyperparathyroidism. This client had a partial parathyroidectomy, so one or more glands remain. Facial and extremity tingling and twitching are associated with hypocalcemia, which can occur in a period following this type of surgery. This can happen because any remaining glands (which may have atrophied because of parathyroid hormone [PTH] overproduction) require several days to several weeks to return to normal function. Without excess PTH, release of calcium and phosphorus is lessened, which can result in hypocalcemia. The client does not have extremity twitching (negative Trousseau's sign), and only has very mild facial movement on percussion over the facial nerve (Chvostek's sign) so they are not experiencing a hypocalcemic crisis. The nurse will check the most recent laboratory reports—especially for the calcium value—and notify the primary health care provider of the positive Chvostek's sign. Early intervention is important to minimize the chance of hypocalcemic crisis. The nurse will continue to trend the serum calcium values and monitor for the onset of tetany, which can indicate worsening hypocalcemia.

Graves' disease is associated with hyperthyroidism. Myxedema coma is a serious complication of undertreated or poorly treated hypothyroidism. The client is not experiencing hypercalcemia because they have undergone a partial parathyroidectomy, which results in less secretion of PTH and thus less release of calcium and phosphorus into the blood.

Infectious thyroiditis is caused by bacterial invasion of the thyroid gland. Symptoms include sudden pain and tenderness on one side of the neck, malaise, and fever. There is no need for the nurse to assess for this because the client's symptoms are not consistent with this disorder. The client has already spoken clearly and without hoarseness. There is no need to further assess vocal patterns. The Rapid Response Team is not needed because this is not an emergent condition at the moment.

Eyeball protrusion is associated with Graves' disease, not hypocalcemia. Hashimoto thyroiditis is not a condition that arises in response to hypocalcemia. Propranolol is not a treatment that would be used for hypocalcemia; this is used when caring for a client during thyroid storm.

## Chapter 56
**Answer Key**
### *Chapter Review*
**Pathophysiology Review**

#1

1. D
2. A
3. J
4. B
5. E
6. G
7. A
8. I
9. C
10. F

#2

1. F
2. T
3. T
4. T
5. T
6. T
7. T
8. T
9. T
10. T
11. T
12. T
13. F
14. T
15. F

## Activities

**Activity #1**

1. E
2. H
3. B
4. I
5. C
6. G
7. A
8. J
9. F
10. D

**Activity #3**

1. E
2. B
3. F
4. H
5. C
6. G
7. A
8. D

**Activity #2**

1. T
2. T
3. T
4. T
5. T
6. F
7. T
8. T
9. F
10. T
11. T
12. T

## Activity #4

Any four of these instructions the nurse would provide to a diabetic patient about how to provide meticulous foot care:

- Inspect your feet daily, especially the area between the toes.
- Wash your feet daily with lukewarm water and soap. Dry thoroughly.
- Apply a moisturizer to your feet (but not between your toes) after bathing.
- Change into clean cotton socks every day.
- Do not wear the same pair of shoes 2 days in a row, and wear only shoes made of breathable materials, such as leather or cloth.
- Check your shoes for foreign objects (pebbles) before putting them on. Check inside the shoes for cracks or tears in the lining.
- Buy shoes that have plenty of room for your toes. Buy shoes later in the day when feet are normally larger. Break in new shoes gradually.
- Wear socks to keep your feet warm.
- Trim your nails straight across with a nail clipper and smooth them with an emery board.
- See your diabetes health care provider immediately if you have blisters, sores, or infections. Protect the area with a dry, sterile dressing. Do not use tape to secure dressing to the skin.
- Do not treat blisters, sores, or infections with home remedies.
- Do not step into the bathtub without checking the temperature of the water with your wrist or thermometer.
- Do not use very hot or cold water. Never use hot-water bottles, heating pads, or portable heaters to warm your feet.
- Do not treat corns, blisters, bunions, calluses, or ingrown toenails yourself.
- Do not go barefooted.
- Do not wear sandals with open toes or straps between the toes.
- Do not cross your legs or wear tight stockings that constrict blood flow.

## Activity #5

| Type/Preparation | Onset of Action (minutes) | Peak Action (hours) | Duration of Action (hours) |
|---|---|---|---|
| Insulin lispro | 15–30 | 0.5–2.5 | 3–6 |
| Regular insulin | 30–60 | 1–5 | 6–10 |
| NPH insulin | 60–120 | 6–14 | 16–24 |
| Insulin detemir | 60–120 | Steady level | 12–24 |
| Insulin degludec | 30–90 | Steady level | 24+ |

## Learning Assessments

### NCLEX Examination Challenge #1

Answer: B

Rationale: The client in the question has severe hypoglycemia as evidenced by a decreased loss of consciousness (LOC) and FSBG of 39 mg/dL (2.16 mmol/L). The normal blood glucose for a nondiabetic client is 74 to 100 mg/dL (4.1–5.6 mmol/L). A client with diabetes is expected to have a blood glucose of 126 mg/dL (7.0 mmol/L) or greater. If this client's blood glucose stays low, the client could go into a coma and likely die. Therefore, the nurse's priority action is to increase the client's glucose by giving glucagon (Choice B). Documenting the client's LOC, reporting the client's condition to the charge nurse, or retaking the client's blood glucose level in 10 minutes are not actions that will help resolve the client's hypoglycemia (Choices A, C, and D).

### NCLEX Examination Challenge #2
Answer: A, B, C, D, E
Rationale: The assessment data in the question supports the client's condition of diabetic ketoacidosis (DKA). Clients who have DKA have a blood glucose level of 300 mg/dL (16.7 mmol/L) or greater and positive ketone bodies. In addition to hyperglycemia, DKA is a condition in which the client also has dehydration. Therefore, interventions are directed at treating these two problems. Hyperglycemia is managed by a bolus of short-acting insulin followed by a continuous IV insulin infusion (Choices C and D). To manage dehydration, the client is encouraged to drink more fluids, and the nurse would initiate peripheral IV fluids (Choice A and B). Laboratory tests would be drawn, especially to assess the serum potassium level (Choice E). Clients who have DKA often have mild to moderate hyperkalemia until insulin is infused. During this infusion, the potassium level decreases and may need to be replaced. Glucagon stimulates conversion of glycogen stored in the liver into glucose. This client does not need more glucose, and, therefore, Choice F is not a correct response.

### NCLEX Examination Challenge #3
Answer: A
Rationale: The client has an infection that can alter the client's glucose level. "Sick day" principles help to manage the client's blood glucose level during this illness. All of the client's statements are correct regarding these principles with the exception of Choice A. The fluid recommendation is 8 to 12 ounces every hour rather than every 3 to 4 hours.

### NGN Challenge
*Item #1*
Answer:

| Vital Signs | Nurses Notes | Orders | Laboratory Results |
|---|---|---|---|

**0805:** Drowsy but easily awakened; disoriented and confused this morning. Able to move all extremities but needs assistance getting out of bed because of weakness. Nursing assistant states that client only eats about half of each meal and needs strong encouragement to drink fluids. Refuses supplemental enteral nutrition between meals. Daily urinary output has decreased since admission. Skin and mucous membranes dry with poor skin turgor over sternum. $S_1$ and $S_2$ present; no abnormal or adventitious breath sounds. VS this morning: T 99.6°F (39.3°C); HR 112 beats/min; RR 21 breaths/min; BP 98/76 mm Hg. Medical Director notified of resident condition and lab results.

| Laboratory Test | Results (from Yesterday's Blood Draw) | Normal Reference Range |
|---|---|---|
| Fasting blood glucose (FBG) | 357 mg/dL (19.81 mmol/L) | 74–106 mg/dL (4.1–5.9 mmol/L) |
| Blood urea nitrogen (BUN) | 68 mg/dL (24.28 mmol/L) | 10–20 mg/dL (3.6–7.1 mmol/L) |
| Serum creatinine (Cr) | 1.5 mg/dL (132.63 mmol/L) | 0.6–1.3 mg/dL (53.05–114.95 mmol/L) |
| Blood osmolality | 325 mOsm/kg $H_2O$ (325 mmol/kg) | 285–295 mOsm/kg $H_2O$ |

Rationale: Older adults have less fluid volume than younger adults. Therefore, they are easily susceptible to dehydration from hypovolemia or other cause. This client has been taking a diuretic for about a week, yet the client's urinary output has decreased. This finding is of immediate concern because the client's body is trying to conserve fluid and eliminating less than earlier in the week. The client also has a decreased level of consciousness, which is likely occurring because of hypoxia from hypovolemia. The client is hypotensive, which is likely from decreased fluid volume. Tachycardia is likely a compensatory mechanism because there is less blood to circulate throughout the body and is not an immediate concern. Laboratory results support hyperosmolar dehydration because the client's BUN and the blood osmolality are elevated. The client's blood glucose is very high and would also be of immediate concern to the nurse. The creatinine level is only slightly elevated, which is typical in older adults. Therefore, that laboratory result is not of immediate concern but would be monitored in the future.

### Item #2

Answer: The client is at high risk for **hyperglycemic-hyperosmolar state** because the client has **type 2 diabetes mellitus** and is prescribed **diuretics**.

Rationale: The client has T2DM and is an older adult. In T2DM, the client has an insulin deficiency. Hyperglycemic-hyperosmolar state (HHS) is a slowly developing complication of this disorder and occurs most often in older adults who have T2DM. Diabetic ketoacidosis occurs more often in clients who have T1DM in which they have no insulin production. In addition to hyperglycemia, these clients usually are positive for ketones. There is no evidence that the client has metabolic syndrome. The client has a history of hypertension (HTN), but HTN does not contribute to the development of HHS. The client

does not have chronic kidney disease as evidenced by only a slightly elevated serum creatinine. HHS is caused by a number of factors. In this client's case, the client was taking diuretics, which initially likely increased urinary output and depleted the client's fluid reserves. Metformin is given to stimulate the pancreas to increase insulin production and should help prevent hyperglycemia, not contribute to causing HHS. Amlodipine is used to control HTN, which did not contribute to the client's HHS.

### Item #3

Answer: A, C

Rationale: The client who has HHS has two major conditions that must be managed as quickly as possible—dehydration and hyperglycemia (Choices A and C). Hypotension and tachycardia are findings that support dehydration, along with unintentional weight loss (Choices B, D, and E). The client does not have chronic kidney disease (CKD) as evidenced by only a slightly elevated serum creatinine. CKD is not a major manifestation of HHS, but acute kidney injury could develop if dehydration is not treated promptly.

### Item #4

Answer:

| Client Condition | Potential Interventions |
|---|---|
| Dehydration | **X** Start a peripheral IV with 0.45% NS.<br>**X** Encourage oral fluids as tolerated.<br>**X** Insert an indwelling urinary catheter. |
| Hyperglycemia | **X** Administer IV insulin.<br>o Increase metformin dosage.<br>o Initiate continuous glucose monitoring. |

Rationale: The *first* priority for fluid replacement in HHS is to increase blood volume. In shock or severe hypotension, normal saline is used. Otherwise, half-normal saline is used. If the client is able to drink oral fluids, they are encouraged to do so. To evaluate the effectiveness of managing hypovolemia, the client would likely have a urinary catheter to accurately measure hourly urinary output. Fluids are typically infused at 1 L/h until central venous pressure begins to rise or until blood pressure and urine output are adequate. The rate is then reduced to 100 to 200 mL/h. Half of the estimated fluid deficit is replaced in the first 12 hours, and the rest is given over the next 36 hours. IV insulin is administered after adequate fluids have been replaced. Usually, an initial bolus dose is given followed by continuous IV infusion until blood glucose levels fall to 250 mg/dL (13.9 mmol/L). Metformin has not controlled the client's glucose levels during the past week and, at this time, would not be given. After the client is stabilized in the next few days, the client's antidiabetic medication would be reevaluated. Continuous blood glucose monitoring is usually used in the community; however, the client's blood glucose would be followed carefully during HHS management.

## Item #5

Answer: A, B, C, D, E

Rationale: The nurse would perform frequent assessments during the client's treatment for HHS. Urine output, kidney function, and the presence or absence of pulmonary congestion and jugular venous distention help determine the rate of fluid infusion (Choices C and D). The patient should be assessed hourly for signs of cerebral edema (i.e., abrupt changes in mental status and level of consciousness). Lack of improvement in level of consciousness may indicate inadequate rates of fluid replacement or reduction in plasma osmolarity. Regression after initial improvement may indicate a too-rapid reduction in plasma osmolarity. A slow but steady improvement in CNS function is the best evidence that fluid management is satisfactory (Choice E). As the blood glucose decreases as a result of insulin administration, potassium enters the cells and the serum potassium level decreases. If the level falls below 5.0 mEq/L (5.0 mmol/L), this electrolyte has to be replaced (Choices A and B). Skin turgor is not a reliable indicator of fluid status in older adults (Choice F).

## Item #6

Answer:

| Admission Client Finding | Current Client Finding | Improved | Not Improved |
|---|---|:---:|:---:|
| Drowsy and disoriented | Alert and oriented ×1 | X | |
| Weight loss of 8 lb (3.6 kg) | Weight gain of 2.2 lb (1 kg) | X | |
| T 99.6°F (39.3°C) | T 98°F (36.7°C) | X | |
| HR 112 beats/min | HR 88 beats/min | X | |
| BP 98/76 mm Hg | BP 122/72 mm Hg | X | |
| FBG 357 mg/dL (19.81 mmol/L) | FBG 146 mg/dL (8.1 mmol/L) | X | |
| BUN 68 mg/dL (24.28 mmol/L) | BUN 25 mg/dL (8.93 mmol/L) | X | |

Rationale: The client's physical condition and laboratory values have all improved since admission because of appropriate and aggressive treatment for HHS. There is no evidence of dehydration because the BUN has markedly decreased, the blood pressure has increased, and the client has gained some of the lost weight. Additionally, the client's body temperature and HR are now within normal range, and the client's level of consciousness has improved.

## Chapter 57

**Answer Key**

*Chapter Review*

**Anatomy & Physiology Review**

#1.
1. E
2. B
3. G
4. D
5. A
6. H
7. C
8. F

#2.
1. Renal Artery
2. Nephron
3. Angiotensin I
4. Renal threshold
5. Angiotensin II
6. Vitamin D
7. Cystitis
8. Concentrate

## Activities

### Activity #1

1. Any three of these renal/urinary physiologic changes of aging:
   - Decreased glomerular filtration rate (GFR)
   - Nocturia
   - Decreased bladder capacity
   - Weakened urinary sphincters and shortened urethra in women
   - Tendency to retain urine

### Activity #2

1. Cystitis
2. Infection
3. Renal colic
4. Uremia
5. Bladder scanners
6. Dull
7. Creatinine
8. Creatinine clearance

### Activity #3

1. T
2. T
3. T
4. T
5. F
6. T
7. F
8. T

### Activity #4

1. B
2. D
3. F
4. A
5. E
6. C

## Learning Assessments

### NCLEX Examination Challenge #1

Answer: C

Rationale: The client having a cystoscopy for tumor removal would be expected to have pink-tinged urine but not gross hematuria. If not treated, bleeding could lead to dehydration and hypovolemia. Therefore, Choice C is the correct answer. Discomfort (Choice A) and increased urinary output (Choice D) as a result of receiving IV fluids during the procedure would be expected. Constipation is not a complication of cystoscopy (Choice B).

### NCLEX Examination Challenge #2

Answer: B, C, D

Rationale: Urine is a sterile fluid that contains few particles. Bilirubin, ketones, and glucose in the urine are abnormal; none of these substances should be found in urine (Choices B, C, and D). A pH of 6 is within normal range (Choice A), and a protein level of less than 8 mg/dL is also normal (Choice E).

**NCLEX Examination Challenge #3**
Answer: B, C, D, E
Rationale: A renal scan is used to examine the perfusion, function, and structure of the kidneys by the IV administration of a radioisotope, not an iodine-based contrast medium (Choice A). All of the other choices are correct and appropriate to include in the nurse's health teaching (Choices B, C, D, and E).

## Chapter 58

**Answer Key**
*Chapter Review*
**Pathophysiology Review**

#1

1. G
2. C
3. I
4. E
5. K
6. B
7. F
8. L
9. A
10. H
11. J
12. D

#2

1. F
2. T
3. T
4. T
5. T
6. F
7. T
8. T

## Activities

### Activity #1

Any three of these factors contribute to urinary incontinence in older adults:

- Drugs, such as diuretics
- Diseases, such as Parkinson's disease or stroke
- Depression
- Inadequate resources, such as personal assistance to help ambulate to the toilet

### Activity #2

Any four of these measures that help minimize CAUTIs:

- Maintain good hand hygiene during insertion and manipulation of the catheter system to avoid contamination.
- Insert urinary catheters for appropriate use only, including:
  - Acute urinary retention or bladder obstruction.
  - Accurate measurement of urine volume in critically ill patients if needed
  - Perioperative situations only as needed, such as urogenital, gynecological, laparoscopic, and orthopedic surgeries. Avoid routine use of indwelling catheters for surgical patients.
  - To assist in healing of open sacral or perineal wounds in incontinent patients. Avoid use of indwelling catheters to manage patients who are incontinent.
  - Consider intermittent catheterization or other alternatives to indwelling catheters for patients with spinal cord injuries or conditions.
  - To provide comfort at end of life.

- Ensure that only properly trained personnel insert and maintain catheters.
- Use routine hygiene to clean periurethral area; antiseptic cleaning solutions are NOT recommended.
- Leave catheters in place *only* as long as needed. The strongest predictor of a CAUTI is the length of time the catheter dwells in a patient.
- Assess the need for urinary catheter daily and document patient needs or indications.
- For example, remove catheters in postanesthesia care or as soon as possible after surgery when intraoperative indications have resolved.
- Use aseptic technique and sterile equipment in the acute care setting when inserting a urinary (intermittent or indwelling) catheter.
- Maintain a closed system by ensuring that catheter tubing connections are sealed securely; disconnections can introduce pathogens into the urinary tract.
- Obtain urine samples aseptically.
- If breaks in the system occur, replace the catheter and entire collecting system.
- Maintain unobstructed urine flow:
  - Keep the catheter and collecting tube free from kinking.
  - Keep the urine collection bag below the level of the bladder and do not rest the bag on the floor.
  - Empty the bag regularly, using a separate, clean container for each patient.
  - Ensure that the drainage spigot does not come into contact with nonsterile surfaces.
- Secure the catheter to the patient's thigh (females) or lower abdomen (males); catheter movement can cause urethral friction and irritation.
- Consider the use of antiseptic or antimicrobial catheters for patients requiring urinary catheters for more than 3 to 5 days. These catheters reduce bacterial colonization (i.e., biofilm) along the catheter.
- Consider appropriate alternatives to an indwelling catheter:
  - External (condom) devices in males without obstruction or urinary retention
  - External PureWick collecting device (females)

  - Intermittent catheterization in patients requiring drainage for neurogenic bladder or postoperative urinary retention
- Use portable ultrasound devices to assess urine volume to reduce unnecessary catheterization.
- Implement best practices in quality improvement to ensure that core recommendations for use, insertion, and maintenance are implemented. Examples of projects that improve patient care and reduce CAUTI include:
  - Nurse-initiated protocols for urinary catheter removal
  - Compliance with hand hygiene
  - Impact of educational programs on CAUTI occurrence
  - Compliance with documentation for catheter placement or maintenance
  - Number of CAUTI per 1000 catheter days or patient days on unit
  - Track number of catheters inserted

**Activity #3**
1. T
2. F
3. T
4. T
5. T
6. F
7. T
8. T
9. T
10. T

**Activity #4**
1. E
2. C
3. F
4. F
5. A
6. D
7. D
8. B

## Learning Assessments

### NCLEX Examination Challenge #1
Answer: D

Rationale: Older adults who are incontinent are often placed in briefs or on pads and told to wet the bed for the convenience of the staff. This action does not demonstrate that the staff is treating the client with dignity and neither Choice A nor B is a correct response. The Crede method is appropriate for clients who retain urine after voiding, such as the client who has overflow incontinence (Choice C). Instead, the staff should follow an individualized toileting schedule, or habit training, to help improve the client's incontinence (Choice D).

### NCLEX Examination Challenge #2
Answer: A, C, D

Rationale: The client will be taking a sulfa-based drug and, therefore, the nurse would double-check that the client does not have any known sulfa allergies (Choice C). A rash may indicate the onset of Stevens-Johnson syndrome, which is a serious condition (Choice A). The nurse should teach clients to drink a full glass of water with each dose and to have an overall fluid intake of 3 L daily because these drugs can form crystals that precipitate in the kidney tubules. Fluids can prevent this complication (Choice D). This drug does not affect heart rate and blood pressure (Choice B) and should effectively treat the UTI (Choice E).

### NCLEX Examination Challenge #3
Answer: A

Rationale: The client's surgery was a month ago, suggesting that if urine leakage, peritonitis, or bowel obstruction were going to occur, these complications would have already happened (Choices B, C, and D). However, urinary infection can occur anytime and is a common complication of this surgery (Choice A).

**NGN Challenge #1**
Answer:

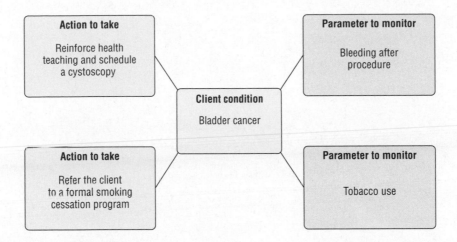

Rationale: The client has had vague urinary symptoms including pain and pressure for more than 2 years with minimal relief from the treatment plan. The urine shows presence of red blood cells, indicating urinary endothelial irritation or damage. There is no evidence that a cystocele is present, and the client is not having the typical severe pain associated with urolithiasis. The client likely does not have a UTI because antibiotic therapy has not been effective. Therefore, the client likely has a bladder lesion, which could be a cancerous tumor. A cystoscopy would provide the urologist the opportunity to visualize the bladder wall and biopsy any lesion for a confirmed diagnosis. After this procedure, the client would be monitored for bleeding and should report bleeding if it occurs later after the procedure. The client is older than 55 years of age and has been smoking for a prolonged period. The client needs to enroll in a formal smoking cessation program to possibly slow any potential cancerous growth. The nurse would want to follow up after the program is completed to determine if the client continues to use tobacco.

**NGN Challenge #2**
Answer:

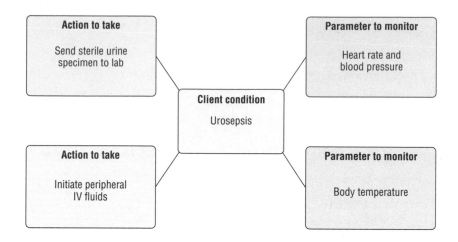

Rationale: Older adults often manifest vague symptoms, including acute confusion, when they have acute infections or other disorders. This client also has new symptoms of urinary incontinence and a low-grade fever. Additionally, the client may be dehydrated because the client has tachycardia, a low blood pressure, and dry mucous membranes and lips. These symptoms indicate possible urosepsis. Bladder cancer does not manifest quickly and is associated with vague symptoms. There is no evidence that the client had a stroke or pneumonia. For urosepsis, the client would need an antibiotic, but the provider would need confirmation of the UTI. The nurse would likely catheterize the client to obtain a sterile specimen for culture and sensitivity. Until those results are available, the client would receive broad-spectrum antibiotics. The client is likely dehydrated and, therefore, would need IV fluids. Skin turgor is not a good measure of dehydration. The peripheral line would also be used for IV antibiotics. An antipyretic drug would not be given because the client's fever is not very high. However, the client's vital signs, including body temperature, would be carefully monitored. An indwelling urinary catheter could worsen the client's infection and would likely not be used. There is no indication that the client needs supplemental oxygen therapy. An $SpO_2$ of 94% without respiratory symptoms is expected in older adults of advanced age.

## Chapter 59

### Answer Key
#### *Chapter Review*
**Pathophysiology Review**

#1
1. C
2. F
3. B
4. E
5. G
6. A
7. D

#2
1. F
2. T
3. T
4. T
5. T
6. F
7. T
8. T
9. F
10. T
11. T

## Activities

### Activity #1
Any four of these common symptoms of acute pyelo-nephritis:
- Fever
- Chills
- Tachycardia and tachypnea
- Flank, back, or loin pain
- Tenderness at the costovertebral angle
- Abdominal, often colicky, discomfort
- Nausea and vomiting
- General malaise or fatigue
- Burning, urgency, or frequency of urination
- Nocturia
- Recent cystitis or treatment for urinary tract infection

### Activity #2
1. sterile
2. Pyelonephritis
3. leukocyte esterase; nitrite
4. blood; protein
5. kidney biopsy
6. high blood pressure
7. ultrasound
8. angiotensin-converting enzyme inhibitors
9. obstruction
10. nephrectomy

### Activity #3
1. T
2. F
3. T
4. T
5. T
6. T
7. T
8. T
9. F
10. T

## Learning Assessments

### NCLEX Examination Challenge #1
Answer: C
Rationale: The purpose of the nephrostomy is to drain urine from the kidney and avoid the ureteral obstruction area. No drainage suggests that the tube is obstructed or kinked and must be addressed immediately. If not, the urine will back up into the kidney and cause hydronephrosis (Choice C). The client is expected to have pain and the pain described is moderate at 5/10 (Choice A). Having dry mucous membranes is a possible indicator of dehydration and could be easily managed by increasing the IV fluid rate (Choice B). The blood pressure of 108/74 mm Hg is within normal range but would be monitored carefully for additional signs of dehydration or bleeding (Choice D).

### NCLEX Examination Challenge #2
Answer: A
Rationale: The client has a blood pressure of 90/50, which is hypotension. Hypotension after removal of a kidney can indicate bleeding, either external or internal, or adrenal insufficiency. Either of these complications is potentially life-threatening and requires the nurse to report this finding to the surgeon immediately (Choice A). The $SpO_2$ of 94% and shallow but regular respirations are likely because of difficulty taking deep breaths from surgical pain (Choices B and C). The glucose level in Choice D is within normal limits (Choice D).

**NGN Challenge #1**
Answer:

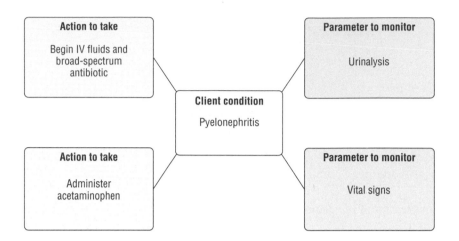

Rationale: The client has classic symptoms of pyelonephritis, or kidney infection. In addition, the urinalysis is positive for leukocyte esterase and nitrites with white blood cells and bacteria present. These laboratory findings confirm the diagnosis of pyelonephritis. The client does not have urolithiasis as evidenced by the KUB results. Although a fever can occur with glomerulonephritis (GN) if the causative agent is infectious, fever and chills with tachycardia is not a typical finding for GN. The appropriate nursing actions for pyelonephritis include acetaminophen for pain and fever and broad-spectrum antibiotics to attack the offending infectious agent. The other options for nursing actions are not appropriate for infection. To determine if the infection is resolving, the nurse would monitor the client's vital signs, especially temperature and HR, and monitor the urinalysis findings for improvement. Urine in a healthy person is sterile. The client's pain should improve as the infection resolves, but pain level is not the best parameter to monitor for client progress. The client's $SpO_2$ is within normal range and does not need monitoring nor does the client need supplemental oxygen.

**NGN Challenge #2**
<u>Answer</u>:

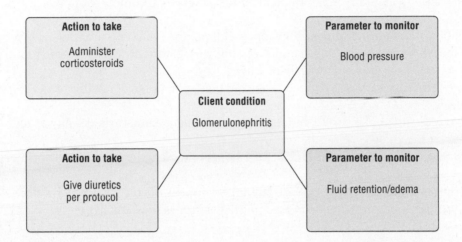

<u>Rationale</u>: The client has a history of systemic lupus erythematosus (SLE), which is an autoimmune condition that can "attack" major organs, especially the kidneys. A major cause of death in clients who have SLE is secondary glomerulonephritis (GN). There is no evidence that the client has a kidney infection, cancer, or stones. To manage this client's GN given that it is caused by an immune response, the client needs corticosteroids or other immunomodulating agent. To reduce edema and high blood pressure, diuretics are typically administered. Antihypertensive drugs may also be needed. The client would likely have a urine sample submitted to the laboratory, but it does not need to be sterile, and an indwelling catheter would likely not be placed to prevent catheter-associated urinary tract infection. An antipyretic is not necessary because the client does not have a fever. Therefore, body temperature does not need to be monitored, but the client's blood pressure and urinary output should be monitored, especially after giving the client diuretics. The client's $SpO_2$ is within normal range. Skin turgor is not a reliable indication of fluid balance, but the client's edema needs to be monitored along with daily weights.

## Chapter 60

**Answer Key**
*Chapter Review*
**Pathophysiology Review**

#1

1. B
2. G
3. E
4. C
5. H
6. A
7. F
8. D

#2

1. T
2. T
3. T
4. F
5. T
6. T
7. F
8. T
9. T
10. T

## Activities

### Activity #1

Any three of these actions that nurses can implement for patients to promote kidney health and prevent acute kidney injury:

- Assess all patients for signs of impending kidney dysfunction including monitoring of laboratory values.
- Accurately measure intake and output and check body weight to identify changes in fluid balance (weight is the most reliable indicator of fluid gain or loss).
- Ensure that all patients are well hydrated by encouraging oral fluids, if feasible, and adjusting IV fluid administration.
- Note the characteristics of the urine and report new sediment, hematuria (smoky or red color), foul odor, or other concerning changes.
- Report a urine output of less than 30 mL/h for 2 hours or dark amber urine to the primary health care provider.
- Assess patients carefully to recognize the signs and symptoms of volume depletion (low urine output, decreased systolic blood pressure, decreased pulse pressure, orthostatic hypotension, thirst, and rising blood osmolarity).

### Activity #2

List at least two of these assessment findings for each body system or process that can be affected by end-stage kidney disease.

| Body System/Process | Assessment Findings |
|---|---|
| Urinary | • Polyuria, nocturia (early)<br>• Oliguria, anuria (later)<br>• Proteinuria<br>• Hematuria<br>• Diluted, straw-colored urine appearance (early)<br>• Concentrated and cloudy urine appearance (later) |
| Neurologic | • Lethargy and daytime drowsiness<br>• Inability to concentrate or decreased attention span<br>• Seizures<br>• Decreased level of consciousness<br>• Slurred speech<br>• Asterixis (jerky movements or "flapping" of the hands)<br>• Tremors, twitching, or jerky movements<br>• Myoclonus<br>• Ataxia (alteration in gait)<br>• Paresthesias from peripheral neuropathy |
| Integumentary | • Decreased skin turgor<br>• Yellow-gray pallor<br>• Dry skin<br>• Pruritus<br>• Ecchymosis<br>• Purpura<br>• Soft-tissue calcifications<br>• Uremic frost (late, not common) |

| Body System/Process | Assessment Findings |
|---|---|
| Cardiovascular | • Cardiomyopathy<br>• Hypertension<br>• Peripheral edema<br>• Heart failure<br>• Uremic pericarditis<br>• Pericardial effusion<br>• Pericardial friction rub<br>• Cardiac tamponade<br>• Cardiorenal syndrome |
| Respiratory | • Uremic halitosis<br>• Tachypnea<br>• Deep sighing, yawning<br>• Kussmaul respirations<br>• Uremic pneumonitis<br>• Shortness of breath<br>• Pulmonary edema<br>• Pleural effusion<br>• Depressed cough reflex<br>• Crackles |
| Musculoskeletal | • Muscle weakness and cramping<br>• Bone pain<br>• Fractures<br>• Renal osteodystrophy |
| Reproductive | • Decreased fertility<br>• Infrequent or absent menses<br>• Decreased libido<br>• Impotence<br>• Sexual dysfunction |
| Hematologic | • Anemia<br>• Abnormal bleeding and bruising<br>• Reduced white blood cell count<br>• Increased risk for infection |
| Gastrointestinal | • Anorexia<br>• Nausea<br>• Vomiting<br>• Metallic taste in the mouth<br>• Changes in taste acuity and sensation<br>• Uremic colitis (diarrhea)<br>• Constipation<br>• Uremic gastritis (possible GI bleeding)<br>• Uremic fetor (breath odor)<br>• Stomatitis |

| Body System/Process | Assessment Findings |
| --- | --- |
| Metabolic | • Hyperparathyroidism<br>• Hyperlipidemia<br>• Alterations in vitamin D, calcium, and phosphorus adsorption and metabolism<br>• Metabolic acidosis<br>• Hyperkalemia |

**Activity #3**

1. Kidney replacement therapy
2. Creatinine
3. Hemodialysis
4. Fluid restriction
5. Pulmonary edema
6. Angiotensin-converting enzyme inhibitors
7. Protein restriction
8. Phosphorus (phosphate)
9. Anemia
10. Renal osteodystrophy

**Activity #4**

1. T
2. T
3. T
4. F
5. T
6. T
7. T
8. T
9. T
10. F

**Activity #5**

1. C
2. D
3. B
4. A
5. E
6. B
7. F
8. A

**Learning Assessments**

**NCLEX Examination Challenge #1**

Answer: A, C, D, E

Rationale: The client who has chronic kidney disease (CKD), especially end-stage disease, has a high serum creatinine and blood urea nitrogen levels (Choice A). These nitrogenous wastes cannot be eliminated by the kidneys because of severe damage and dysfunction. Phosphorus (phosphate) is a large molecule that cannot be eliminated by the diseased kidneys and therefore accumulates in the blood (Choice D). Phosphorus and calcium have an inverse relationship meaning that an increased phosphate level would decrease the calcium in the blood (Choice C). Additionally, the damaged kidneys are not able to release erythropoietin, a hormone that stimulates the bone marrow to produce red blood cells that carry hemoglobin. Therefore, decreased RBC production results in decreased hemoglobin (Choice E). The potassium level usually increases in conjunction with metabolic acidosis; therefore, Choice B is an incorrect response.

**NCLEX Examination Challenge #2**

Answer: B

Rationale: Clients who have chronic kidney disease have damaged kidneys that cannot excrete hydrogen (acid) or control the reabsorption of bicarbonate (alkaline). Therefore, these clients typically have metabolic acidosis (Choice B) instead of metabolic alkalosis (choice A). CKD is not a respiratory problem and, therefore, the acid-base imbalance is not of respiratory origin (Choices C and D).

### NCLEX Examination Challenge #3
Answer: A, B, C, D, E
Rationale: All of these choices are correct to protect the integrity of the arteriovenous (AV) fistula or graft. Both types of vascular access connect a vein with an artery to allow for inflow of dialysate and removal of fluid and toxins during hemodialysis. Circulation to the extremity where the access is established is essential because the access site could clot. Therefore, any action to limit or restrict circulation must be avoided (Choices A, B, E). The nurse should hear a bruit over the AV fistula to indicate its integrity (Choice D) and check distal pulses and other indicators of perfusion frequently (Choice C).

### NCLEX Examination Challenge #4
Answer: A, B, D, E
Rationale: All of these choices are important nursing actions for the client who is receiving hemodialysis. During this procedure, the dialyzer removes excess fluid and toxins from the body. Therefore, weighing the client before and after the procedure is important to ensure weight loss corresponding to fluid removal (Choice A). Vital signs need to be monitored carefully, especially pulse and blood pressure because the BP would decrease as fluid volume decreases (Choice B). If too much fluid is removed too quickly, the client may experience hypotension, not hypertension (Choice C). The client's heart rate would likely increase to

compensate for decreased fluid volume. If the fluid is removed too quickly, the client may experience a headache, nausea, and/or vomiting for which the nurse would monitor (Choice D). Bleeding during the procedure at the insertion site could occur because heparin is added to the dialysate to prevent clotting (Choice E).

### NGN Challenge #1
Answer: A, E
Rationale: All five of the client's selected laboratory results are abnormal, but Choices A and E are the most significant and immediately concerning to the nurse. Serum creatinine is the primary and most specific indicator of accumulating wastes from protein metabolism. An increasing creatinine indicates that the client's kidneys are not adequately functioning, which could be potentially life-threatening (Choice A). An increasing BUN can occur when a client is dehydrated, has extensive tissue damage, or has increased protein catabolism. This client was admitted with dehydration, which may account for the increased BUN (Choice B). An elevated potassium is very concerning because potassium is needed for proper cardiac functioning. Hypo- or hyperkalemia can cause potentially life-threatening cardiac dysrhythmias. Therefore, Choice E is also a correct response to this question. An elevation in phosphorus usually results in a decrease in calcium. At this time, there are only slight changes in these laboratory results and would not be of immediate concern to the nurse (Choices C and D). However, these values need to be monitored as the client's condition progresses.

NGN Challenge #2
Answer:

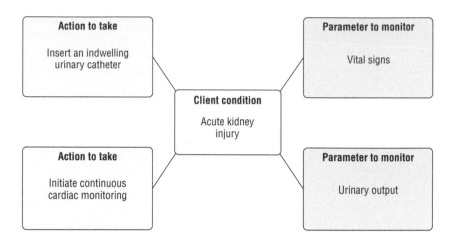

Rationale: The most current definition of AKI is an increase in serum creatinine by 0.3 mg/dL (26.2 mcmol/L) or more within 48 hours; or an increase in serum creatinine to 1.5 times or more from baseline, which is known or presumed to have occurred in the previous 7 days; or a urine volume of less than 0.5 mL/kg/h for 6 hours. The client's serum creatinine has increased quickly and significantly during the past several days, but the client's exact urinary output is unknown. This rapid change is not common in clients who have chronic kidney disease. There is no evidence that the client has pyelonephritis, such as fever. If the client had urolithiasis, the client would likely be restless and perhaps shout out from intense pain. To obtain accurate urinary output measurement, the nurse would insert an indwelling urinary catheter, even though the client was admitted with urosepsis. Urinary output would be the most important parameter to monitor for this client. The client's hyperkalemia increases the risk for cardiac dysrhythmias and, therefore, the client's heart needs to be monitored. Vital sign monitoring would help determine fluid overload if the kidneys continue to deteriorate because blood pressure would likely increase and the pulse would become bounding. The client already has beginning crackles, which could worsen if fluid overload worsens.

## Chapter 61

**Answer Key**

*Chapter Review*

**Anatomy & Physiology Review**

#1.

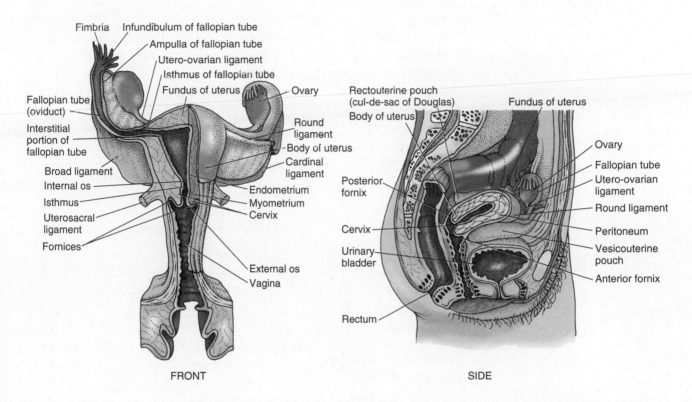

#2.

1. B
2. D
3. G
4. A
5. H
6. C
7. E
8. F

## Activities

### Activity #1

Answers may include any five of these common reproductive system changes associated with aging, and nursing interventions:

| Physiologic Change | Nursing Interventions | Rationales |
|---|---|---|
| **Women** | | |
| Graying and thinning of pubic hair<br>Decreased size of labia majora and clitoris | Reassure that these are normal and expected changes. | Education helps patients know which normal physiologic changes associated with aging to expect, and that other findings need to be reported to their health care provider. This action can also decrease problems associated with body image by understanding that these changes occur in most older adults. *(This rationale about education applies when teaching all people about age-related body changes.)* |
| Drying, smoothing, and thinning of vaginal walls | Provide information about vaginal estrogen therapy (if desired by the patient and recommended by the health care provider) and water-soluble lubricants to minimize discomfort associated with intercourse. | Education enables the patient to make informed decisions about how or whether to treat vaginal dryness. |
| Decreased uterine size<br>Atrophy of the endometrium<br>Decreased size and marked convolution of the ovaries<br>Loss of tone and elasticity of the pelvic ligaments and connective tissue | Teach Kegel exercises to strengthen pelvic muscles. | Strengthening exercises can prevent or reduce pelvic relaxation and incidences of urinary incontinence. |
| Decreased firmness, which allows breasts to hang lower on the chest wall; decreased erection of the nipples; increased incidence of fibrosis | Teach (1) how to be self-aware of potential breast changes and (2) the evidence-based recommendations for clinical breast examination and mammography based on the patient's age. | These methods can serve to detect masses or other changes that may indicate the presence of cancer. The sooner a change is noted and examined, the sooner intervention—if the patient desires—can take place. |

| Physiologic Change | Nursing Interventions | Rationales |
|---|---|---|
| **Men** | | |
| Graying and thinning of pubic hair | Reassure that this is a normal and expected change. | Education helps patients know which normal physiologic changes associated with aging to expect, and that other findings need to be reported to their health care provider. This action can also decrease problems associated with body image by understanding that these changes occur in most older adults. *(This rationale about education applies when teaching all people about age-related body changes.)* |
| Increased relaxation of the scrotum with loss of rugae | Teach how to be self-aware of potential testicular changes based on evidence-based recommendations for testicular self-examination (TSE). | TSE can serve to detect masses or other changes that may indicate the presence of cancer. The sooner a change is noted and examined, the sooner intervention – if the patient desires – can take place. |
| Prostate enlargement, with increased likelihood of urethral obstruction | Teach about symptoms associated with urethral obstruction and the importance of prostate cancer screening. | Education helps the patient detect prostate enlargement and/or obstruction, which may indicate the presence of benign prostatic hyperplasia (BPH) or cancer. The sooner a change is noted and examined, the sooner intervention – if the patient desires – can take place. |

**Activity #2**
1.   Orchitis
2.   Salpingitis
3.   Prostatitis
4.   Orchitis
5.   Peritonitis

**Activity #3**
1.   F
2.   F
3.   T
4.   T
5.   T
6.   T
7.   F
8.   F
9.   F
10.   T

## Activity #4

Pertinent teaching points the nurse will provide to a patient who has undergone cervical biopsy include, but are not limited to:

- Do not lift any heavy objects until the site is healed (about 2 weeks).
- Rest for 24 hours after the procedure.
- Report any excessive bleeding (more than that of a normal menstrual period) to your health care provider.
- Report signs of infection (fever, increased pain, foul-smelling drainage) to your primary health care provider right away.
- Do not douche, use tampons, or have vaginal intercourse until the site is healed (about 2 weeks).
- Keep the perineum clean and dry by using antiseptic solution rinses (as directed by your health care provider) and changing pads frequently.

## Activity #5

1. Circumcision
2. Acidic
3. Fallopian tubes
4. Prostate
5. *BRCA1, BRCA2*
6. Human papillomavirus
7. Red
8. Anxiolytic (benzodiazepine also is acceptable)
9. Antibiotic
10. 24

## Learning Assessments

### NCLEX Examination Challenge #1

Answer: A, B, C, D, E

Rationale: The nurse will assess for all of these factors when a male client reports a decrease in libido. A poor diet can contribute to this symptom (Choice A). Tobacco use (Choice B), alcohol use (Choice D), and illicit drug use (Choice E) can all contribute to a decreased libido, impaired sperm production, and the ability to obtain or sustain an erection. Prescription drugs can also inhibit the libido (Choice C).

### NCLEX Examination Challenge #2

Answer: C

Rationale: After prostate biopsy, the nurse will remind the client that he may experience slight soreness, light rectal bleeding that is bright red for a few days, and moderate hematuria that should resolve in a few days (Choice C). Seminal fluid may be discolored red or rust for several weeks, not a day after the procedure (Choice A). A low-grade fever and bright red penile discharge for several days are not expected findings (Choice B), nor are swelling of the biopsy area and difficulty urinating (Choice D); these should be reported to the health care provider.

### NCLEX Examination Challenge #3

Answer: D

Rationale: The nurse will teach the client who is going to have a mammogram to refrain from using lotions, creams, or powder on the day of the study (Choice D). These products can be visible on the mammogram and contribute to misdiagnosis. The client does not need to observe any type of dietary restriction (Choice A), abstain from sexual relations (Choice B), or wear a supportive bra (Choice C).

## Chapter 62

**Answer Key**
*Chapter Review*
**Pathophysiology Review**
#1

1. G
2. J
3. F
4. A
5. I
6. B
7. H
8. C
9. D
10. E

#2

| Risk Factor | How Risk Factor is Significant |
|---|---|
| Gender | Most breast cancer occurs in __**women**_____. |
| Age | Risk increases with aging, especially after the age of ___**55**_____. |
| Genetic factors | Inherited mutations of _**BRCA1**_____ and/or _**BRCA2**_____ increase risk. |
| Race | Overall, __**White**_____ women are more likely to develop breast cancer than __**Black**_____ women; however, in women younger than __**40**_____ years old, breast cancer is more common in _**Black**_____ women. |
| Heritage | Women of ____**Ashkenazi Jewish**_____ heritage have higher incidences of *BRCA1* and *BRCA2* genetic mutations, which raises the risk. |
| Personal history of certain benign breast conditions | Choice for benign breast conditions that slightly raise the risk for breast cancer can include two of these five options:<br>• Fibroadenoma<br>• Papillomatosis<br>• Radial scar<br>• Sclerosing adenosis<br>• Usual ductal hyperplasia (without atypia)<br>One benign breast condition that significantly raises the risk for breast cancer:<br>• Atypical ductal hyperplasia (ADH)<br>• Atypical lobular hyperplasia (ALH)<br>• Lobular carcinoma in situ (LCIS) |
| Breast density | Dense breasts contain more ___**glandular**___ and ___**connective tissue**___, which increases the risk for developing breast cancer. |
| Family history of breast cancer | Having a ____**first**_____-degree relative with breast or ovarian cancer increases risk. |
| Menstrual history | The risk for breast cancer rises if the patient had early menstruation (younger than ___**12**___ years old) or late menopause (at the age of __**55**___ or older), or both. |

## Activities

### Activity #1

1. T
2. F
3. F
4. F
5. T
6. F
7. F
8. F
9. T
10. F

### Activity #2

Things the nurse will teach to a male client diagnosed with gynecomastia can include:

- It is a condition in which there is a benign ridge of glandular tissue within the breast.
- It is caused by an increase in ratio of estrogen to androgen activity.
- It can occur bilaterally or unilaterally with a palpable mass at least 0.5 cm in diameter.
- Many men are asymptomatic.
- Some men may report tenderness or sensitivity when clothing touches the nipple or affected area.
- Certain drugs (e.g., spironolactone) can cause this condition; those drugs may be discontinued if this condition arises.
- Conditions such as hyperthyroidism or hypogonadism can contribute to this condition.
- Selective estrogen receptor modulators (SERMs) such as tamoxifen, aromatase inhibitors, and androgens may also be used for treatment.
- Surgery can be considered for men who have unresolved gynecomastia where nonsurgical management does not resolve the condition.

### Activity #3

| Breast Disorder | Incidence |
|---|---|
| Fibroadenoma | During teenage years into the 30s (most commonly) |
| Fibrocystic changes (FCCs) | Onset late teens and 20s; usually subsides after menopause |
| Ductal ectasia | Women approaching menopause |
| Intraductal papilloma | Women 40-55 years of age |

### Activity #4

1. Massage
2. Aromatherapy, ginger, progressive muscle relaxation
3. Massage, yoga
4. Black cohosh, flaxseed
5. Aromatherapy, massage, progressive muscle relaxation, yoga
6. Aromatherapy, progressive muscle relaxation, yoga

**Learning Assessments**

## NCLEX Examination Challenge #1

Answer: B

Rationale: Before surgery, a large tumor is sometimes treated with chemotherapy, called neoadjuvant therapy, to shrink the tumor before it is surgically removed (Choice B). An advantage of this therapy is that cancer then can be removed by lumpectomy rather than mastectomy. This type of therapy is not done after surgery (Choice A), with radiation (Choice C), or during surgery (Choice D).

## NCLEX Examination Challenge #2

Answer: C

Rationale: Women with large breasts may experience recurrent fungal infections under the breasts during hot or humid conditions because of the difficulty in keeping skin in this area dry (Choice C). This is the most likely finding the nurse will observe in this client. The presence of peau d'orange (Choice A), drainage from one or both nipples (Choice B), and multiple instances of fibrocystic changes (Choice D) are not likely to be present when a client has larger breasts; however, recurrent fungal infections are quite common.

## NCLEX Examination Challenge #3

Answer: C

Rationale: It is important to teach the client who had a mastectomy how to check the surgical site for infection or bleeding (Choice C) because these can be potential complications of surgery. Ambulation is begun the day after surgery—not 1 week later (Choice A)—as is consumption of a regular diet (Choice B). The affected arm should be elevated on a pillow—not lowered—to promote drainage (Choice D).

## NGN Challenge #1

Answer:

The nurse analyzes the assessment data and determines that the client is most likely experiencing **sepsis** as evidenced by **decreasing blood pressure** and **decreased level of consciousness**.

Rationale: Sepsis is a complication that can follow surgery. It is characterized by changes in consciousness, disorientation, increasing heart rate and respiratory rate, fever, shivering, and chills. This client has a blood pressure that is decreasing over the 48-hour period, as well as a decline in change of consciousness. A transient ischemic attack is unlikely, given the onset of fever. Although the client is hypotensive, that is not the only concern that is occurring as noted by other trended vital signs including temperature and an increase in heart rate. The client's orientation ×3 in the earlier periods of time is favorable. Urinary output is normal. The variance in $SpO_2$ is not of concern, as results are normal. Respiratory rate is also normal.

**NGN Examination Challenge #2**
Answer:

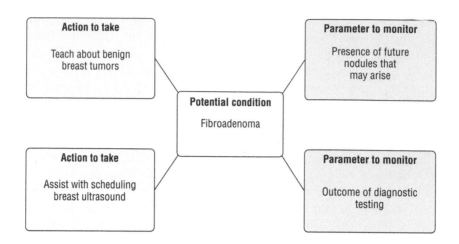

**Rationale:** The client's presentation is characteristic of fibroadenoma, a common benign tumor that occurs in women usually in their 20s and 30s. A fibroadenoma is a well-defined solid mass of connective tissue that is unattached to the surrounding breast tissue and is usually discovered personally by the patient or during mammography. Although the immediate fear is that of breast cancer, these changes are generally not associated with an increased risk for such. On clinical examination, these various-sized tumors are oval, freely mobile, and rubbery. The nurse will teach about benign breast tumors and assist with scheduling a breast ultrasound, which is often performed for diagnostic purposes. The nurse will monitor for the presence of any future nodules, as more fibroadenomas may arise, and the outcome of diagnostic testing that will likely confirm the condition. Atypical hyperplasia is usually found on biopsy, not general palpation. Gynecomastia can occur in female clients; however, it is a benign ridge of glandular tissue in the breast—not nodules. Ductal carcinoma in situ is a noninvasive form of breast cancer usually found during mammography, as the cancer cells are located in within the duct. They have not invaded the surrounding fatty breast tissue, so palpation is unlikely. Back pain is associated with large breasts, not fibroadenomas. Tamoxifen therapy will not be prescribed for fibroadenomas. Because fibroadenomas are not cancerous, there is not a concern for lymphatic metastasis.

# Chapter 63

**Answer Key**
## Chapter Review
**Pathophysiology Review**

#1

1. E
2. F
3. D
4. C
5. A
6. B

#2

1. F
2. F
3. T
4. F
5. F
6. T
7. F
8. T
9. T
10. F

# Activities

## Activity #1

1. D
2. E
3. F
4. B
5. G
6. A
7. H
8. C

## Activity #2

Things the nurse will assess and monitor for a client who has had a hysterectomy should include any of these components.

- Vital signs, including pain level
- Activity tolerance level
- Temperature and color of the skin
- Heart, lung, and bowel sounds
- Incision characteristics
  - Presence or absence of bleeding at the site (a small amount is normal)
  - Intactness of incision
  - Pain at site of incision
- Dressing and drains for color and amount of drainage
- Fluid intake (via IV until peristalsis returns and oral intake is tolerated)
- Urine output
- Red blood cell, hemoglobin, and hematocrit levels
- Vaginal discharge and/or bleeding

## Activity #3

1. Superabsorbent
2. 3-6
3. Sanitary napkins
4. Insertable contraceptive devices
5. Contact primary health care provider

## Activity #4

Examples of things the nurse would teach a patient about preventing vulvovaginitis include, but are not limited to:

- Wear cotton underwear; nylon and other fabrics retain heat and moisture, which increases the risk for infection.
- Avoid wearing tight clothing because it can cause chafing. You can also get hot and sweaty, which can increase the risk for infection.
- Always wipe front to back after having a bowel movement or urinating.
- Use fragrance-free laundry detergent.
- During a bath or shower, cleanse the inner labial mucosa with water, not soap.
- Do not douche or use feminine hygiene sprays.
- Choose other methods of contraception instead of spermicide or vaginal sponges, which can irritate the condition.
- If your sexual partner has an infection of the sex organs, do not have intercourse with them until you both have been treated.
- You are more likely to get an infection if you are pregnant, have diabetes, take oral contraceptive drugs, or are menopausal. Make

sure your primary health care provider is aware of any preexisting health conditions.

• If irritation is due to a yeast or parasitic infection, take or apply the prescribed drug treatment as ordered by the primary health care provider.

• Applying cool compresses several times a day can be helpful in minimizing itching.

## Learning Assessments

### NCLEX Examination Challenge #1

Answer: A

Rationale: The nurse anticipates that a client admitted with uterine leiomyomas most likely has presented with heavy vaginal bleeding (Choice A). Many women with leiomyomas report painful menstruation, often with heavy flow and the presence of clots, which cause them to seek medical care. Pelvic pain—not abdominal pain— is sometimes associated with leiomyomas (Choice B). Urinary stress incontinence (Choice C) and foul-smelling vaginal discharge (Choice D) are not normally associated with leiomyomas.

### NCLEX Examination Challenge #2

Answer: C

Rationale: An anterior colporrhaphy (anterior repair) tightens the pelvic muscles for better bladder support, so verbalization of good urination control indicates this procedure was successful (Choice C). It is usually only performed after the client has unsuccessfully tried conservative management and continues to have bothersome symptoms. Resolution of constipation (Choice A), abdominal pain (Choice B), or vaginal bleeding (Choice D) do not demonstrate efficacy of an anterior colporrhaphy.

### NCLEX Examination Challenge #3

Answer: D

Rationale: The main symptom of endometrial cancer is abnormal uterine bleeding (AUB), especially in postmenopausal women; therefore, the 64-year-old client reporting bleeding after menopause should be evaluated for endometrial cancer at this time (Choice D). The client who is 22 may be pregnant or may have another condition such as anorexia nervosa (which occurs primarily in the teen years and early 20s) that can contribute to amenorrhea (Choice A). Having multiple sexual partners, such as reported by the 37-year-old client, is a risk factor for sexually transmitted infections but not for endometrial cancer (Choice B). The 50-year-old client is likely entering menopause because of having irregular menses for 6 months (Choice C).

**NGN Challenge #1**

Answer:

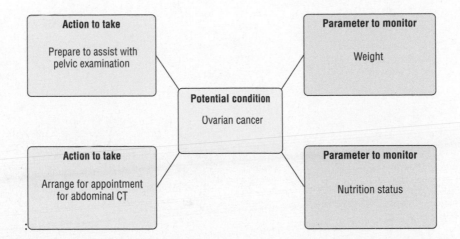

Rationale: The client's symptoms are characteristic of ovarian cancer. Common symptoms include bloating or abdominal fullness; weight gain; constipation; urinary urgency or frequency; difficulty eating, anorexia, or feeling full after a few bites of food. Abdominal or pelvic pain is often experienced very early in the disease process. The nurse will assist the health care provider by setting up and witnessing the pelvic examination; during the examination, the provider will assess for the presence of a palpable mass, which may or may not be present. The nurse will also assist with arranging an appointment for an abdominal CT (as ordered by the provider), which will be done to assess for metastasis and ascites. It will be important to monitor the client's weight; weight can increase in the presence of ovarian cancer, yet it can also decrease if the client is not eating well. Therefore, nutrition status is another parameter the nurse will monitor over time. The Gardasil 9 vaccination is for prevention of human papillomavirus (HPV) not ovarian cancer. Using perineal pads instead of tampons is important in the prevention of toxic shock syndrome. Calcium carbonate will not help the client's abdominal discomfort. There is no need to monitor antibiotic therapy because this will not be prescribed based on the client's presentation. A cone biopsy and the LEEP procedure may be done in the presence of cervical cancer, not ovarian cancer.

**NGN Examination Challenge #2**

Activity:

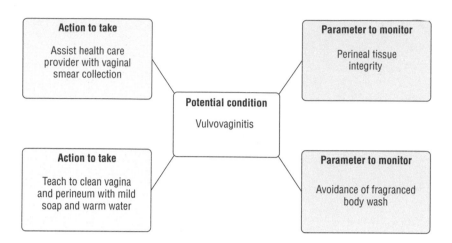

Rationale: The client's presentation is characteristic of vulvovaginitis, which includes symptoms such as itching and unusual discharge. Vulvovaginitis that is nonsexually transmitted is often related to the use of spermicides, vaginal sponges, feminine hygiene sprays, bubble baths, soaps, and lotions. The nurse will assist the health care provider with collection of vaginal smears during a pelvic examination and teach the client to carefully cleanse the vagina and perineum with mild soap and warm water. It is important to monitor tissue integrity, as some women develop an *itch-scratch-itch cycle* in which the itching leads to scratching, which causes excoriation that then must heal. As healing takes place, itching occurs again. If the cycle is not interrupted, the chronic scratching may lead to the white, thickened skin of lichen planus. This dry, leathery skin cracks easily, increasing the risk for infection. The nurse will also monitor the client's use of hygiene products to confirm the avoidance of irritating chemicals such as those in bubble baths, soaps, and lotions. There are no symptoms present that are characteristic of toxic shock syndrome, leiomyoma, or cervical cancer. The client does not need to be recommended the Gardasil 9 vaccination because the health record states she is current on immunizations. Douching should be avoided because this introduces unnecessary chemicals into the vagina. Cotton underwear should be worn. Nylon underwear retains moisture and heat, which increases the risk for infection. There is no need to monitor for the onset of fever or rash; these are associated with other infectious agents or toxic shock syndrome. The client does not need to be screened for endometrial cancer.

# Chapter 64

## Answer Key

### *Chapter Review*

**Pathophysiology Review**

#1

1. A
2. F
3. D
4. B
5. C
6. G
7. E

#2

1. F
2. T
3. F
4. F
5. T
6. T
7. T
8. F
9. T
10. F

## Activities

### Activity #1

Any four of these nonmodifiable risk factors associated with the development of benign prostatic hyperplasia (BPH) are acceptable:

- Race
  - o Black men younger than 65 need treatment more often than White men
  - o LUTS is more common in Black men than White men
  - o Asian men have BPH less often than Black and White men
  - o Asian men are less likely to need surgery for BPH than White men
- Genetic susceptibility—Variants in the *GATA3* gene have been associated with development of BPH/LUTS.
- Family history of cancer—Men with a family history of bladder cancer (not prostate cancer) are at higher risk to develop BPH.

### Activity #2

1. F
2. T
3. T
4. F
5. T
6. T
7. T
8. F
9. T
10. T

### Activity #3

1. D
2. F
3. C
4. G
5. A
6. E
7. B

**Activity #4**

Answers should resemble these descriptions.

| Procedure | Description |
|---|---|
| Phosphodiesterase-5 (PDE5) inhibitors (drug therapy including avanafil, sildenafil, tadalafil, vardenafil) | Relaxes the smooth muscles in the corpora cavernosa so blood flow to the penis is increased.<br>The veins exiting the corpora are compressed, limiting outward blood flow and resulting in penile swelling. |
| Intraurethral alprostadil injections | Self-administered pellet is placed into urethra immediately after urination; penis is rolled between hands for 10 seconds to complete administration. |
| Penile injections | Self-injection into the shaft of the penis.<br>Patient uses an insulin syringe with prostaglandin E1. |
| Penile prostheses | Semirigid or inflatable options:<br>• Semirigid option results in permanent erection.<br>• Inflatable option involves placement of two hollow cylinders in the corpora cavernosa, and a saline reservoir. Use of a pump moves the saline from the reservoir to the penile cylinders, causing an erection. |
| Vacuum-assisted erection device | A cylinder is placed over the penis, sitting firmly against the body.<br>Using a pump, a vacuum is created to draw blood into the penis to maintain an erection.<br>A rubber ring (tension band) is placed around the base of the penis to maintain the erection, and the cylinder is removed. |

**Activity #5**

Any five of these potential treatment measures for erectile dysfunction (ED) are acceptable for the nurse to share with a client.

• Lifestyle modifications (e.g., smoking cessation, weight loss, management of hypertension)
• Management of medications that may cause ED (e.g., antidepressants)
• Penile self-injection with prostaglandin E1
• Phophodiesterase-5 (PDE5) drug therapy
• Psychotherapy
• Testosterone and PDE5 drug therapy (for men with hypogonadism)
• Surgery (prosthesis)
• Vacuum-assisted erection devices

## Activity #6

Descriptions and signs/symptoms of each condition should resemble this information.

| Condition | Description | Signs and Symptoms |
|---|---|---|
| Hydrocele | Swelling in the scrotum where fluid has collected around one or both testicles | Painless testicle swelling; often the sensation is described as "heaviness" of the scrotum |
| Spermatocele | A cyst that develops in the epididymis; usually is painless | Usually asymptomatic; sometimes pain and/or heaviness occurs in the affected testicle |
| Varicocele | Vein enlargement inside the scrotum (usually on the left side), which can cause low sperm production | Can be asymptomatic; pain, if experienced, may be dull or sharp, worsening with activity and throughout the day |
| Paraphimosis | The foreskin (of an uncircumcised male) cannot be pulled over the penis tip, resulting in the foreskin becoming stuck, impeding blood flow to the penile tip and lymphatic drainage | Enlargement and congestion of glans and foreskin, with a band of constrictive tissue that prevents moving the foreskin forward over the penile tip (glans) |
| Priapism | Persistent, painful erection (usually >4 hours initially) not associated with sexual stimulation; is common in patients with sickle cell disease, and can be associated with use of certain drugs | Painful erection unrelated to sexual stimulation that lasts >2 to 4 hours (patients with recurrent priapism may have shorter duration of erection) |
| Testicular torsion | Twisting of the spermatic cord that results in ischemia from decreased arterial inflow and venous outflow obstruction; can occur spontaneously or as a result of trauma | Nausea<br>Vomiting<br>Lower abdominal pain<br>Tender mass or knot above the testis |
| Epididymitis | Inflammation or infection of the epididymis; often caused by *Neisseria gonorrhoeae* or *Chlamydia trachomatis* in men younger than 35 years of age; in older men, it often occurs in association with obstructive uropathy from benign prostatic hyperplasia (BPH). For men of any age who practice insertive anal intercourse, this condition is often associated with exposure to rectal coliform bacteria. | Localized testicular pain<br>Tenderness and swelling on palpation of the epididymis<br>May have scrotal erythema<br>Advanced cases may include testicular swelling |
| Phimosis | Tightness that results in the inability to retract the foreskin | Swelling and pain at the head of the penis, causing difficulty in retraction of the foreskin<br>Is often associated with hygienic concerns (neglecting to replace the foreskin after cleaning, intercourse, or urination) or body piercing of the glans or foreskin |

**Learning Assessments**

**NCLEX Examination Challenge #1**

Answer: 1140 mL

Rationale: The client has had 1100 mL of bladder irrigating solution infused, and there is 2240 mL of fluid in the urinary drainage bag. 2240 mL – 1100 mL = 1140 mL, which represents the amount of urinary output that the client has produced.

**NCLEX Examination Challenge #2**

Answer: A, B, C, E

Rationale: For a client with BPH, most of these criteria indicate the need for surgery: hematuria (Choice A), hydronephrosis (Choice B), acute urinary retention resulting from obstruction (which is a medical emergency) (Choice C); and chronic urinary tract infections secondary to residual urine in the bladder (Choice E). Usually, another antibiotic will be tried when a client has an acute urinary tract infection that does not respond to first-line antibiotics (Choice D).

**NCLEX Examination Challenge #3**

Answer: D

Rationale: As the client's prostate gland enlarges, it extends upward into the bladder and inward, causing bladder outlet obstruction. Because of this, the nurse expects the symptom of difficulty in starting and continuing urination (Choice D). Constipation (Choice A), scrotal discomfort (Choice B), and erectile dysfunction (Choice C) are not frequently associated with benign prostatic hypertrophy.

**NGN Challenge #1**

<u>Answer:</u>

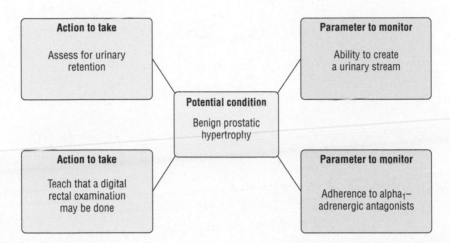

<u>Rationale:</u> A client who has difficulty urinating, or starting or stopping the urinary stream, or continuing a urinary stream with expected force, likely has benign prostatic hyperplasia (BPH). BPH is characterized by urinary difficulty, a sensation of incomplete bladder emptying, straining to begin urinating, and postvoid dribbling. It is critical to assess for acute urinary retention, which can occur if the prostate has enlarged to the point that the client cannot void at all. The nurse will teach that a digital rectal examination, in addition to the physical assessment, may be performed so the provider can determine the consistency and size of the prostate. The client will likely be prescribed an alpha$_1$-adrenergic antagonist to reduce the prostate size, so adherence to this drug therapy will be monitored. As the prostate shrinks during drug therapy, the nurse will also monitor the client's ability to create a urinary stream. Difficulty starting, maintaining, and stopping a urinary stream is not characteristic of erectile dysfunction or prostate cancer. The grouping of symptoms the client reports is less likely to be reflective of a urinary tract infection, particularly because the symptoms have been present for 4 months and no burning or pain is reported. There is no need for prostate artery embolism at this time; that type of procedure is considered after drug therapy fails. External beam radiation therapy is used to treat cancer, not BPH. An antibiotic will not resolve BPH; therefore, monitoring for adherence to antibiotic therapy is not necessary. The client has no fever, so monitoring for such is unnecessary. It is not necessary to have a culture and sensitivity test monitored because this is unlikely to be performed since the client does not have an infectious process.

**NGN Challenge #2**
<u>Answer</u>:

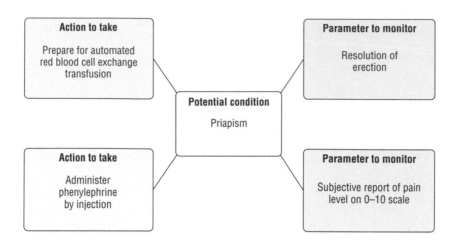

<u>Rationale</u>: The client who has an erection that will not resolve likely has a priapism. Because of the history of sickle cell disease, the client may need an automated red blood cell exchange transfusion in addition to expected therapy (injected phenylephrine to reduce the erection). A nonresolving erection is not associated with paraphimosis, epididymitis, or spermatocele. This condition will not resolve on its own. Elevating the scrotum will not reduce the erection. This is not an infectious condition, so IV antibiotics will not be given, and adherence to antibiotic therapy is unnecessary. Proper hygiene is needed when a client has a paraphimosis, which is often associated with not keeping oneself clean. This condition is not infectious so purulent penile drainage is not anticipated.

## Chapter 65
### Answer Key
*Chapter Review*
**Terminology Review**
#1

1. E
2. F
3. I
4. C
5. B
6. A
7. D
8. H
9. G

*Review of Nursing Care for Patients with Sexually Transmitted Infections*
#2

1. T
2. T
3. F
4. T
5. F
6. T
7. F
8. F
9. F
10. F

## Activities

### Activity #1
1. C
2. G
3. A
4. F
5. D
6. B
7. E

### Activity #2
Examples of questions the nurse would ask when taking a history of a patient who may have a sexually transmitted infection (STI) include, but are not limited to:

- For women: "Do you have any symptoms, such as vaginal discharge, dysuria, pelvic pain, or irregular bleeding?"
- For men: "Do you have any symptoms, such as penile discharge or burning or discomfort on urination?"
- For any patient:
  - "Do you have a history of STIs?"
  - "Are you aware whether your current or past sexual partners have had symptoms or a history of STIs?"
  - "Do you have any new sexual partners, specifically those that you do not know about their sexual history?"
  - "Have you had recent unprotected intercourse?"

### Activity #3
The conditions shown in **bold** are nationally notifiable.

1. **HIV**
2. **Syphilis**
3. **Chancroid**
4. **Gonorrhea**
5. **Chlamydia**
6. Genital herpes
7. Condylomata acuminata
8. Pelvic inflammatory disease

### Activity #4
Examples of things the nurse would teach a patient about the proper use of condoms include, but are not limited to:

- Use external latex or polyurethane condoms.
- Do not use natural membrane condoms because they provide much less protection against STIs.
- Use a new condom with each sexual encounter (including oral, vaginal, and anal), even with the same person.
- The efficacy of internal condoms ("female condoms")—polyurethane or nitrile sheaths placed in the vagina or anus—have not been studied as closely as traditional male condoms.
- Do not use an external condom with an internal condom; this causes friction and can cause a condom to break.
- Replace broken condoms immediately.

- Keep condoms (especially latex ones) in a cool, dry place, out of direct sunlight.
- Do not use condoms that are in damaged packages or are brittle or discolored.
- Handle a condom with care to avoid damaging it with fingernails, teeth, or other sharp objects.
- Put condoms on before any genital contact.
- To apply a condom, hold it by the tip and unroll it on the penis. Leave a space at the tip to collect semen.

- Ensure that lubricant, if used, is water based and washes away with water.
- Do not use oil-based products for lubrication, as these damage latex condoms.
- Recognize that nonoxynol-9 does not protect against sexually transmitted diseases; it can actually increase the risk for HIV transmission in women.
- After ejaculation, withdraw the erect penis carefully, holding the condom at the base of the penis to prevent the condom from slipping off.

## Learning Assessments

### NCLEX Examination Challenge #1
Answer: C
Rationale: Clients with pelvic inflammatory disease (PID) can develop perihepatitis, inflammation of the liver capsule and peritoneal surfaces on the anterior right upper quadrant. This condition is characterized by right upper quadrant pain with a pleuritic component (often the right shoulder) (Choice C), which needs to be reported by the nurse. Other symptoms such as yellowish vaginal discharge (Choice A), temperature 101.2°F (38.4°C) (Choice B), and spotting 2 weeks after a period (Choice D) are associated with PID for which the client has just begun treatment. These are expected findings and do not need to be reported to the health care provider unless they worsen during treatment with antibiotics and pain medication.

### NCLEX Examination Challenge #2
Answer: A
Rationale: The nurse needs to provide further teaching when the client thinks that the condition is resolved when the chancre goes away (Choice A). It is common for a chancre to disappear; however, the organism that causes syphilis is still present in the body. Statements about neurosyphilis involving the loss of hearing or vision (Choice B), the disease being contagious even if the client is without symptoms (Choice C), and the need to contact the health care provider if a rash develops (Choice D) indicate understanding of the condition, and do not require further nursing teaching.

**NGN Challenge #1**

<u>Answer:</u>

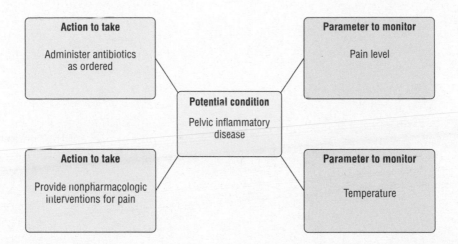

| Action to take | | Parameter to monitor |
|---|---|---|
| Administer antibiotics as ordered | | Pain level |
| | **Potential condition** | |
| | Pelvic inflammatory disease | |
| Action to take | | Parameter to monitor |
| Provide nonpharmacologic interventions for pain | | Temperature |

<u>Rationale:</u> The client has reported classic symptoms associated with pelvic inflammatory disease (PID) including abdominal pain, fever, dysuria, and vaginal discharge. PID is likely because the client also reports having had unprotected intercourse with several people recently, which increased her risk of contracting an infection that often accompanies PID. The client's blood pressure and respirations are slightly elevated, most likely from pain associated with PID. The nurse will administer antibiotics as ordered to address infection and will provide pain interventions (pharmacologic and nonpharmacologic). The client's pain level should be monitored to determine if interventions to address pain are successful, and the temperature must be monitored to determine the efficacy of antibiotic treatment. Syphilis is characterized by a chancre (or can be asymptomatic); Mpox is characterized by fever, myalgias, and lymphadenopathy. Although the client has a fever, there is no indication of myalgias or lymphadenopathy. Gonorrhea if often asymptomatic in women. Placing the client in a prone position will put pressure on the abdomen. Antiviral treatment is not used for PID, so teaching about this type of medication is not necessary. A nasogastric tube is contraindicated; the client's abdominal pain is not due to a gastrointestinal condition. For the same reason, it is not necessary to monitor the client's ALT/AST or abdominal girth. Capillary refill will not provide information about the efficacy of treatment for PID.

**NGN Examination Challenge #2**
Answer:

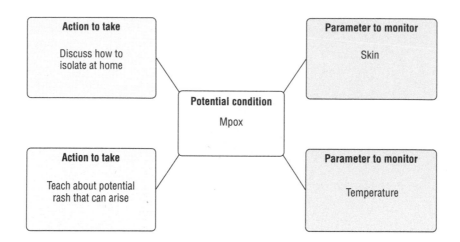

Rationale: Mpox is a poxlike disease that is part of the virus family that causes smallpox. It is characterized by an incubation period of 7 to 14 days, which leads to viral spread; the second viremia includes 1 to 2 days of fever and lymphadenopathy followed by the eruption of lesions in the oropharynx and skin that continue to expand over the body. Recognizing that the client had unprotected intercourse with another person about 10 days ago, the likelihood of these symptoms being Mpox (versus influenza) is high. There is no indication of a chancre, which is an indication of syphilis, or of anal warts, which are known as condylomata acuminata. This client is experiencing fever and lymphadenopathy and may experience the eruption of lesions soon; therefore, the nurse will teach about this as a priority. The nurse will also discuss how to isolate at home so the client does not spread Mpox to others. Because Mpox is viral in nature, antibiotics are not indicated. Although HPV vaccination is recommended for people, this is not a priority intervention at this time; the immediate need is to treat the client for Mpox and avoid spread of the infection. There is no indication of the need for a sputum specimen. Treatment for Mpox is supportive in nature. The nurse will teach the client to monitor their skin, in case the rash erupts, and temperature, which can indicate that the infection is subsiding or worsening. Culture and sensitivity for a bacterial result is not needed because Mpox is viral in nature. This condition is not marked by genital warts, so monitoring for those is unnecessary. Topical antifungal therapy is not prescribed for Mpox.